Advances in Molecular and Cellular Microbiology 26

Meningitis

Cellular and Molecular Basis

Edited by

Myron Christodoulides

Neisseria Research Group, Molecular Microbiology,
Clinical and Experimental Sciences,
University of Southampton Faculty of Medicine

www.cabi.org

amcm **Advances in Molecular and Cellular Microbiology**

Through the application of molecular and cellular microbiology, we now recognize the diversity and dominance of microbial life forms on our planet, which exist in all environments. These microbes have many important planetary roles, but for us humans a major problem is their ability to colonize our tissues and cause disease. The same techniques of molecular and cellular microbiology have been applied to the problems of human and animal infection during the past two decades and have proved to be immensely powerful tools in elucidating how microorganisms cause human pathology. This series has the aim of providing information on the advances that have been made in the application of molecular and cellular microbiology to specific organisms and the diseases that they cause. The series is edited by researchers active in the application of molecular and cellular microbiology to human disease states. Each volume focuses on a particular aspect of infectious disease and will enable graduate students and researchers to keep up with the rapidly diversifying literature in current microbiological research.

Series Editor

Professor Michael Wilson
University College London

Titles Available from CABI

17. *Helicobacter pylori* in the 21st Century
Edited by Philip Sutton and Hazel M. Mitchell

18. Antimicrobial Peptides: Discovery, Design and Novel Therapeutic Strategies
Edited by Guangshun Wang

19. Stress Response in Pathogenic Bacteria
Edited by Stephen P. Kidd

20. Lyme Disease: an Evidence-based Approach
Edited by John J. Halperin

21. Tuberculosis: Laboratory Diagnosis and Treatment Strategies
Edited by Timothy McHugh

22. Antimicrobial Drug Discovery: Emerging Strategies
Edited by George Tegos and Eleftherios Mylonakis

24. Bacteriophages in Health and Disease
Edited by Paul Hyman and Stephen T. Abedon

26. Meningitis: Cellular and Molecular Basis
Edited by Myron Christodoulides

Titles Forthcoming from CABI

Microbial Metabolomics
Edited by Silas Villas-Bôas and Katya Ruggiero

The Human Microbiota and Microbiome
Edited by Julian Marchesi

Earlier titles in the series are available from Cambridge University Press (www.cup.cam.ac.uk).

CABI is a trading name of CAB International

CABI
Nosworthy Way
Wallingford
Oxfordshire, OX10 8DE
UK

Tel: +44 (0)1491 832111
Fax: +44 (0)1491 833508
E-mail: info@cabi.org
Website: www.cabi.org

CABI
Chauncey Street
Suite 1002
Boston, MA 02111
USA

T: +1 800 552 3083 (toll free)
T: +1 (0)617 395 4051
E-mail: cabi-nao@cabi.org

A catalogue record for this book is available from the British Library, London, UK.

Library of Congress Cataloging-in-Publication Data

Meningitis : cellular and molecular basis / Myron Christodoulides, editor.
p. ; cm. -- (Advances in molecular and cellular microbiology ; v. 26)
Includes bibliographical references and index.
ISBN 978-1-78064-162-1 (alk. paper)
I. Christodoulides, Myron. II. C.A.B. International. III. Series: Advances in molecular and cellular microbiology ; v. 26.
[DNLM: 1. Meningitis--microbiology. 2. Meningitis--pathology. 3. Meninges--microbiology. 4. Meninges--pathology. WL 200]

RC376
616.8'2--dc23

2013002769

ISBN-13: 978 1 78064 162 1

Commissioning editor: Rachel Cutts
Editorial assistant: Alexandra Lainsbury
Production editor: Lauren Povey

Typeset by Columns Design XML Ltd, Reading, UK.
Printed and bound in the UK by CPI Group (UK) Ltd, Croydon, CR0 4YY.

Contents

Contributors

Wim Ang, Department of Medical Microbiology and Infection Control, VU University Medical Center, PO Box 7057, 1007 MB, Amsterdam, the Netherlands. E-mail: w.ang@vumc.nl

Ronny Beer, Neurological Intensive Care Unit, Department of Neurology, Innsbruck Medical University, 6020 Innsbruck, Anichstr. 35, Austria. E-mail: ronny.beer@i-med.ac.at

Sandrine Bourdoulous, Université Paris Descartes, Sorbonne Paris Cité, Faculté de médecine; INSERM, U1016, Institut Cochin; CNRS, UMR8104, Paris, France. E-mail: sandrine.bourdoulous@inserm.fr

Michael S. Bronze, Department of Medicine, University of Oklahoma Health Sciences Center, Oklahoma City, OK, USA. E-mail: michael-bronze@ouhsc.edu

Diego Cadavid, Center for Immunology and Inflammatory Diseases, Massachusetts General Hospital, Boston, MA, USA; Neurology Clinical Development, Biogen Idec, Cambridge, MA, USA. E-mail: cadavid.diego@gmail.com

Myron Christodoulides, Neisseria Research Group, Molecular Microbiology, Clinical and Experimental Sciences, University of Southampton Faculty of Medicine, Southampton General Hospital, Southampton, SO16 6YD, UK. E-mail: mc4@soton.ac.uk

Mathieu Coureuil, INSERM, unité U1002; Université Paris Descartes, Sorbonne Paris Cité, Faculté de médecine, Paris, France. E-mail: mathieu.coureuil@inserm.fr

Sarah Curtis, Department of Pediatrics, Division of Pediatric Emergency Medicine, Edmonton Clinic Health Academy (ECHA), 11405–87 Avenue, Edmonton, Alberta T6G 1C9, Canada. E-mail: scurtis@ualberta.ca

Kelly S. Doran, Department of Biology and Center for Microbial Sciences, San Diego State University, 5500 Campanile Drive, San Diego, CA 92182, USA. E-mail: kdoran@mail.sdsu.edu

Douglas A. Drevets, Department of Medicine, WP-1160, 920 Stanton L. Young Blvd., University of Oklahoma Health Sciences Center, Department of Veterans Affairs Medical Center, Oklahoma City, OK 73104, USA. E-mail: douglas-drevets@ouhsc.edu

Nahuel Fittipaldi, Department of Pathology and Genomic Medicine, The Methodist Hospital Research Institute, Houston, TX, USA. E-mail: nvfittipaldi@tmhs.org

Nancy E. Freitag, Department of Microbiology and Immunology, University of Illinois at Chicago, Chicago, IL, USA. E-mail: nfreitag@uic.edu

Marcelo Gottschalk, Faculty of Veterinary Medicine, University of Montreal, 3200 Sicotte, St-Hyacinthe, Québec, Canada, J2S 2M2. E-mail: marcelo.gottschalk@umontreal.ca

Sven Hammerschmidt, Department Genetics of Microorganisms, Interfaculty Institute for Genetics and Functional Genomics, Ernst Moritz Arndt University of Greifswald, Greifswald, Germany. E-mail: sven.hammerschmidt@uni-greifswald.de

Raimund Helbok, Neurological Intensive Care Unit, Department of Neurology, Innsbruck Medical University, 6020 Innsbruck, Anichstr. 35, Austria. E-mail: raimund.helbok@uki.at

Darryl J. Hill, School of Cellular and Molecular Medicine, University of Bristol, Medical Sciences Building, Bristol, BS8 1TD, UK. E-mail: darryl.j.hill@bristol.ac.uk

David N. Irani, Department of Neurology, University of Michigan Medical School, BSRB Room 4007, 109 Zina Pitcher Place, Ann Arbor, MI 48109-2200, USA. E-mail: davidira@med.umich.edu

Olivier Join-Lambert, INSERM, unité U1002; Université Paris Descartes, Sorbonne Paris Cité, Faculté de medicine; Assistance Publique – Hôpitaux de Paris, Hôpital Necker Enfants Malades, Paris, France. E-mail: olivier.join-lambert@inserm.fr

Kwang Sik Kim, Division of Pediatric Infectious Diseases, Johns Hopkins University School of Medicine, 200 North Wolfe Street, Room 3157, Baltimore, MD 21287, USA. E-mail: kwangkim@jhmi.edu

Matthias Klein, Department of Neurology, Klinikum Großhadern, Ludwig-Maximilian University, Munich, Germany. E-mail: matthias.klein@med.uni-muenchen.de

Uwe Koedel, Department of Neurology, Klinikum Großhadern, Ludwig-Maximilian University, Munich, Germany. E-mail: uwe.koedel@med.uni-muenchen.de

Hervé Lécuyer, INSERM, unité U1002; Université Paris Descartes, Sorbonne Paris Cité, Faculté de medicine; Assistance Publique – Hôpitaux de Paris, Hôpital Necker Enfants Malades, Paris, France. E-mail: herve.lecuyer@inserm.fr

Stefano Marullo, Université Paris Descartes, Sorbonne Paris Cité, Faculté de medicine; INSERM, U1016, Institut Cochin; CNRS, UMR8104, Paris, France. E-mail: stefano.marullo@inserm.fr

Florence Miller, INSERM, unité U1002; Université Paris Descartes, Sorbonne Paris Cité, Faculté de médecine, Paris, France. E-mail: florence.miller@inserm.fr

Xavier Nassif, INSERM, unité U1002, Pathogeny of systemic infections, Université Paris Descartes – Faculté de médecine Necker, 156 rue de Vaugirard, 75015 Paris, France. E-mail: xavier.nassif@inserm.fr

Victor Nizet, Department of Pediatrics, University of California at San Diego, School of Medicine, La Jolla, CA 92093, USA. E-mail: vnizet@ucsd.edu

Bettina Pfausler, Neurological Intensive Care Unit, Department of Neurology, Innsbruck Medical University, 6020 Innsbruck, Anichstr. 35, Austria. E-mail: b.pfausler@i-med.ac.at

Erich Schmutzhard, Neurological Intensive Care Unit, Department of Neurology, Innsbruck Medical University, 6020 Innsbruck, Anichstr. 35, Austria. Email: erich.schmutzhard@i-med.ac.at

Mariela Segura, Faculty of Veterinary Medicine, University of Montreal, 3200 Sicotte, St-Hyacinthe, Québec, Canada, J2S 2M2. E-mail: mariela.segura@umontreal.ca

Guy Thwaites, Centre for Clinical Infection and Diagnostic Research, Kings College London, St Thomas' Hospital, Westminster Bridge Road, London, SE1 7EH, UK. E-mail: guy.thwaites@btinternet.com

Roy O. Weller, Clinical Neurosciences, Mail Point 806, South Pathology and Laboratory Block, University of Southampton Faculty of Medicine, Southampton General Hospital, Southampton SO16 6YD, UK. E-mail: row@soton.uk

Preface

Meningitis is defined as inflammation of the meninges, the membranes that surround the brain within the skull and the spinal cord within the spinal canal. In this book, our current knowledge of the molecular and cellular basis of meningitis is presented. This knowledge is presented on an individual pathogen basis, enabling the reader to compare and contrast the variety of different mechanisms that lead to invasion of the cerebrospinal fluid and meningeal irritation. To varying degrees, based on our current understanding – and for many pathogens, still the surprisingly significant lack of understanding – each chapter presents the particular pathology and mechanisms of pathogen interactions with specific host barriers. These barriers include primary mucosal surfaces, immune clearance mechanisms in the blood and especially the blood vessel endothelial cells that constitute the blood–brain barrier (BBB) and blood–cerebrospinal fluid barrier (BCSFB). Accordingly, emphasis is given to the nature of pathogen-specific ligands and their host cell recognition receptors, if known, and the resulting host cell responses and cellular rearrangements that are stimulated. Where appropriate, information from *in vivo* animal models and *ex vivo* cell culture-based models is provided to explain the human pathology.

This book begins with a chapter on the history of bacterial meningitis as a disease recognized from antiquity, and the roster of famous microbiologists and clinician scientists who discovered the major causative organisms. Fundamental to understanding meningitis, the following chapter describes the structural and functional aspects of the meninges and the nature of the BBB and BCSFB. This is followed by the third introductory chapter, which presents a review of the evidence-based clinical and diagnostic features of meningitis. Before considering bacterial meningitis, an overview of viral meningitis is included, in acknowledgement that most cases of meningitis are indeed viral in origin, aseptic and more often resolving. Next, we consider the major organisms causing pyogenic meningitis and infection that can occur in epidemic form, i.e. *Neisseria meningitidis*, *Streptococcus pneumoniae* and *Haemophilus influenzae.* These chapters are followed by reviews of the two major causative organisms of neonatal meningitis, *Escherichia coli* and Group B *Streptococcus.* By contrast to the descriptions of epidemic meningitis, we also recognize the chronic condition: a chapter is included that provides an overview of chronic meningitis, with mention of bacterial, fungal (e.g. *Cryptococcus neoformans*, a significant opportunistic pathogen of immune-compromised patients), protozoan and helminthic causes. This is followed by chapters that go into greater detail on specific pathogens, two of which are historical scourges of humankind, *Mycobacterium tuberculosis* and *Treponema pallidum.* Next follows a series of chapters that describe particularly interesting zoonotic pathogens that can cause meningitis, namely *Streptococcus suis, Listeria monocytogenes* and *Borrelia burgdorferi.* A chapter is dedicated to nosocomial infections and the organisms that can cause meningitis associated with hospital-acquired infection and microbial contamination of intracranial biomaterials. The book ends with a description of the molecular and cellular constitution of 'pus' within the subarachnoid space.

Before the advent of antibiotics, the mortality rate for bacterial meningitis was >90% (Swartz, 2004). Indeed, if one reads historical reports of epidemic meningitis from the mid-19th century to the early decades of the 20th century, often mention is made of only single survivors! As W.W. Herrick remarked in 1919: 'No other infection so quickly slays' (Herrick, 1919). Yet no other infection has responded so remarkably to antibiotic chemotherapy. Nevertheless, the disease burden associated with bacterial meningitis in the 21st century can still be compared with sexually transmitted diseases (gonorrhoea, syphilis, chlamydia and others, but excluding human immunodeficiency virus (HIV)) combined; and is also comparable to a set of tropical diseases (trypanosomiasis, Chagas disease, schistosomiasis, leishmaniasis, lymphatic filariasis, onchocerciasis, leprosy and dengue fever) combined (Mathers *et al.*, 2006). This is a significant burden of disease worldwide. Although outside the remit of this particular book, the development of meningitis vaccines, especially against organisms causing major pyogenic meningitis, has made a significant impact on reducing, indeed virtually eliminating, some infection in those countries with vaccination programmes. Understanding the cellular and molecular basis of meningitis is fundamental to vaccine development, and this is emphatically shown by the success of vaccines introduced against *H. influenzae, S. pneumoniae* and *N. meningitidis* (Giuliani *et al.*, 2006; Morris *et al.*, 2008; Lynch and Zhanel, 2009; Granoff, 2010; Gruber *et al.*, 2012; Khatami *et al.*, 2012). Vaccine research programmes are now established for other meningitis-causing organisms (Cullen and Cameron, 2006; Brockstedt and Dubensky, 2008; Cozzi *et al.*, 2011; Nuccitelli *et al.*, 2011; Schuijt *et al.*, 2011; Bottomley *et al.*, 2012; Cassone and Casadevall, 2012; Ottenhoff and Kaufmann, 2012), but, as this book clearly shows, there still remain many challenging and elusive organisms.

This book would not have been possible without the enthusiastic contributions of many, and I would like to express my gratitude to the authors of these chapters, clinicians and basic scientists, who are all acknowledged experts with their respective pathogens and fields, and who have shown patience with my editing and questions. Gratitude is also expressed to the staff of CABI, for commissioning this book and for all their support during its preparation. Finally, this book emphasizes that meningitis can be caused by a wide variety of different organisms (indeed, many more chapters could be written on the less common organisms causing meningitis, than the major ones presented herein), and that the pathophysiological mechanisms involved are complex and teach us a great deal not only about microbial biology, but also about human biology.

Myron Christodoulides

References

Bottomley, M.J., Serruto, D., Palazzi Safadi, M.A. and Klugman, K.P. (2012) Future challenges in the elimination of bacterial meningitis. *Vaccine* 30, B78–B86.

Brockstedt, D.G. and Dubensky, T.W. (2008) Promises and challenges for the development of *Listeria monocytogenes*-based immunotherapies. *Expert Review of Vaccines* 7, 1069–1084.

Cassone, A. and Casadevall, A. (2012) Recent progress in vaccines against fungal diseases. *Current Opinion in Microbiology* 15, 427–433.

Cozzi, R., Telford, J.L. and Maione, D. (2011) Toward the development of a universal vaccine against Group B Streptococcus. In: Rappuoli, R. and Bagnoli, F. (eds) *Vaccine Design: Innovative Approaches and Novel Strategies.* Norwich, Caister Academic Press, pp. 289–302.

Cullen, P.A. and Cameron, C.E. (2006) Progress towards an effective syphilis vaccine: the past, present and future. *Expert Review of Vaccines* 5, 67–80.
Giuliani, M.M. *et al.* (2006) A universal vaccine for serogroup B meningococcus. *Proceedings of the National Academy of Sciences USA* 103, 10834–10839.
Granoff, D.M. (2010) Review of meningococcal Group B vaccines. *Clinical Infectious Diseases* 50, S54–S65.
Gruber, W.C., Scott, D.A. and Emini, E.A. (2012) Development and clinical evaluation of Prevnar 13, a 13-valent pneumococcal CRM(197) conjugate vaccine. *Annals of the New York Academy of Sciences* 1263, 15–26.
Herrick, W.W. (1919) Extrameningeal meningococcus infections. *Archives of Internal Medicine* 23, 409–418.
Khatami, A. *et al.* (2012) Persistence of the immune response at 5 years of age following infant immunisation with investigational quadrivalent MenACWY conjugate vaccine formulations. *Vaccine* 30, 2831–2838.
Lynch, J.P. and Zhanel, G.G. (2009) *Streptococcus pneumoniae*: epidemiology, risk factors, and strategies for prevention. *Seminars in Respiratory and Critical Care Medicine* 30, 189–209.
Mathers, C.D., Lopez, A.D. and Murray, C.J.L. (2006) The burden of disease and mortality by condition: data, methods, and results for 2001. In: Lopez, A.D., Mathers, C.D., Ezzati, M., Jamison, D.T. and Murray, C.J.L. (eds) *Global Burden of Disease and Risk Factors*. Disease Control Priorities Project, World Bank, Washington, DC. For updates, visit http://www.ncbi.nlm.nih.gov/books/NBK11812/
Morris, S.K., Moss, W.J. and Halsey, N. (2008) *Haemophilus influenzae* type b conjugate vaccine use and effectiveness. *Lancet Infectious Diseases* 8, 435–443.
Nuccitelli, A., Cozzi, R., Gourlay, L.J., Donnarumma, D., Necchi, F., Norais, N., Telford, J.L., Rappuoli, R., Bolognesi, M., Maione, D., Grandi, G. and Rinaudo, C. (2011) Structure-based approach to rationally design a chimeric protein for an effective vaccine against Group B *Streptococcus* infections. *Proceedings of the National Academy of Sciences USA* 108, 10278–10283.
Ottenhoff, T.H. and Kaufmann, S.H. (2012) Vaccines against tuberculosis: where are we and where do we need to go? *PLoS Pathogens* 8, e1002607.
Schuijt, T., Hovius, J., van der Poll, T., van Dam, A. and Fikrig, E. (2011) Lyme borreliosis vaccination: the facts, the challenge, the future. *Trends in Parasitology* 27, 40–47.
Swartz, M.N. (2004) Bacterial meningitis – a view of the past 90 years. *New England Journal of Medicine* 351, 1826–1828.

1 A History of Bacterial Meningitis from Antiquity to Modern Times

Myron Christodoulides*
University of Southampton Faculty of Medicine, Southampton General Hospital, Southampton, UK

1.1 Introduction

The history of central nervous system (CNS) infections is as old as humankind itself, and tantalizing evidence of CNS infections can be found in collections of anthropological specimens and archaeological artefacts dating back to the Neolithic Revolution (10,000–3000BC). The first known description of the word 'brain' is to be found in the Edwin Smith Papyrus, an Egyptian medical and surgical text, dating from *c.*1500BC. The papyrus was bought by the Egyptologist Edwin Smith in 1862 and eventually translated by James H. Breasted in 1930 (Breasted, 1930). The papyrus contains 27 cases of head injury, six cases of throat and neck injury and one case of spinal injury: significantly for neuroanatomists, it also contains the earliest descriptions of cranial sutures, the meninges, cerebrospinal fluid and the external surface of the brain (Wilkins, 1964).

1.2 From Hippocrates to the Renaissance

There were primitive discussions about the nervous system in pre-Hippocratic Greece by 'philosopher-physicians', but this medical literature only survives in fragments or in the quotations and testaments of later scribes (Rose, 1994). It is Hippocrates (*c.*460–370BC) that scholars of history and medicine turn to for the first recorded descriptions of CNS afflictions. The *Corpus Hippocraticum* contains the surviving medical treatises attributed to Hippocrates, to his students and to his followers since antiquity. Between 1839 and 1861, the French physician and philologist Maximilien Paul Emile Littré (1801–1881) provided a Greek edition and a French translation interpreted with authority (Littré, 1839). Contemporaneously and with a heavy debt to Littre, the English physician Francis Adams (1796–1861) was commissioned by the Sydenham Society to translate 'the genuine works of Hippocrates', which was invaluable in reinforcing the Hippocratic tradition in England and America (Adams, 1849).[1]

Within the *Corpus Hippocraticum* (Section VII) are the Seven Books of Epidemics, which consist mainly of histories and cases of diseases, many ending with fatality. Although his descriptions cannot be taken as conclusive proof of meningism, particular cases are compelling. Fever is a constant, and nuchal rigidity is suggested. In The First Book of

*mc4@soton.ac.uk

Epidemics, Section II, Year 2, Hippocrates describes:

> Pains and heavinesses about the head and neck, with or without a fever, in phrenitic cases denote convulsions; and æruginous vomitings succeed. Some of these die presently. But in burning fevers and others, a pain of the neck, a heaviness of the temples, a dimness of the sight … Children are generally attacked thus, and mostly affected with convulsions in these cases.

In The Third Book of Epidemics:

> He that had a phrensy and was laid up the fifth day … and had a weight and pain in the head and neck … was very feverish ... and at night was convulsed. The third (day), was worse in all respects. The fourth, died.

The son of Cydis exhibited a suppurative ear discharge with 'fever, headache, vomiting, mental confusion, intense neck rigidity …', which has been suggested to describe meningitis secondary to otitis (Nutton, 1986).

Although Hippocrates was aware of the membranes surrounding the brain – as was the Greek polymath Aristotle (384–322BC) in his anatomical studies of animals (*The History of Animals*) – it was Herophilus of Calcedon (330–260BC; the 'Father of Anatomy') and his pupil Erasistratus of the School of Alexandria who named precisely the dura mater and pia mater of the meninges (von Staden, 1989; Rose, 1994). Hippocrates was also aware of the importance of not damaging the meninges during the treatment of head injuries. In 'On Wounds of the Head' in the *Corpus Hippocraticum*, Hippocrates describes the necessary cleansing steps to prevent infection and inflammation of head wounds, and he was equally clear on the method of trepanning.

Medical teaching in Europe ceased after the fall of the Roman Empire, but the Hippocratic tradition extended by Claudius Galen (129–217AD) and others was collected, preserved and added to by Arab scholars. Galen gave an accurate description of the dura and pia mater and is credited with using the term 'meninx' to specifically mean the coverings of the brain, rather than the membranes that generally covered all organs. The most famous Arab physician, Abu Ali al-Husayn ibn Abd Allah ibn Sina (Latin: Avicenna 980–1037AD), described meningitis in his Kitab al-Qanun fi al-tibb (The Canon of Medicine) as an 'inflammation or tumour of the envelopes of the brain'. The Canon was compulsory reading through the Renaissance to the 17th century. It is also worth noting the publication *De Contagione et Contagiosis Morbis et Eorum Curatione* (1546) by the Italian physician and poet Girolamo Fracastoro (1478–1553), which contains remarkable insight into the transmission of infectious disease and presents the first evidence of a 'germ theory'. In his lifetime, Fracastoro's fame would not relate to meningitis directly but to his poem of 1530, *Syphilis sive morbus Gallicus* ('Syphilis or The French Disease'). In the *Libri Tres* of the poem, Fracastoro's eponymous hero is the shepherd boy Syphilus, who unfortunately is made to suffer with the disease that bears his name.[2]

1.3 Phresny and Dropsy

The *Corpus Hippocraticum* frequently referred to patients who suffered phrensy or who were phrenitic, from which we derive our modern word 'frenzy'. In Greco-Roman times, these terms were given to patients with 'acute inflammation of the mind and body', i.e. exhibiting fever and chill, nuchal rigidity and headache, and voiding scanty urine. In particular, continuous delirium attended phrensy prior to death. The English physician Thomas Willis (1621–1675), in his *London Practice of Physick* (posthumously published in 1685), in a section titled 'Of the phrensy', offered 'meningitis' as the modern diagnosis of phrensy/phrenitis. Moreover, Willis clearly described the pathology of compression of the brain as a consequence of meningeal inflammation and also mentions an epidemic of meningitis in the chapter 'An account of an epidemic fever, reigning An.1661, which chiefly infested the brain and the genus nervosum' (Willis, 1685). In his magnus opus, *De Sedibus et Causis Morborum per Anatomen Indagatis* (1761),[3] the Italian anatomist Giovanni Battista Morgagni (1682–1771) presented and analysed 640 autopsies. In one autopsy, he recognized how the infectious process in otitis media and mastoiditis advanced to the meninges and produced meningitis (Klotz, 1932).

In 'On Diseases' (Section V, Book II, *De Morbis*), Hippocrates writes of 'water upon the brain' (and suggests, as a last resort, an opening of the cranium in order to discharge the fluid), which we recognize today as hydrocephalus or dropsy that can be acute or chronic. In 1768, the Scottish physician Robert Whytt (1714–1766) published a seminal book *Observations on the Dropsy in the Brain*[4] in which he related the history of dropsy and described cases that appeared to result from tuberculous (chronic) meningitis. Whytt's Scottish physician colleagues and contemporaries (the 'Edinburgh School'), David MacBride (1726–1778), John Cheyne (1777–1836), John Fothergill (1712–1780), William Cullen (1710–1790) and John Abercrombie (1781–1844) (Tyler, 2010), all made contributions to the study of hydrocephalus.

1.4 The Swiss and the French

Major contributions towards understanding meningitis were made by the Swiss-Geneva physicians Jean-Francois Coindet (1774–1834), Louis Odier (1748–1814), Gaspard Vieusseux (1746–1814), Jacques-Andre Matthey (1778–1842), Francois-Louis Senn (1799–1873) and Frederic Rillet (1814–1861) (Mullener, 1965), and by the French clinicians Francois Herpin (dates unknown), Louis Guersent (1777–1848) and Antoine Bayle (1799–1858). In his thesis, the French army surgeon Herpin (1803) described cases of CNS infection complicating head injuries in soldiers, particularly noting the presence of pus (suppuration) in the meninges at autopsy. Herpin termed the infection 'meningitis' to describe this 'inflammation of the membranes of the brain' and distinguished this from 'phrenitis' due to the absence of delirium in many of the patients. Back in Edinburgh, the neuropathologist Abercrombie (1828) recognized that meningeal inflammation was the primary pathology in meningitis and was centred specifically on the arachnoid and pia mater and did not involve the dura mater.

1.5 Pathological Subtypes of Meningitis

Abercrombie, in 1828, also recognized that several pathological subtypes of meningitis could present, with inflammation involving the base of the brain (basilar), the surface of the brain (classical) and extending into the ventricles (ventriculitis). In 1839, Louis Guersent proposed a classification of meningitis into (i) tuberculous and (ii) simple, non-tuberculous, which encompassed acute meningitis, chronic meningitis, meningitis following trauma, epidemic meningitis and general paresis of the insane (also known as syphilitic meningitis) (Guersent, 1839). In 1822, the French physican Antoine Laurent Bayle (1799–1858) was the first to comprehensively describe general paresis or 'maladie de Bayle' (Mullener, 1965).

In 1779, Odier described an 'epidemic of meningitis' that occurred in Geneva, with 16 cases and 12 deaths, commenting that this disease occurred every year with this frequency (Odier, 1779). In 1789, Odier described post-mortem results on a boy and a girl, on whom dissection showed hydrocephalus and 'green and yellow pus between the meninges' ('hydrocephale combine avec l'inflammation des meninges'). But Vieusseux is generally credited with the first detailed description of epidemic meningitis, occurring in the environs of Geneva in January 1805, with 33 deaths during a 3-month period. His cases showed classical clinical signs of *Neisseria meningitidis* (meningococcal) meningitis in children with rapid onset and death within 24–48 h (Vieusseux, 1805). Vieusseux also noted at post-mortem that the brain was the only organ that showed pathological changes. But it was his colleague Matthey, reporting on the same epidemic in 1806, who described the archetypal pathology in detail, i.e. congestion of the vessels of the meninges, a blood-tinged gelatinous 'humour' (infiltrate) covering the surface of the brain, ventricular hydrocephalus and the basilar accumulation of suppuration (yellow pus) extending down the spinal canal, without obvious changes in the underlying cerebral tissue (Matthey, 1806). Contemporary accounts of epidemic meningitis were not restricted to Europe, and Lothario Danielson and Elias Mann reported in 1806 an outbreak in Medfield, Massachusetts, that affected nine individuals (Danielson and Mann, 1806). Among the cases, the doctors recorded 'livid spots resembling petechiae' in a child of 15 months old and after 'examination by dissection was had on five bodies' they also recorded that 'Between the dura and pia mater was effused a fluid resembling pus, both over the cerebrum and cerebellum ...', a clear description of purulent meningitis. Elisha North (1771–1843) described the outbreak in Connecticut (1807) as a 'spotted (i.e. petechial) fever' (North, 1811), and in 1810, Nathan Strong (1781–1837) reported on the same outbreak and described cardinal signs of nuchal rigidity (Strong, 1810; Grady, 1965). These clinical presentations in affected children and post-mortem findings are identical to those of Vieusseux (1805) and Matthey (1806).

If the historical records have no antecedents, it appears that epidemic meningitis is a recent phenomenon, appearing with regularity only over the past two centuries. The literature is replete with records of large-scale outbreaks and epidemics in both industrialized countries and Third World countries. An excellent review was published in 1898 by William T. Councilman (1854–1933) and colleagues, of the European and American history of cases, outbreaks and first reports of cerebrospinal meningitis dating back to the 1750s (Councilman *et al.*, 1898).[5] In 1886, August Hirsch (1817–1894) described the occurrence of four major cycles of epidemic cerebrospinal meningitis during the preceding 50 years (Hirsch, 1886). Tellingly, Hirsch noted that infection was seasonal, affected children and soldiers, and occurred in waves with a peak of incidence every 10 years. More modern accounts of epidemic meningococcal meningitis are remarkably similar (Rolleston, 1919; Greenwood, 2006; Leimkugel *et al.*, 2009). In 1922, the American virologist Thomas M. Rivers (1888–1962) published arguably the first comprehensive review of over 220 cases of 'influenzal meningitis' in Baltimore, Chicago and New York (Rivers, 1922). In 2002, the World Health Organization published a scientific analysis of data abstracted from 229 studies of *Haemophilus influenzae* type b (Hib) meningitis published worldwide since the 1940s, before the introduction of the Hib vaccine. Nearly 30,000 cases of Hib meningitis were reported in children under 5 years of age and more than 2100 deaths (Bennett *et al.*, 2002). The written records of pneumococcal meningitis date back to as early as 1868, when the German physicians Immerman and Heller described nine cases of purulent meningitis in 30 cases of croupous pneumonia during an epidemic in Erlangen (Drummond, 1912).

By contrast to these descriptions of epidemic meningitis, several other physicians appreciated a more chronic condition, which we know today is due mainly to disseminated *Mycobacterium tuberculosis* infection. The French physician Francois Lois Senn (1799–1825) described cases of meningitis in children, which he classified as a 'complicated basilar' and chronic tuberculous meningitis, distinct from a 'simple' meningitis (after Guersent) (Senn, 1825). A year later, the English physician Robert Hooper (1773–1835) clearly illustrated basilar meningitis in his *Morbid Anatomy of the Human Brain* (Hooper, 1826).

1.6 Kernig's and Brudzinski's Signs

Evidently, by the mid-19th century, medical science was familiar with the cardinal signs of meningeal irritation and the pathology of meningitis. Understanding that early diagnosis and treatment were critical to patient survival, the Latvian physician Vladimir Kernig (1840–1917) and the Polish physician Jozef Brudzinski (1874–1917) described several clinical signs that now bear their names. Kernig was familiar with neck stiffness in meningitis patients and in 1882 described his cardinal sign (Kernig, 1884). Brudzinski described several different signs of meningitis, including a 'cheek sign', a 'symphisis sign', an 'arm sign', an 'identical contralateral sign' and a 'reciprocal contralateral sign' (Verghese and Gallemore, 1987), but his most well-known sign is the 'nape of the neck sign' (Brudzinski, 1909).

Yet arguably, the first description of a diagnostic test for head flexion is from the Flemish anatomist and physician Andreas Vesalius (1514–1564), author of the influential *De Humani Corporis Fabrica*. On 30 June 1559, Henry II of France was wounded by a jousting lance in the head and subsequently died as a result of his injuries on 10 July. This historical tragedy is interesting for the witness account of Adam Henricpetri, who describes Vesalius using a test to elicit the head flexion sign, leading some commentators to suggest meningitis secondary to head trauma. However, although suppuration was observed post-mortem, Henry's death was probably due to cerebral compression additional to concussion following a contre-coup injury to the brain and subdural haemorrhage.

1.7 A History of the Microbiological Identification of Bacteria Causing Meningitis

The isolation and identification of organisms causing meningitis owes a debt, in part, to the introduction of lumbar puncture as a means of examining cerebrospinal fluid (CSF). The modern and facile technique was introduced by the German physician Heinrich Quincke (1855–1923) in 1891 (Quincke, 1891a,b). Drawing CSF allowed H. Houston Merritt (1902–1979) and Frank Fremont-Smith (1895–1974), in their classic profiling study in 1937 of CSF taken from patients with infectious and other neurological diseases (21,000 fluids examined), to correlate purulent bacterial meningitis, identified by smear or culture, with cardinal signs of low CSF glucose and pleocytosis (Merritt and Fremont-Smith, 1937).

The majority of the recorded epidemics and cases of community-acquired pyogenic bacterial meningitis are due principally to infection with *N. meningitidis* (meningococcus), *Haemophilus influenzae* type B and *Streptococcus pneumoniae* (pneumococcus). Remarkably, these and many other organisms were discovered and identified with association to meningitis between 1881 and 1893, a true 'golden age' in microbiology. In 1887, the Austrian pathologist and bacteriologist Anton Weichselbaum (1845–1920) identified a *Diplococcus intracellularis meningitidis* from the CSF of patients with 'epidemic cerebrospinal meningitis' (Weichselbaum, 1887a,b). The organism was later reclassified as a member of the genus *Neisseria*, named after the German physician Albert Neisser (1855–1916). He discovered in 1879 the causative agent of gonorrhoea, the diplococcus known as *Neisseria gonorrhoeae*, which is also a rare cause of meningitis arising from disseminated infection. In 1884, the Italian physicians and zoologists Ettore Marchiafava (1847–1935) and Angelo Celli (1857–1914) described the presence of oval micrococci within leucocytes in the CSF of patients dying with meningitis (Marchiafava and Celli, 1884). In 1896, the German physicians and microbiologists Johann Heubner (1843–1926) and F. Kiefer independently isolated meningococci from the CSF and throat of living patients (Heubner, 1896; Kiefer, 1896; Goodwin and von Sholly, 1905). The story of the American immunologist George D. Heist (1886–1920) is particularly significant in the history of meningococcal research. His posthumously published seminal paper describes how the author died from meningococcal infection due to a lack of serum bactericidal activity (Heist *et al.*, 1922).

H. influenzae was first isolated by the German physician and bacteriologist Richard Pfeiffer (1858–1945) in 1892 from specimens of lung and sputum taken from patients dying from viral influenza during the pandemics of 1889–1892 (Pfeiffer, 1892). Mistakenly, Pfeiffer attributed the organism as the causative agent of influenza. However, the connection between meningitis and *H. influenzae* (Pfeiffer's bacillus) was made by Slawyk in 1899, who isolated 'influenza-bacillen' from the CSF of patients by lumbar puncture and from the brains of children post-mortem (Slawyk, 1899). In 1931, the American bacteriologist Margaret Pittman (1901–1995) identified six capsular polysaccharides of *H. influenzae*, of which Pittman type B was invariably isolated from cases of human systemic infection (Pittman, 1931).

The remarkable French chemist and microbiologist Louis Pasteur (1822–1895) identified a 'microbe septicemique de la salive' from the saliva of a child who had died of rabies (Pasteur, 1881). Pasteur showed that inoculation of rabbits with infectious saliva could induce septicaemia, fulfilling in part the postulates of his contemporary H.H. Robert Koch (1843–1910) (Koch, 1884, 1890). The same organism, *Micrococcus pasteuri*, was also discovered in 1881 by the American microbiologist and Brigadier General George Sternberg (1838–1915) (Sternberg, 1881). Both these microbiologists alluded to the pneumococcus, but the studies of Albert Fraenkel (1864–1938) and Anton Weichselbaum in 1886 provided definite identification, assigning the bacterium initially to the genus *Diplococcus*. The organism was later reclassified as *S. pneumoniae*.

In 1884, the German physician and microbiologist Friedrich Rosenbach (1842–1923) described the streptococcus of wound infections and gave it the specific name *Streptococcus pyogenes* (Rosenbach, 1884). In 1933, the American microbiologist Rebecca C. Lancefield (1895–1981) published a serological classification of haemolytic streptococci into different groups based on the presence of a group-specific polysaccharide (Lancefield, 1933). Thus, *S. pyogenes* isolates were all serogroup A (GAS) and *Streptococcus agalactiae* or *Streptococcus mastitidis* was classified as Lancefield Group B (GBS). *S. mastiditis* was the name given to the organism associated with bovine mastitis (Hansen, 1935), although it appears to have been recorded by V. Trevisan in 1889 by a different name, *Streptococcus nocardi*. The exact identity of *S. mastiditis* probably dates from the studies of S. Henry Ayers and colleagues from 1918 to 1922 (Ayers *et al.*, 1918; Ayers and Mudge, 1922; Ayers and Rupp, 1922), who differentiated the organism from *S. pyogenes*, and Lancefield and others, between 1933 and 1937, who reported on organisms identical in physiology and serology, i.e. Lancefield Group B (*agalactiae*), isolated from human sources including the nose and throat, vagina and from faeces (Hare, 1935; Lancefield and Hare, 1935; Plummer, 1935; Sherman, 1937).

Before the introduction of antibiotics, the incidence of pyogenic streptococcal meningitis was between 10 and 20%, but the incidence of GAS meningitis was unknown, as Lancefield grouping was not reported in these studies (Murphy, 1983). However, many reports of GAS meningitis have been published more recently (Berner *et al.*, 2000; Mathur *et al.*, 2004). The earliest reports of GBS meningitis appear to be from Leonard Colebrook and Anthony W. Purdie, who included two cases in a description of 106 cases of puerperal fever (Colebrook and Purdie, 1937), and from R.M. Fry (1938), Brown (1939) and Nyhan and Fousek (1958). The other significant member of the genus *Streptococcus* that can cause meningitis is the zoonotic pathogen *Streptococcus suis*; the first human cases of *S. suis* meningitis and sepsis were diagnosed in Denmark in 1968 by Perch *et al.* (1968).

The Scottish military surgeon Sir Alexander Ogston (1844–1929) first discovered *Staphylococcus aureus* in 1883 during his studies on 'acute suppuration' in abscess formation. Ogston has been credited with the naming of *Staphylococcus*, struck by the resemblance between staphylococcal clumps and bunches of grapes (Ogston, 1880, 1883). Subsequently, Rosenbach (1884) distinguished between *S. aureus* and *Staphylococcus albus*, later renamed as *epidermidis*, on the basis of the bacteria forming white and yellow colonies, respectively.

Several other important organisms that can cause meningitis are noted in Table 1.1 and range from the common to the very rare. Murray, Webb and Swann in 1924 isolated an organism, which they called *Bacterium monocytogenes*, from laboratory animals presenting with septicaemia and an intense monocytosis (Murray *et al.*, 1926). The organism was renamed *Listeria monocytogenes*, in honour of Joseph Lister (1827–1912), by James Pirie in 1940 (Pirie, 1940). The first case of listeriosis hominis was reported in 1929 by A. Nyfeldt in Denmark (Nyfeldt, 1929), but C.G. Burn in 1934 established a causal link between *Listeria* 'granulomatous septicaemia' and meningitis in newborn infants and adults (Burn, 1934).

In 1882, C. Gessard first reported that 'blue pus' was caused by the chromogenic Gram-negative organism *Bacillus pyocyaneus*, later named *Pseudomonas aeruginosa* (Gessard,

Table 1.1. Causative organisms of bacterial meningitis.

Type of meningitis	Causative organisms
Major, pyogenic	*Haemophilus influenzae*
	Neisseria meningitidis
	Streptococcus pneumoniae
Neonatal, Gram-positive	*Bacillus* spp. (*B. cereus*, *B. circulans*, *B. alvei*)
	Clostridium perfringens
	Listeria monocytogenes, *seeligeri*
	Staphylococcus aureus
	Staphylococcus coagulase-negative, e.g. *S. epidermidis*, *S. capitis*
	Streptococcus bovis (*gallolyticus*)
	Streptococcus pyogenes (Group A)
	Streptococcus agalactiae (Group B)
	Streptococcus dysgalactiae subsp. *equisimilis*/(Group C)
	Streptococcus pneumoniae
Neonatal, Gram-negative	*Achromobacter xylosoxidans*
	Acinetobacter calcoaceticus (*Mima polymorpha*; *Herellea vaginolica*)
	Burkholderia pseudomallei
	Citrobacter spp. (*diversus-koseri*, *freundii*, *sedlakii*)
	Elizabethkingia (*Flavobacterium*) *meningosepticum*
	Enterobacter spp., *Chronobacter sakazakii* (Gram-negative bacillary meningitis)
	Escherichia coli K1
	Haemophilus influenzae, *parainfluenzae*, type C
	Klebsiella pneumoniae
	Moraxella (*Branhamella*) *catarrhalis*
	Pasteurella multicoda, *ureae*, *gallinarum*
	Proteus mirabilis
	Pseudomonas aeruginosa
	Salmonella spp. (rare include *S. berta* (Kauffman group D) (Brendan), *S. pomona* (Ahmad), *S. poona* (G), *S. virchow* (C), *S. oslo*, *S. stanley* (B), *S. hadar*, *S. oranienberg* (C), *S. maltopeni*, *S. carmel*, *S. enteriditis dublin*, *S. thompson* (C))
	Serratia marcesens
Neonatal, other	*Mycoplasma hominis*
	Ureaplasma urealyticum
Actinomycetales (typical and atypical)	*Mycobacterium avium-intracellulare*, *kansasii*, *fortuitum*
	Mycobacterium tuberculosis
	Nocardia spp. (*N. asteroides*, *N. brasiliensis*, *N. caviae*, *N. farcinica*, *N. transvalensis*)
	Oerskovia xanthineolytica (*Nocardia*-like)
	Tropheryma whippelii
Spirochaetales	*Borrelia* spp. (*B. burgdorferi*, *B. duttonii*, *B. recurrentis*, *B. turicatae*)
	Leptospira spp. (*L. interrogans*, *L. australis*, *L. panama*, *L. hardjo*, *L. grippotyphosa*, *L. wolffi*)
	Treponema pallidum

Continued

Table 1.1. Continued

Type of meningitis	Causative organisms
Other acquired (uncommon/ opportunistic/nosocomial/ zoonotic/head trauma, neurosurgical procedures)	*Acinetobacter* spp. (*A. baumannii*, *A. calcoaceticus* (*Mima polymorpha*; *Herellea vaginicola*), *anitratum*, *lwoffii*) *Bacillus anthracis*, *B. sphericus*, *B. cereus* *Bacteroides* spp. (*B. distasonis*, *B. fragilis*, *B. melanogenicus*, *B. ovatus*, *B. thetaiotamicron*, *B. ureolyticus*; *Bacillus funduliformis*; *Eggerthella convexa*; *Eikenella corrodens*; *Ristella convexa*) *Bergeyella zoohelcum* (CDCIIj) *Branhamella catarrhalis* *Brucella* spp. (*melitensis*, *abortus*, *suis*) *Burkholderia* (*Pseudomonas*) *pseudomallei*, *picketii* *Capnocytophaga canimorsus* *Clostridium* spp. (*C. ramosum*, *C. welchii*, *C. perfringens*, *C. septicum*, *C. cadaveris*, *C. tertium*) *Corynebacterium acnes* *Edwardsiella tarda* *Enterobacter* spp. (*E. aerogenes*, *E. cloacae*, *E. agglomerans*) *Fusobacterium necrophorum*, *aquatile*, *nucleatum* *Haemophilus influenzae*, non-typeable *Kingella kingae* *Klebsiella oxytoca*, *K. ozaenae*, *K. aerogenes* *Morganella morganii* *Mycoplasma pneumoniae* *Neisseria gonorrhoeae* *Pasteurella* spp. *(P. multicoda*, *P. haemolytica*, *P. pestis*, *P. tularensis*, *P. ureae*, *P. septica)* *Proteus mirabilis/vulgaris* *Providentia stuartii* *Pseudomonas putida* *Pseudomonas* spp. (*P. pyocyanea*, *P. cepacia*, *P. maltophilia*, *P. paucimobilis*, *P. stutzeri*, *P. putrefaciens*, *P. denitrificans*) *Ralstonia mannolytica* *Serratia marcesens* *Staphylococcus* and coagulase-negative *Staphyloccus* spp. (*S. aureus*, *S. haemolyticus*, *S. warneri*, *S. cohnii*, *S. capitis*, *S. epidermidis*, *S. lugdunensis*) *Stenotrophomonas* (*Xanthomonas*) *maltophila* *Streptococcus bovis* *Streptococcus suis*, *S. zooepidemicus*, *S. milleri*, *S. salivarius* *Yersinia* (*enterocolitica*, *pestis*)
Polymicrobial, feculent	*Enterococcus faecalis* *Peptostreptococcus* spp. *Prevotella* *Slackia exigua* *Streptococcus constellatus*, *faecium* *Veillonella* spp.

1882). In 1890, E. Ehlers published the first reports of meningitis, in a brother and sister aged 11 and 12 years, due to *P. aeruginosa* infection (Ehlers, 1890), and in 1893–1894, Kossel isolated pure bacteria from the pia mater and blood of a 6-week-old infant who had died from meningitis secondary to middle ear infection (Kossel, 1893, 1894). In an early review of the case literature, J.W. Epstein and A.B. Grossman in 1936 had already noted that infection of the meninges by *P. aeruginosa* generally arose by direct extension and was rarely haematogenous (Epstein and Grossman, 1933).

Salmonella spp. represent a leading cause of Gram-negative bacterial meningitis, predominantly in neonates in the developing world but also affecting infants and older children. Adult meningitis is reported but less common. The first *Salmonella* species (*Salmonella enterica* var. *choleraesuis*) was discovered in 1885 by the American epidemiologist and pathologist Theobald Smith (1859–1934), during his tenure as a research assistant to the veterinary surgeon Daniel Elmer Salmon (1850–1914). The genus *Salmonella* was named by J. Lignieres in 1901 in honour of Salmon, and he used 'le microbe du hog-cholera de Salmon' as the type species (Lignieres, 1901). (Erroneously, the organism isolated by Smith and Salmon was, in fact, not the causative organism of hog cholera.) Today, the genus *Salmonella* consists of two species, *Salmonella enterica* (containing six subspecies) and *Salmonella bongori*, which together contain 2463 different serovars (Brenner *et al.*, 2000). New serovars are reported annually in the journal *Research in Microbiology* as supplements to the Kauffmann–White–Le Minor scheme (Kauffmann, 1931).

The first cases of *Salmonella* meningitis were reported by A. Ghon in 1907 (Ghon, 1907). Siegbert Bornstein in 1943 remarked that all types of *Salmonella* may produce pathological changes in man (Bornstein, 1943), and this would appear to hold true for meningeal infection. For example, *Salmonella enteriditis* (isolated by A. Gartner, 1888), *Salmonella typhi* (isolated by G. Gaffky (1850–1918), 1884), *Salmonella paratyphi A* (isolated by N.B. Gywn and G.E. Wantz, 1898), *Salmonella paratyphi B* (isolated by E.C. Achard (1856–1914) and R. Bensaude (1866–1938) in 1896 as the 'Bacille paratyphique'), *Salmonella havana*, *Salmonella panama* (isolated by E.O. Jordan, 1931), *Salmonella typhimurium* (isolated by F.A. Loeffler (1852–1915) in 1892), *Salmonella choleraesuis*, *Salmonella montevideo* and *Salmonella enterica* subsp. *arizonae* and subsp. *houtenae* have all been reported as causing meningitis. Other rare salmonellae have been isolated from cases (Table 1.1). The generally accepted pathogenesis begins with ingestion of virulent *Salmonella*, entry into the blood to produce bacteraemia and septicaemia, and penetration into the leptomeninges to establish acute purulent inflammation. In addition to nosocomial transmission, zoonotic transmission can also occur. Interestingly, *S. enterica* subsp. *arizonae*, first discovered by M.E. Caldwell and D.L. Ryerson in 1939 (Caldwell and Ryerson, 1940), was initially considered a reptile pathogen, particularly of snakes (Hinshaw and McNeil, 1945) but is now recognized as a significant meningeal pathogen in young children and immunocompromised individuals.

In 1882, the German pathologist and microbiologist Carl Friedländer (1847–1887) discovered the microorganism that he believed caused bacterial pneumonia (Friedländer, 1882), following the observations of the German-Swiss pathologist Edwin Klebs (1834–1913) who had seen bacteria in the airways of individuals who died from pneumonia in 1875. The organism was named *Bacillus friedlanderi* or Freidlander's bacillus, now included in the genus *Klebsiella*, to honor the work of Klebs. In 1888, Anton Weichselbaum described the first case of Friedlander's bacillus meningitis (Weichselbaum, 1888), and, although rare in the literature that followed (Holland, 1950), today we recognize that *Klebsiella* spp. frequently cause nosocomial septicaemia and meningitis in newborns in neonatal intensive care units and other infections in hospitalized patients (Podschun and Ullmann, 1998).

The genus *Escherichia* was discovered by the German-Austrian paediatrician Theodor Escherich (1857–1911) in 1885 (Escherich, 1885a,b). Escherich described in his thesis an intestinal bacterium that he called 'bacterium coli commune' (Escherich, 1886). The organism was later reclassified as *Bacillus coli* in 1895 by Walter Migula (1863–1938), the German pioneer of systematics (Migula, 1895) and then renamed in 1919 by A. Castellani and A.J. Chalmers as the type genus *Escherichia* and type species *coli*, after its original discoverer (Castellani and Chalmers, 1919). Bacteria expressing the K (Kapsel) 1 (Kauffmann and Vahlne, 1945) polysaccharide are predominantly isolated in cases of *E. coli* neonatal meningitis. The first record of *E. coli* neonatal infection was made by M. Macaigne in Paris in 1892 (Macaigne, 1892).

Members of the order *Spirochaetales* are also well-known causative agents of meningitis. *Treponema pallidum* subsp. *pallidum*, the causative agent of syphilis with its many varied presentations, was co-discovered in 1905 by the German zoologist Fritz Richard Schaudinn (1871–1906) and the German dermatologist Erich Hoffmann (1868–1959) during their research at the Charité Clinic in Berlin. They isolated a spirochaete from a papula in the vulva of a patient with secondary syphilis and aptly named it *Spirochaeta pallida* (Schaudinn and Hoffmann, 1905). The German bacteriologist August Paul von Wassermann (1866–1925), working at the Robert Koch Institute for Infectious Diseases in Berlin, developed an antibody-dependent complement fixation test with Albert Neisser in 1906, which has become known as the Wassermann test for diagnosing early syphilis (Wassermann *et al.*, 1906). In 1913, the Japanese bacteriologist Hideyo Noguchi (1876–1928) and his colleague J.W. Moore used Wassermann's test to unequivocally demonstrate for the first time the presence of *T. pallidum* in brain specimens taken from individuals with general paresis of the insane, also known as general paralysis or paralytic dementia (Noguchi and Moore, 1913). Syphilitic meningitis and meningovascular syphilis are usually recognized as symptoms of tertiary neurosyphilis although involvement of the meninges can sometimes be observed in early (acute) infection with unusual manifestations and in the (partially) chronic form (Ho and Lukehart, 2011).

In 1982, the Swiss-American entymologist and zoologist Willy Burgdorfer isolated a treponeme-like spirochaete from adult *Ixodes scapularis* (formerly *dammini*), a tick vector of Lyme disease (Burgdorfer *et al.*, 1982). With his colleagues, he also showed that serum from patients with Lyme disease contained antibodies reactive with the isolated organism, which was subsequently named *Borrelia burgdorferi* in his honour. However, prior to isolation of the causative organism, the *erythema migrans* rash typical of Lyme disease was first reported in 1921 by A. Afzelius (1921), and the classic neurologic syndrome of lymphocytic meningitis and involvement of the peripheral nervous system (painful polyradiculoneuropathy) was clearly described first by B. Garin in 1922. It is worth noting that Garin stated succinctly in the title of his paper that paralysis was mediated by ticks (Garin, 1922).

Meningitis is also a characteristic feature of advancing Weil's disease, which is caused by the spirochaete *Leptospira interrogans* (serovar *icterohaemorrhagiae*). The disease is named after the German physician Adolf Weil (1848–1916), who in 1886 described the classical signs and symptoms associated with acute leptospiral infection such as splenomegaly, jaundice and nephritis (Weil, 1886). A spirochaete was noted by A.M. Stimson in 1907 in post-mortem renal tissue and named *Spirochaeta interrogans* because the organism had 'hooked ends' (Stimson, 1907). The first recorded cases of meningitis with jaundice in Weil's disease were reported by C. Laubry and M. Parvu (1910), Laubry and G. Foy (1910), G. Gullain and C. Richet (1910) and M. Rist (1910), in Paris. The causative organism of Weil's disease was finally isolated in 1915 by Ryokichi Inada and Yutaka Ido and named *Spirochaeta icterohaemorrhagiae* (Inada and Ido, 1915). The key role of the rat as a primary reservoir for the pathogen was discovered in 1917 by Ido and colleagues (Ido *et al.*, 1917), and the association between bathing (in contaminated waters) and 'spirochetose meningee pure' was observed later in the 1930s (Schuffner and Walch-Sorgdrager, 1936; Lavergne and Accoyer, 1937). The French clinicians S. Costa and J. Troisier demonstrated in 1916 that *Spirochaeta* (*Leptospira*) *icterohaemorrhagiae* was the causative organism of meningitis in Weil's disease and that meningitis could also present without jaundice (Costa and Troisier, 1916a,b). Subsequently, historical reports of meningitis in Weil's disease became more frequent both in Europe and the USA (Clapper and Myers, 1943). Although meningitis usually presents in the early acute phase, in 1936 F. Murgatroyd presented a case of chronic late-onset meningitis in Weil's disease (Murgatroyd, 1937).

Members of the order *Actinomycetales* are also important causes of bacterial meningitis. A scourge of mankind from earliest recorded history, *M. tuberculosis* was unequivocally identified by Koch in tuberculous lesions in infected human tissues in 1882. Koch announced his findings in a famous lecture to the Berlin Physiological Society on 24 March 1882 (Koch, 1882). In 1933, the pioneering studies of post-mortem tuberculous meningitis brains by the renowned American pathologists Arnold Rice Rich (1893–1968) and Howard McCordock (1895–1938) suggested that, in the majority of cases, bacilli entered the subarachnoidal space from a caseous focus in either the brain cortex or the meninges (Rich and McCordock, 1933). The caseous focus was named the 'Rich focus' and their formation is dependent on haematogenous (miliary) spread of bacilli (Schaaf, 2009). *Nocardia* and *Tropheryma* are also worth noting as rare causes of meningitis. In 1888, the French veterinarian and microbiologist Edmond Nocard (1850–1903) isolated an organism from a case of bovine lymphadenitis, which was named *Nocardia* (Nocard, 1888). In 1889, V. Trevisan characterized the organism and named it *Nocardia farcinica* (Trevisan, 1889), which became the type species to be replaced by *Nocardia asteroides* as a result of phenotypic and taxonomic studies by Ruth Gordon and Joan Mihm in 1962 (Gordon and Mihm, 1962). *Nocardia* infection can vary from cutaneous to severe pulmonary nocardiosis, which is usually observed in immunocompromised individuals with underlying chronic respiratory conditions (Brown-Elliott *et al.*, 2006). However, in 50% of patients with pulmonary nocardiosis, dissemination of the organism is apparent and can be manifested as meningitis and abscess. Involvement of the meninges has been hypothesized to occur by the haematogenous route, disseminating from the primary site, the infected lung; by rupture of cerebral abscess into the ventricles; or by non-haematogenous routes, including direct inoculation from the *Nocardia*-infected ear or mastoid (Bross and Gordon, 1991).

In 1907, the American physician and pathologist George Hoyt Whipple (1878–1976) reported a 'hitherto undescribed disease' that he named 'intestinal lipodystrophy', but which we know today as 'Whipple's disease' (Whipple, 1907). This rare systemic illness, predominantly of middle-aged white men, is a chronic granulomatous disease with mainly gastrointestinal manifestions, but it can affect every major organ, including the CNS. Although case reports in the literature are rare, meningitic features and encephalitis have been noted (Schwartzova *et al.*, 1967; Thompson *et al.*, 1978; Schneider *et al.*, 2008). Whipple originally noted the presence of a bacillus in lymph nodes from the patient but, despite repeated attempts, the organism cannot be cultured *in vitro*. *Tropheryma whippeli* was eventually identified by David Relman and colleagues in 1992 by amplification of the bacterial 16S ribosomal RNA in infected tissue from patients with the disease (Relman *et al.*, 1992).

1.8 Conclusions

Meningitis is defined as inflammation of the meninges, the membranes that surround the brain within the skull and the spinal cord within the spinal canal. Meningitis can be caused by a plethora of different bacteria across all age groups (Table 1.1) and no doubt this list is incomplete as more rare causes are reported. Thus, it seems reasonable to conclude that any organsism that can enter the subarachnoidal space has the potential to cause meningitis.

Notes

1 For the reader interested in the Hippocratic tradition and Galen's Hippocraticism, Wesley D. Smith's book (1979) is judicious reading and is available online at http://www.biusante.parisdescartes.fr/medicina/Hippo2.pdf. Adams' translation is also available at http://www.archive.org/details/genuineworkship02hippgoog

2 The original Latin text is available from the Harvard Medical School Library at http://ia700406.us.archive.org/7/items/hieronymifracast00frac/hieronymifracast00frac.pdf

3 The original Latin text is available at http://www.archive.org/details/desedibusetcaus06adelgoog

4 Available from Harvard Medical School at http://www.archive.org/details/observationsondr00whyt

5 Available from http://www.archive.org/details/epidemiccerebros1898mass

References

Abercrombie, J. (1828) Inflammation of the arachnoid and pia mater. In: *Pathological and Practical Researches on Diseases of the Brain and the Spinal Cord.* Waugh and Innes, Edinburgh, pp. 49–71.

Adams, F. (1849) *The Genuine Works of Hippocrates.* Sydenham Society, London.

Afzelius, A. (1921) Erythema chronicum migrans. *Acta Dermato Venereologica (Stockholm)* 2, 120–125.

Ayers, S.H. and Mudge, C.S. (1922) The streptococci of the bovine udder. IV. Studies of the streptococci. *Journal of Infectious Diseases* 31, 40–50.

Ayers, S.H. and Rupp, P. (1922) Differentiation of hemolytic streptococci from human and bovine sources by the hydrolysis of sodium hippurate. *Journal of Infectious Diseases* 30, 388–399.

Ayers, S.H., Johnson, W.T. and Davis, B.J. (1918) The thermal death point and limiting hydrogen-ion concentration of pathogenic streptococci. *Journal of Infectious Diseases* 23, 290–300.

Bennett, V., Platonov, A.E., Slack, M.P.E., Mala, P., Burton, A.H. and Robertson, S.E. (2002) Haemophilus Influenzae *Type b (Hib) Meningitis in the Pre-vaccine Era: A Global Review of Incidence, Age Distributions, and Case-fatality Rates.* Department of Vaccines and Biologicals, World Health Organization, Geneva, Switzerland.

Berner, R., Herdeg, S., Gordjani, N. and Brandis, M. (2000) *Streptococcus pyogenes* meningitis: report of a case and review of the literature. *European Journal of Paediatrics* 159, 527–529.

Bornstein, S. (1943) Review: the state of the *Salmonella* problem. *Journal of Immunology* 46, 439–496.

Breasted, J.H. (1930) *The Edwin Smith Surgical Papyrus* (trans.). University of Chicago Press, Chicago.

Brenner, F.W., Villar, R.G., Angulo, F.J., Tauxe, R. and Swaminathan, B. (2000) *Salmonella* nomenclature (Guest commentary). *Journal of Clinical Microbiology* 38, 2465–2467.

Bross, J.E. and Gordon, G. (1991) Nocardial meningitis – case reports and review. *Reviews of Infectious Diseases* 13, 160–165.

Brown, J.H. (1939) Double-zone beta-hemolytic streptococci: their cultural characteristics, serological grouping, occurrence and pathogenic significance. *Journal of Bacteriology* 37, 133–144.

Brown-Elliott, B.A., Brown, J.M., Conville, P.S. and Wallace, R.J. (2006) Clinical and laboratory features of the *Nocardia* spp. based on current molecular taxonomy. *Clinical Microbiology Reviews* 19, 259–282.

Brudzinski, J. (1909) Un signe nouveau sur les membres inferieurs dans les meningites chez les infants (signe de la nuque). *Archives de Médecine des Enfants* 12, 745–752.

Burgdorfer, W., Barbour, A.G., Hayes, S.F., Benach, J.L., Grunwaldt, E. and Davis, J.P. (1982) Lyme disease – a tick-borne spirochetosis. *Science* 216, 1317–1319.

Burn, C.G. (1934) Unidentified Gram-positive bacillus associated with meningoencephalitis. *Proceedings of the Society for Experimental Biology and Medicine* 31, 1095–1097.

Caldwell, M.E. and Ryerson, D.L. (1940) A new species of the genus *Pseudomonas* pathogenic for certain reptiles. *Journal of Bacteriology* 39, 323–336.

Castellani, A. and Chalmers, A.J. (1919) *Manual of Tropical Medicine.* Williams Wood and Co., New York.

Clapper, M. and Myers, G.B. (1943) Clinical manifestations of Weil's disease with particular reference to meningitis. *Archives of Internal Medicine* 72, 18–30.

Colebrook, L. and Purdie, A.W. (1937) Treatment of 106 cases of puerperal fever by sulphanilamide (streptocide). *Lancet* 230, 1237–1242.

Costa, S. and Troisier, J. (1916a) Meningite avec subictere dans la spirochetose icterhemorragique. *Bulletins et Mémoires de la Société Médicale des Hôpitaux de Paris* 40, 1928–1931.

Costa, S. and Troisier, J. (1916b) Reactions meningees dans la spirochetose ictero-hemorragique: virulence du liquid cephalorachiden. *Bulletins et Mémoires de la Société Médicale des Hôpitaux de Paris* 40, 1802–1806.

Councilman, W.T., Mallory, F.B. and Wright, J.H. (1898) *Epidemic Cerebrospinal Meningitis and its Relation to other Forms of Meningitis. A Report by the State Board of Health of Massachusetts.* Wright and Potter, Boston.

Danielson, L. and Mann, E. (1806) The history of a singular and very mortal disease, which lately made its appearance in Medfield. Manning and Loring, Boston, pp. 65–69. Reprinted in *Reviews of Infectious Diseases* 5, 969–972 (1983).

Drummond, H. (1912) Pneumococcal meningitis. *British Medical Journal* 1, 179–180.

Ehlers, E. (1890) To tilfaelde af echthyma gangraenosum maladie pyocyanique, hos mennesket. *Hospitale Tidende, Copenhagen* 8, 517.

Epstein, J.W. and Grossman, A.B. (1933) *Bacillus pyocyaneus* in children. *American Journal of Diseases of Children* 46, 132–147.

Escherich, T. (1885a) Die Darmbakterien des Neugeborenen und Siiuglings. *Fortschritte der Medizin* 3, 515–522.
Escherich, T. (1885b) Die Darmbakterien des Neugeborenen und Siiuglings. *Fortschritte der Medizin* 3, 547–554.
Escherich, T. (1886) *Die Darmbakterien des Säuglings und ihre Beziehungen zur Physiologie der Verdauung.* Verlag von Ferdinand Enke, Stuttgart.
Friedländer, C. (1882) Über die Schizomyceten bei der acuten fibrösen Pneumonie. *Virchow's Archive für Pathologische Anatomie und Physiologie* 87, 319–324.
Fry, R.M. (1938) Fatal infections by haemolytic *Streptococcus* Group B. *Lancet* 231, 199–201.
Garin, B. (1922) Paralysie par les tiques. *Journal of Medicine (Lyon)* 71, 765–767.
Gessard, C. (1882) Sur des colorations bleue et verte des linges a pansements. *Comptes Rendus de l'Académie des Science, Paris* 94, 563.
Ghon, A. (1907) Die banillen der typhusgrueppe. Bericht uber den XIV Internationalen Kongress fur Hygiene und Dermographie. IV, 21–23. Berlin.
Goodwin, M.E. and von Sholly, A.I. (1905) The frequent occurrence of meningococci in the nasal cavities of meningitis patients and of those in direct contact with them. *Public Health Papers and Reports* 31, 21–34.
Gordon, R.E. and Mihm, J.M. (1962) The type species of the genus *Nocardia*. *Journal of General Microbiology* 27, 1–10.
Grady, F.J. (1965) Some early American reports on meningitis with special reference to the inaugural dissertation of Nathan Strong. *Journal of the History of Medicine and Allied Sciences* 20, 27–32.
Greenwood, B. (2006) Editorial: 100 years of epidemic meningitis in West Africa – has anything changed? *Tropical Medicine & International Health* 11, 773–780.
Guersent, L.B. (1839) Meningite. In: Nysten, P.H. (ed.) *Dictionnaire de Medecine.* J.S. Chaude, Paris, pp. 387–440.
Gullain, G. and Richet, C. (1910) Etude sur une maladie infectieuse caracterisee par de l'ictere et un syndrome meningee. *Bulletins et Mémoires de la Société Médicale des Hôpitaux de Paris* 30, 289–299.
Hansen, P.A. (1935) *Mastitis III. The Identity of* Streptococcus Agalactiae. *New York Agricultural Experiment Station Technical Bulletin No. 232.* New York Agricultural Experiment Station, Geneva (New York).
Hare, R. (1935) The classification of haemolytic streptococci from the nose and throat of normal human beings by means of precipitin and biochemical tests. *Journal of Pathology and Bacteriology* 41, 499–512.
Heist, G.D., Solis-Cohen, S. and Solis-Cohen, M. (1922) A study of the virulence for man and of human susceptibility to meningococcal infection. *Journal of Immunology* 7, 1–33.
Herpin, F. (1803) Meningitis ou inflammation des membranes de l'encephale précédé de quelques considérations physiologiques sur ces membranes, et suivi de plusieurs observations recueillies à l'armée du Rhin, essai présenté et soutenu à l'Ecole de Médecine de Paris, le 20 vendémiaire an XII. Paris: Impr. didot jeune, 80 pp.
Heubner, J.O.L. (1896) Beobachtungen und versuche über den meningokokkus intracellularis (Weichselbaum-Jaeger). *Jb Kinderheilk* 43, 1–22.
Hinshaw, W.R. and McNeil, E. (1945) Salmonella types isolated from snakes. *American Journal of Veterinary Research* 6, 264–266.
Hirsch, A. (1886) Epidemic cerebro-spinal meningitis. *Hirsch's Handbook of Geographical and Historical Pathology* (translated from the 2nd German edition by Charles Creighton). New Sydenham Society, London, pp. 547–594.
Ho, E.L. and Lukehart, S.A. (2011) Syphilis: using modern approaches to understand an old disease. *Journal of Clinical Investigation* 121, 4584–4592.
Holland, C.W. (1950) Friedlander's bacillus meningitis. *Canadian Medical Association Journal* 63, 131–134.
Hooper, R. (1826) *The Morbid Anatomy of the Human Brain: Being Illustrations of the Most Frequent and Important Organic Diseases to which that Viscus is Subject.* Longman, Ress, Orme, Brown and Green, London.
Ido, Y., Hoki, R., Ito, H. and Wani, H. (1917) The rat as a carrier of *Spirochaeta icterohaemorrhagiae*, the causative agent of Weil's disease (spirochaetosis icterohaemorrhagica). *Journal of Experimental Medicine* 26, 341–353.
Inada, R. and Ido, Y. (1915) A report of the discovery of the causal organism (a new species of spirocheta) of Weil's disease. *Tokyo Ijishinshi* 1908, 351–360.
Kauffmann, F. (1931) Der heutige Stand der Paratyphusforschung. Kritisches ßbersichtsreferat. *Zentralblatt für die gesamte Hygiene* 25, 273.
Kauffmann, F. and Vahlne, G. (1945) Uber die Bedeutung des serologischen Formenwechsels fur de Bakteriophagenwirkung in der Coli-Gruppe. *Acta Pathologica Microbiologica Scandinavica* 22, 119–137.

Kernig, V.M. (1884) Uber ein wenig bemerktes Meningitis-Symptom. *Berlin Klinische Wochenschrift* 21, 829–832.

Kiefer, F. (1896) Zur differentialdiagnose des erregers der epidemischen cerebrospinalmeningitis und der gonorrhoe. *Berlin Klinische Wochenschrift* 33, 628–630.

Klotz, O. (1932) Giovanni Battista Morgagni. *Canadian Medical Association Journal* 27, 298–303.

Koch, R. (1882) Die Aetiologie der Tuberculose. *Berlin Klinische Wochenschrift* 19, 221–230.

Koch, R. (1884) Die Aetiologie der Tuberculose. *Mitt Kaiser Gesundh* 2, 1–88.

Koch, R. (1890) Ueber bakteriologische Forschung: Vortrag in der 1. allgemeinen Sitzung des X. Internationalen Medicinischen Congresses am 4 August 1890, 35.

Kossel, H. (1893) Zur frage der pathogenitat des *Bacillus pyocyaneus* fur menschen. *Charite Ann* 18, 498.

Kossel, H. (1894) Zur frage der pathogenitat des *Bacillus pyocyaneus* fur menschen. *Zeitschrift für Hygiene und Infektionskrankheiten* 16, 368.

Lancefield, R.C. (1933) A serological differentiation of human and other groups of hemolytic streptococci. *Journal of Experimental Medicine* 57, 571–595.

Lancefield, R.C. and Hare, R. (1935) The serological differentiation of pathogenic and non-pathogenic strains of hemolytic streptococci from parturient women. *Journal of Experimental Medicine* 61, 335–349.

Laubry, C. and Foy, G. (1910) Syndrome méningé avec polynucleose rachidienne d'origine indeterminée. *Bulletins et Mémoires de la Société Médicale des Hôpitaux de Paris* 30, 230.

Laubry, C. and Parvu, M. (1910) Syndrome meninge avec lymphocytose rachedienne d'origine indeterminee. *Bulletins et Mémoires de la Société Médicale des Hôpitaux de Paris* 30, 236–244.

Lavergne, V. de and Accoyer, H. (1937) Mémoires originaux. La spirochétose méningée pure. Considérations épidémiologiques et pathogéniques. *Revue d'Hygiène et de Médecine Preventive*, 59, 339–352.

Leimkugel, J., Racloz, V., da Silva, L.J. and Pluschke, G. (2009) Global review of meningococcal disease. A shifting etiology. *Journal of Bacteriology Research* 1, 6–18.

Lignieres, M.J. (1901) Contribution a l'étude et à la classification sépticemies hémorragiques les "pasteurelloses". *Annales de l'Institut Pasteur* 15, 734–736.

Littré, E. (1839) *Oeuvres complètes d'Hippocrate,* 10 volumes. *(1839–1881).* J.B. Bailliere, Paris.

Macaigne, M. (1892) Le Bacterium coli commune son role dans la pathologic. (Thesis, Paris no. 1974). Paris, Societe d'Editons Scientifiques.

Marchiafava, E. and Celli, A. (1884) Spra i micrococchi della meningite cerebrospinale epidemica. *Gazzetta Ospedale* 5, 59.

Mathur, P., Arora, N., Kapil, A. and Das, B. (2004) *Streptococcus pyogenes* meningitis. *Indian Journal of Pediatrics* 71, 423–426.

Matthey, A. (1806) Recherches sur une maladie particuliere qui a regne a Geneve en 1805. *Journal de Médecine, de Chirurgie, et de Pharmacie Militaires* 11, 243–253.

Merritt, H.H. and Fremont-Smith, F. (1937) *The Cerebrospinal Fluid.* WB Saunders, Philadelphia.

Migula, W. (1895) Bacteriaceae (Stäbchenbacterien). In: Engler, A. (ed.) *Die Natürlichen Pflanzenfamilien. Teil I, Abteilung Ia.* W. Engelmann, Leipzig, pp. 20–30.

Mullener, E.R. (1965) Six Geneva physicians on meningitis. *Journal of the History of Medicine* 20, 1–26.

Murgatroyd, F. (1937) Chronic meningitis in Weil's disease. *British Medical Journal* 1, 7–11.

Murphy, D.J. (1983) Group A streptococcal meningitis. *Pediatrics* 71, 1–5.

Murray, E.G.D., Webb, R.A. and Swann, M.B.R. (1926) A disease of rabbits characterized by large mononuclear leukocytes, caused by a hitherto undescribed bacillus: *Bacterium monocytogenes* (n.sp.). *Journal of Pathology and Bacteriology* 29, 407–439.

Nocard, E. (1888) Note sur la maladie des boeufs de la Gouadeloupe connue sous le nom de farcin. *Annales de l'Institut Pasteur* 2, 293–302.

Noguchi, H. and Moore, J.W. (1913) A demonstration of *Treponema pallidum* in the brain in cases of general paralysis. *Journal of Experimental Medicine* 17, 232–238.

North, E. (1811) A treatise on a malignant epidemic commonly called spotted fever. T. & F. Swords, New York.

Nutton, V. (1986) The legacy of Hippocrates: Greek medicine in the library of the Medical Society of London. *Transactions of the Medical Society of London* 103, 21–30.

Nyfeldt, A. (1929) Etiologie de la mononucleose infectieuse. *Comptes Rendus des Séances et Mémoires de la Société de Biologie* 101, 590–591.

Nyhan, W.L. and Fousek, M.D. (1958) Septicemia of the newborn. *Pediatrics* 22, 268–278.

Odier, L. (1779) Memoire sur l'hydrocephale interne, ou hydropisie des ventricles du cerveau.

Histoire de la Société Royale de Médecine, avec les Mémoires de Médecine et de Physique Médicale pour la même année 3, 194–323.
Ogston, A. (1880) Ueber Abscesse. *Archiv für Klinische Chirurgie* 225, 588–600.
Ogston, A. (1883) Micrococcus poisoning. *Journal of Anatomy and Physiology, London,* 17, 24–58.
Pasteur, L. (1881) Note sur la maladie nouvelle provoquee par la salive d'enfant mort de la rage. *Bulletin of the Académie Nationale de Médecine, Paris* 10, 94–103.
Perch, B., Kristjansen, K. and Skadhauge, K. (1968) Group R streptococci pathogenic for man. Two cases of meningitis and one fatal case of sepsis. *Acta Pathologica et Microbiologica Scandinavica* 74, 69–76.
Pfeiffer, R. (1892) Vorlaufige Mittheilungen uber die erreger der influenza. *Deutsche Medicinische Wochenschrift (Berlin)* 18, 28.
Pirie, J.H.H. (1940) Listeria: change of name for a genus of bacteria. *Nature* 145, 264.
Pittman, M. (1931) Variation and type specificity in the bacterial species *Haemophilus influenzae. Journal of Experimental Medicine* 53, 471–493.
Plummer, H. (1935) A serological study of haemolytic streptococci. *Journal of Bacteriology* 30, 5–20.
Podschun, R. and Ullmann, U. (1998) *Klebsiella* spp. as nosocomial pathogens: epidemiology, taxonomy, typing methods, and pathogenicity factors. *Clinical Microbiology Reviews* 11, 589–603.
Quincke, H.I. (1891a) Die lumbalpunction des hydrocephalus. *Berlin Klinische Wochenschrift* 28, 929–933.
Quincke, H.I. (1891b) Ueber hydrocephalus. *Verhandlung des Congress Innere Medizin (X)* 1891, 321–339.
Relman, D.A., Schmidt, T.M., MacDermott, R.P. and Falkow, S. (1992) Identification of the uncultured bacillus of Whipple's disease. *New England Journal of Medicine* 327, 293–301.
Rich, A.R. and McCordock, H.A. (1933) The pathogenesis of tuberculous meningitis. *Bulletin of Johns Hopkins Hospital* 52, 2–37.
Rist, M. (1910) *Bulletins et Mémoires de la Société Médicale des Hôpitaux de Paris* 30, 299.
Rivers, T.M. (1922) Influenzal meningitis. *American Journal of Public Health (NY)* 12, 476–477.
Rolleston, H. (1919) The Lumleian Lectures on Cerebro-Spinal Fever: delivered before the Royal College of Physicians of London. *British Medical Journal* 1, 406, 536, 573–408, 540, 575.
Rose, F.C. (1994) The neurology of Ancient Greece – an overview. *Journal of the History of the Neurosciences* 3, 237–260.
Rosenbach, F. (1884) *Mikro-Organismen bei den Wund-infections-krankheiten des Menschen.* J.F. Bergmann, Wiesbaden.
Schaaf, H.S. (2009) *Tuberculosis. A Comprehensive Clinical Reference.* Elsevier, Oxford.
Schaudinn, F.R. and Hoffmann, E. (1905) Vorläufiger Bericht über das Vorkommen von Spirochaeten in syphilitischen Krankheitsprodukten und bei Papillomen. *Arbeiten aus dem kaiserlichen Gesundheitsamtes (Berlin)* 22, 527–534.
Schneider, T., Moos, V., Loddenkemper, C., Marth, T., Fenollar, F. and Raoult, D. (2008) Whipple's disease: new aspects of pathogenesis and treatment. *Lancet Infectious Diseases* 8, 179–190.
Schuffner, W.A.P. and Walch-Sorgdrager, B. (1936) Meningitis bij ziekte van Weil (meningitis leptospirosa). *Nederlands Tijdschrift voor Geneeskunde* 80, 3000–3007.
Schwartzova, K., Schwartz, A. and Marek, J. (1967) Whipplova choroba s. neurologickou symptomatologii. *PlzenskyP lek Sborn* 28, 99–106.
Senn, L. (1825) *Recherches anatomico-pathologiques sur la meningite aigue des enfants, et ses principales complications (hydrocephale aigue des auteurs).* Gabon et Compagnie Libraires, Paris.
Sherman, J.M. (1937) The streptococci. *Microbiology and Molecular Biology Reviews* 1, 3–97.
Slawyk, E. (1899) Ein fall von Allgemeininfecktion mit influenzabacillen. *Zeitschrift für Hygiene Infektionskrankheiten* 32, 443–448.
Sternberg, G.M. (1881) A fatal form of septicaemia in the rabbit, produced by the subcutaneous injection of human saliva. An experimental research. *National Board of Health Bulletin* 2, 781–783.
Stimson, A.M. (1907) Note on an organism found in yellow-fever tissue. *Public Health Report* 22, 541.
Strong, N. (1810) An inaugural dissertation on the disease termed petechial or spotted fever. Peter B. Gleason, Hartford.
Thompson, D.G., Ledingham, J.M., Howard, A.J. and Brown, C.L. (1978) Meningitis in Whipple's disease. *British Medical Journal* 2, 14–15.
Trevisan, V. (1889) *Generi e le specie delle Batteriacee.* Zanaboni and Gabuzzi, Milan, Italy.
Tyler, K.L. (2010) A history of bacterial meningitis. In: Finger, S., Boller, K. and Tyler, K.L. (eds) *Handbook of Clinical Neurology,* Volume 95. *History of Neurology.* Elsevier, Oxford, pp. 417–433.
Verghese, A. and Gallemore, G. (1987) Kernig and Brudzinski signs revisited. *Reviews of Infectious Diseases* 9, 1187–1192.

Vieusseux, G. (1805) Memoire sur la maladie qui a regne a Geneve au printemps de 1805. *Journal de Médecine, Chirurgie et Pharmacie.* 11, 163–182.

von Staden, H. (1989) *Herophilus: The Art of Medicine in Early Alexandria* (ed. trans). Cambridge University Press, Cambridge.

Wassermann, A., Neisser, A. and Bruck, C. (1906) Eine serodiagnostische reaktion bei syphilis. *Deutsche Medicinische Wochenschrift (Berlin)* 32, 745–746.

Weichselbaum, A. (1887a) Uber die atiologie der akuten meningitis cerebrospinalis. *Fortschritte der Medizin* 5, 573–583.

Weichselbaum, A. (1887b) Uber die atiologie der akuten meningitis cerebrospinalis. *Fortschritte der Medizin* 5, 620–626.

Weichselbaum, A. (1888) Ueber eine von einer otitis media suppurativa ausgehende und durch den *Bacillus pneumoniae* (Friedlander) bedingte allgemeininfection. *Monatsschrift für Ohrenheilkunde und Laryngo-Rhinologie* 22, 200–205.

Weil, A. (1886) Ueber eine eigenthumlich, mit milztumor, icterus und nephritis einhergehende, acute infectionskrankheit. *Deutsches Archiv für Klinische Medizin* 39, 209–232.

Whipple, G.H. (1907) A hitherto undescribed disease characterized anatomically by deposits of fat and fatty acids in the intestinal and myenteric lymphatic tissues. *Bulletin of the Johns Hopkins Hospital* 18, 382–391.

Wilkins, R.H. (1964) Neurosurgical Classic – XVII. *Journal of Neurosurgery* 21, 240–244.

Willis, T. (1685) *The London Practice of Physick, Or The Whole Practical Part of Physick.* Thomas Basset and William Crooke, London.

2 Anatomy of the Meninges: Structural and Functional Aspects

Roy O. Weller*
University of Southampton, Southampton, UK

2.1 Introduction

The meninges that surround the brain in the cranial cavity and the spinal cord and nerve roots in the vertebral column comprise the pachymeninges, or dura mater, and the leptomeninges (Weller, 1995, 2005). Although grouped together under the general heading of meninges, the dura mater and the leptomeninges, consisting of the arachnoid and pia mater, have distinctly different structures and functions. The leptomeninges, in particular, exhibit structural and functional heterogeneity; they not only coat the surface of the brain and intracranial blood vessels but the leptomeningeal cells also extend into the brain around arteries, constitute the stroma of the choroid plexus, and form an important part of the arachnoid granulations and villi through which cerebrospinal fluid (CSF) drains from the subarachnoid space (SAS) into venous sinuses.

Although the anatomy of the meninges in other mammals has many similarities to the human meninges, there are differences among the species. This chapter deals for the most part with the structure and functional aspects of the human meninges. But as some of the functional aspects are derived from experimental studies, mention will be made of meninges in other species.

The meninges originate embryologically from paraxial mesenchyme in the spinal regions and more caudal parts of the head, and from the neural crest in the skull anterior to the midbrain (O'Rahilly and Muller, 1986). Pia mater is derived from mesenchymal cells of the rostral end of the notochord and coats the brain by 24 days of human embryonic development. By 41 days of embryonic life, the dura mater can be recognized in the basal areas of the skull, and the arachnoid mater has become separate from the dura mater (O'Rahilly and Muller, 1986).

2.2 Dura Mater

The dura mater coats the inside of the cranial cavity and extends as a tube to invest the spinal cord and spinal nerve roots; it is a pliable fibrous sheet composed of interwoven bundles of collagen fibres.

2.2.1 Cranial dura mater

The cranial dura mater is closely applied to the bones of the skull and forms the inner periostium. On its inner aspect, the dura mater is intimately associated with the arachnoid mater, although the two structures

*row@soton.ac.uk

can be easily separated. Composed of a tough sheet of fibrous tissue, the dura mater encompasses major venous sinuses, particularly the superior sagittal sinus, lateral and sigmoid sinuses, the cavernous sinus at the base of the skull and several other smaller venous channels (Weller, 1995). The cranial dura mater at the top of the skull extends a semi-rigid sheet, the falx cerebri, between the cerebral hemispheres. Posteriorly, the falx cerebri is attached to the tentorium cerebelli that separates the brain stem and cerebellum in the posterior fossa from the cerebral hemispheres in the middle and anterior fossae (Weller, 1995).

Pathology

In infants, before the cranial sutures have closed, the dura mater is adherent to the suture lines between skull bones. In young adults, the dura mater separates easily from the inside of the skull bones and following head injuries may be separated by extradural haemorrhages that result from injuries to the middle meningeal arteries that run between the dura and the bones of the skull (Blumbergs *et al.*, 2008). Major cerebral veins extend from the superior aspect of the cerebral hemispheres to join the superior sagittal sinus, and they may rupture in the course of a head injury and result in a subdural haemorrhage. A semi-circular opening or aditus in the anterior aspect of the tentorium cerebelli allows the midbrain to connect with the cerebral hemispheres (Weller, 1995). As a space-occupying lesion, such as a subdural or extradural haematoma, expands, the medial aspects of the temporal lobe may be forced into the aditus (transtentorial herniation) to compress the midbrain, often with a fatal result (Blumbergs *et al.*, 2008). Infection may spread into the subdural space, mostly from the frontal sinuses, to produce a subdural abscess, commonly situated between the cerebral hemispheres (Brown and Gray, 2008).

2.2.2 Spinal dura mater

In the vertebral column, the dura mater is divided into two layers: the outer layer forms the periostium of the vertebral bones, and the inner layer forms a dural tube that encompasses the spinal cord, spinal nerve roots and the surrounding SAS filled with CSF. The spinal dura is attached to the bone surrounding the foramen magnum at the base of the skull and to the posterior longitudinal ligament, particularly at the caudal end of the spinal column. Between the outer and inner layers of spinal dura, there is an extradural space filled with adipose tissue (Weller, 1995).

Pathology

A variety of mass lesions may form in the extradural space between the spinal dura and the bones of the vertebral column, resulting in compression of the spinal cord and the neurological deficits of paralysis and loss of sensation (Blumbergs *et al.*, 2008). Chief among spinal space-occupying lesions are metastatic tumours, mainly carcinomas, and extradural haematomas and extradural abscesses that arise from infection in neighbouring bone (Brown and Gray, 2008). Although meningiomas are tumours derived from the arachnoid mater, they are frequently adherent to the inner aspect of the spinal dura and may compress the spinal cord (Ironside *et al.*, 2002; Louis *et al.*, 2007).

2.3 Leptomeninges

Cranial and spinal leptomeninges are composed of two closely connected sheets of cells, the arachnoid mater and the pia mater. The arachnoid mater forms a translucent, waterproof sheet that encompasses the SAS containing CSF; this parietal layer of arachnoid mater is closely applied to the cranial and spinal dura mater. The arachnoid mater both in the cranial and spinal compartments forms trabeculae that traverse the SAS, surround arteries and veins and connect with the pia mater on the surface of the brain and spinal cord.

2.3.1 Cranial arachnoid and pia mater

As a surgeon opens the skull and reflects the dura mater, the thin translucent arachnoid mater is revealed and the surface of the brain can be seen through the layer of CSF in the SAS (Fig. 2.1). In histological sections, the parietal arachnoid mater on the surface of the brain spans the sulci between the cerebral gyri, and sheet-like trabeculae extend from the inner aspect of the arachnoid to traverse the SAS and join the pia mater both over the surface of the gyri and in the depths of the sulci (Hutchings and Weller, 1986; Weller, 2005). The SAS is thus divided into compartments that vary in size. Over much of the surface of the cerebral hemispheres the compartments are small, but at the base of the brain and posterior to the fourth ventricle, there are large cisterns containing CSF. These include the cisterna magna and cisterns over the anterior surface of the brainstem and inferior surface of the hypothalamus (Weller, 1995).

By electron microscopy, the parietal arachnoid has distinct layers (Alcolado *et al.*, 1988). Where it abuts on to the dura mater, the arachnoid is formed from a layer of loosely packed cells – the border or grenz layer – that is easily separated from the inner aspect of the dura. Below the grenz layer, arachnoid cells are joined by tight intercellular junctions, and this layer forms the waterproof barrier that contains the CSF within the SAS. The main body of the arachnoid is composed of cells with pale cytoplasm and interconnected by

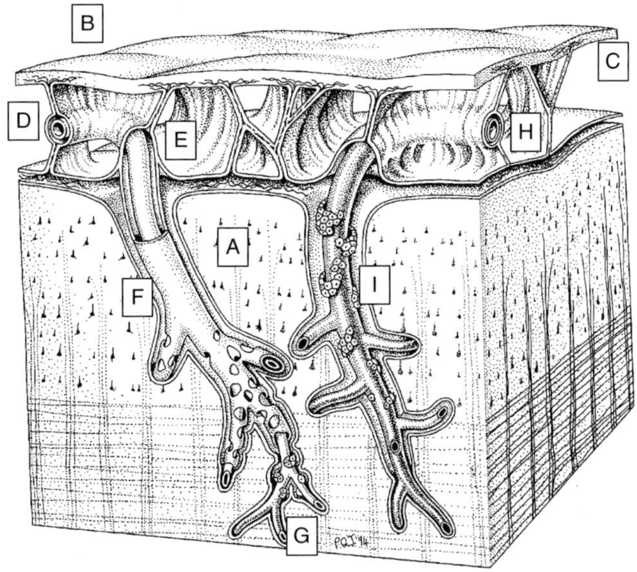

Fig. 2.1. Anatomical arrangement of the arachnoid and pia mater on the surface of the cerebral hemispheres. (A) The brain is coated by pachymeninges (dura mater) and leptomeninges (arachnoid and pia mater). Arteries and veins penetrate the brain from its surface. (B) The dura mater has been removed from the diagram to expose the arachnoid mater. (C) A continuous sheet of waterproof arachnoid mater encompasses the outer aspect of the SAS and is connected to the pia mater on the surface of the brain by numerous sheet-like trabeculae. (D) Arteries within the SAS are coated by a layer of leptomeninges and are suspended between the arachnoid and pia mater by the trabeculae. (E) As an artery enters the brain, the pia mater is reflected from the surface of the brain on to the artery, thus separating the SAS from the subpial space. (F) Each artery carries a sheath of pia mater with it as it enters the brain; over much of the artery this sheath of leptomeningeal cells is continuous. (G) As the artery forms its capillary bed, the leptomeningeal sheath becomes discontinuous and few if any leptomeningeal cells surround capillaries. (H) Veins in the SAS are also coated by leptomeninges. (I) However, veins within the brain lack a continuous leptomeningeal sheath so that only isolated leptomeningeal cells are associated with veins within the brain itself. (Modified and reproduced with permission from Zhang *et al.*, 1990.)

desmosomes (Alcolado *et al.*, 1988). There is no collagen or connective tissue within the arachnoid, so it can be easily distinguished from fibrous tissue through its lack of staining for collagen and reticulin. Leptomeningeal cells in the arachnoid and pia mater express vimentin intermediate filaments, epithelial membrane antigen and, through the presence of intercellular junctions, desmosomal proteins (Parrish *et al.*, 1986). All these proteins can be identified by immunocytochemistry and are useful for detecting thin layers of leptomeninges associated with normal CNS and for identifying meningiomas (Ironside *et al.*, 2002; Louis *et al.*, 2007).

Trabeculae that extend from the inner aspect of the arachnoid mater to cross the SAS are formed from a core of collagen coated by arachnoid cells; these trabeculae encompass and coat arteries and veins within the SAS and ultimately fuse with the pia mater and subpial collagen on the surface of the brain (Alcolado *et al.*, 1988) (Fig. 2.1).

The pia mater is a delicate sheet of leptomeningeal cells that is often only one or two layers thick (Alcolado *et al.*, 1988). It is continuous with the arachnoid mater through the trabeculae that cross the SAS. Originally, it was thought that the SAS connected directly with the perivascular spaces around arteries and veins in the brain. However, by scanning electron microscopy, it is clear that the pia mater is reflected from the surface of the brain on to the surface of arteries and veins (Hutchings and Weller, 1986; Zhang *et al.*, 1990), thus cutting off any direct connection between the SAS and perivascular spaces of the brain. Although the pia mater appears to form a regulatory interface between the SAS and the surface of the brain, the exact functions of the pia mater are not totally clear. Particulate matter such as red blood cells does not appear to cross the pia mater following subarachnoid haemorrhage (Hutchings and Weller, 1986). Monolayer cultures of meningioma cells have been used as a surrogate for leptomeningeal cells. In such preparations, leptomeningeal cells phagocytose particulate matter (Feurer and Weller, 1991) but do not permit the passage of bacteria (*Neisseria meningitidis*) (Hardy *et al.*, 2000). However, the pia mater does not form a barrier to macrophages as they cross freely between the subpial and subarachnoid spaces (Krahn, 1981; Hutchings and Weller, 1986). Leptomeningeal cells produce cytokines (Christodoulides *et al.*, 2002) and the enzyme catechol-*O*-methyltransferase that catabolizes neurotransmitters (Kaplan *et al.*, 1981), which suggests that these cells have a role in inflammation and that the pia mater may form a barrier to access of some pharmacological agents from the CSF into the surface of the brain.

In addition to the reflection of pia mater cells on to the surface of blood vessels in the SAS, a layer of pia mater cells accompanies arteries into the brain (Zhang *et al.*, 1990) (Fig. 2.1). No similar coating of pial cells is present around veins in the brain. At the base of the brain, where branches of the middle cerebral artery penetrate the basal ganglia, two layers of pia mater accompany arteries into brain tissue and form an expandable perivascular space (Pollock *et al.*, 1997) that may enlarge to form lacunae around arteries in the basal ganglia (Salzman *et al.*, 2005). The relationship of the sheath of pial cells to arteries in the brain shows regional variation. In the cerebral cortex, pial cells are closely associated with the smooth muscle layer of the tunica media of cortical arteries (Zhang *et al.*, 1990), and expansion of the perivascular space is rarely, if ever, seen. In the white matter, basal ganglia and midbrain, the arrangement of perivascular leptomeninges differs from that in the cortex, and expansion of the perivascular spaces is frequently seen in these regions (Salzman *et al.*, 2005), particularly in the elderly.

Separating the pia mater from the surface of the brain is a subpial space that contains bundles of collagen of varying fibre size and blood vessels as they enter or leave the brain (Alcolado *et al.*, 1988; Zhang *et al.*, 1990). Collagen bundles within the cores of trabeculae that cross the SAS are continuous with collagen in the subpial space and may thus form an anchor for the arachnoid and blood vessels in the SAS (Alcolado *et al.*, 1988). Abutting on to the subpial space is the *glia limitans* on the surface of the brain; it is formed from tightly packed layers of astrocyte processes and a basement membrane that separates the subpial collagen from the astrocyte layer (Alcolado *et al.*, 1988).

Pathology

Pathology of the leptomeninges results mainly from haemorrhage or infection in the SAS or from the presence of primary and metastatic tumours. The major consequences of haemorrhage and bacterial infection are spasm and damage to the blood vessels in the SAS and consequent infarction of the underlying central nervous system (CNS) (Weller, 1999; Brown and Gray, 2008). In the acute stages, haemorrhage and infection may obstruct the flow of CSF whereas the development of more significant hydrocephalus may result from subsequent scarring and fibrosis of the arachnoid (Weller, 1998). Whereas infections do not usually invade the surface of the brain, metastatic tumours and primary tumours such as medulloblastoma may track alongside arteries into the brain or directly invade the surface of the brain itself (Ironside *et al.*, 2002). Meningiomas are primary tumours of arachnoid cells and as they increase in size they may compress the brain, or, if large, they may distort the brain. Anaplastic, malignant meningiomas may directly invade the surface of the brain (Ironside *et al.*, 2002).

2.3.2 Spinal arachnoid and pia mater

The arrangement of the arachnoid mater in the spinal column is more complicated than that over the surface of the brain. A parietal, waterproof layer of arachnoid encompasses the outer aspect of the SAS, the spinal cord and the nerve roots; this layer is closely associated with the inner aspect of the dura mater (Fig. 2.2) (Nicholas and Weller, 1988). There are also highly perforated intermediate layers of arachnoid, particularly over the dorsal aspect of the spinal cord; the intermediate layers contribute to the dorsal,

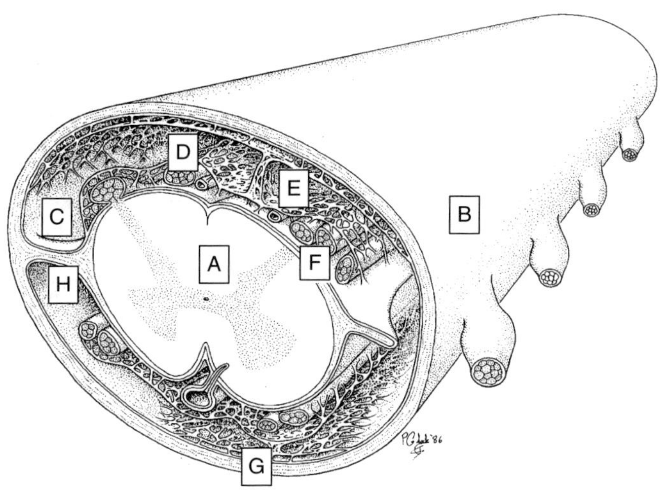

Fig. 2.2. Anatomical arrangement of the spinal meninges. (A) The spinal cord is at the centre of a tube filled with CSF and coated on its outer aspect by (B) the dura mater. (C) The parietal arachnoid mater adheres to the inner aspect of the dura mater, although they can be easily separated. (D) Perforated sheets of arachnoid mater form intermediate layers of leptomeninges on the dorsal aspect of the spinal cord. (E) The dorsal ligament and other ligaments (e.g. dorsolateral ligaments) of the spinal cord are formed by sheets of perforated arachnoid as they connect intermediate layers of arachnoid together. (F) Dorsal nerve roots lie close to the surface of the spinal cord and are coated on their dorsal aspect by perforated sheets of arachnoid. (G) A similar arrangement of intermediate sheets of arachnoid is present on the anterior aspect of the spinal cord, but here they are less substantial. (H) Dentate ligaments on the lateral aspects of the spinal cord are formed from sheets of collagen that connect the subpial collagen on the surface of the spinal cord with the dura mater. The dentate ligaments are thought to stabilize the spinal cord within the SAS. (Modified and reproduced with permission from Nicholas and Weller, 1988.)

dorsolateral and ventral spinal cord ligaments. It is probable that the ligaments stabilize the spinal cord within the subarachnoid fluid, and that the intermediate sheets of arachnoid baffle any waves in the CSF that pass up and down the spinal column. There are prominent, lateral dentate ligaments that also stabilize the spinal cord throughout its length (Fig. 2.2). Each dentate ligament has a thick collagenous core that connects the dura mater to the substantial layer of subpial collagen that surrounds the spinal cord (Nicholas and Weller, 1988); dentate ligaments are coated by a layer of arachnoid cells. The arachnoid mater also coats the surface of nerve roots within the SAS and extends to the exit zones in the intervertebral foramina.

Histologically, the arachnoid mater coating the spinal cord resembles that of cranial arachnoid with a grenz layer abutting the dura. In the parietal waterproof layer of the spinal arachnoid, the cells form tight junctions and desmosomes that bind cells within the main thickness of the arachnoid. As with the cranial arachnoid, trabeculae between the arachnoid and pia mater in the spinal column are derived from the inner aspect of the parietal arachnoid and have cores of collagen. The pia mater is reflected from the surface of the spinal cord on to blood vessels and nerves in the SAS, thus separating the CSF in the SAS from the spinal cord (Nicholas and Weller, 1988).

Pathology

The spinal arachnoid and pia mater may be damaged by subarachnoid haemorrhage, infections and inflammation in the SAS, leading to subsequent fibrosis and spinal arachnoiditis. Syringomyelia with cyst formation in the cervical cord may complicate spinal arachnoiditis, especially in the region of the foramen magnum (Fernandez *et al.*, 2009). Metastatic tumours, including lymphomas and leukaemias, and primary tumours of the CNS may invade the SAS and damage the leptomeninges, spinal cord and nerve roots. Meningiomas arise from the spinal arachnoid and frequently cause spinal cord or nerve root compression (Ironside *et al.*, 2002).

2.3.3 Meninges in experimental animals

Both the dura mater and the leptomeninges in smaller experimental animals, such as rats and mice, are less substantial than in humans. The SAS over the cerebral hemispheres is mainly confined to perivascular regions around major branches of the cerebral arteries but expands over the base of the brain to form basal cisterns (Zhang *et al.*, 1992). Drainage of CSF in rodents is mainly through the cribriform plate into nasal lymphatics (Kida *et al.*, 1993); CSF from the basal portions of the rat brain drains along the perivascular SAS on the inferior aspects of the olfactory bulbs (Zhang *et al.*, 1992). Trabeculae join the parietal arachnoid to the pia mater across the cisterns associated with the base of the rat brain (Kida *et al.*, 1993).

2.4 Fluid Compartments of the CNS

There are four major fluid compartments in the CNS: (i) blood; (ii) CSF, (iii) interstitial (extracellular) fluid; and (iv) intracellular fluid. This chapter concentrates mainly on (i), (ii) and (iii) and the interrelations between these three fluids. For intracellular fluid, levels are largely regulated by sodium and potassium ATPase pumps and by voltage- and ligand-gated channels. Intracellular (cytotoxic) oedema develops when there is energy depletion, failure of the ATPase pumps and the entry of sodium into cells with the outflow of potassium. In the CNS, swelling of astrocytes following tissue damage also occurs due to the sustained uptake of osmotically reactive solutes such as serum proteins.

2.4.1 Blood

Blood flows into the CNS along arteries and capillaries and flows out of the CNS via venules and veins. There are several features that are almost unique to the CNS: the distinct blood–brain barrier (BBB), the production and drainage of CSF, the pathways for the elimination of interstitial fluid and the concept of immunological privilege for the CNS. All these features are discussed in the sections below.

BBB

The concept of the BBB (the blood–CNS barrier as the spinal cord is also involved) originated from the observation during the 19th century that, under normal circumstances, dyes bound to serum proteins did not pass from the blood into the CNS. This was tested by the intravenous injection of blue-coloured dyes that bound to serum albumin and showed that all tissues in the body were stained blue except for the brain, spinal cord and peripheral nerves. The modern concept of the BBB is of a number of regulatory mechanisms that control the entry of: (i) solutes from blood into brain; and (ii) inflammatory cells from blood into brain. Solutes appear to enter the brain via the endothelium of capillaries, whereas inflammatory cells migrate into the brain via the endothelium of post-capillary venules (Ge *et al.*, 2005).

Endothelial cells of arterioles, capillaries and venules have different characteristics that reflect the different functions of the three types of vessel. The site of the BBB for solutes is in capillaries (Fig. 2.3a). A close investment of capillaries by astrocytes induces the BBB, which depends upon the presence of tight junctions between endothelial cells; specific transport mechanisms for solutes, such as glucose and amino acids; and enzymes that degrade substances such as neurotransmitters and mechanisms by which xenobiotic substances can be extruded from the brain into the blood (Ge *et al.*, 2005). Pericytes are involved in a number of key functions in relation to the BBB and the contractile nature, suggesting that they play a role in the constriction of capillaries (Liu *et al.*, 2012). In Fig. 2.3a, processes of pericytes can be seen embedded in the capillary basement membrane. These mechanisms are essential for maintaining homeostasis of the interstitial fluid in the brain.

In addition to the specificity of the BBB for solutes in capillary endothelial cells, there are specific mechanisms for the migration of inflammatory cells, mainly lymphocytes and monocytes, from the blood into the brain. The major site for migration of inflammatory cells is the venules (Fig. 2.3b); lymphocytes destined to enter the brain express a combination of integrins that are recognized by receptors on the venular endothelium (Engelhardt, 2008). Lymphocytes then migrate either between or through endothelial cells to accumulate initially in the perivenular space and then migrate through the astrocyte basement membrane into CNS tissue. In inflammatory disorders, such as viral infections and multiple sclerosis, lymphocytes may be observed around venules and expanding the perivascular spaces around larger veins. There is some restriction on the entry of inflammatory cells into the brain. Polymorphonuclear leucocytes (PMNLs) only enter brain tissue in substantial numbers when pyogenic bacteria are present, whereas after cerebral infarction the small numbers of PMNLs that enter the brain are soon replaced by monocytes.

2.4.2 CSF

Blood–CSF barrier (BCSFB)

CSF is produced from the blood by the choroid plexuses in the cerebral ventricles (Fig. 2.3c). Embryologically, the choroid plexus is derived from leptomeninges that invaginate into the ventricles through the dorsal aspect of the developing brain. Thus, the stroma of the choroid plexus is composed of arachnoid cells that produce collagen bands or collagen spheres that may calcify to form the calcospherites typical of the aged choroid plexus (Alcolado *et al.*, 1986). The ventricular surface of the choroid plexus is coated by epithelium derived from ependyma, although the two types of cell can be distinguished by their cytological and immunocytochemical characteristics. Ependymal cells have cilia on their ventricular surfaces and express glial fibrillary acidic protein (GFAP); choroid plexus epithelium, on the other hand, is coated mainly by microvilli, and, in addition to GFAP, the cells express the enzyme carbonic anhydrase C. The site of the BCSFB is at the choroid plexus

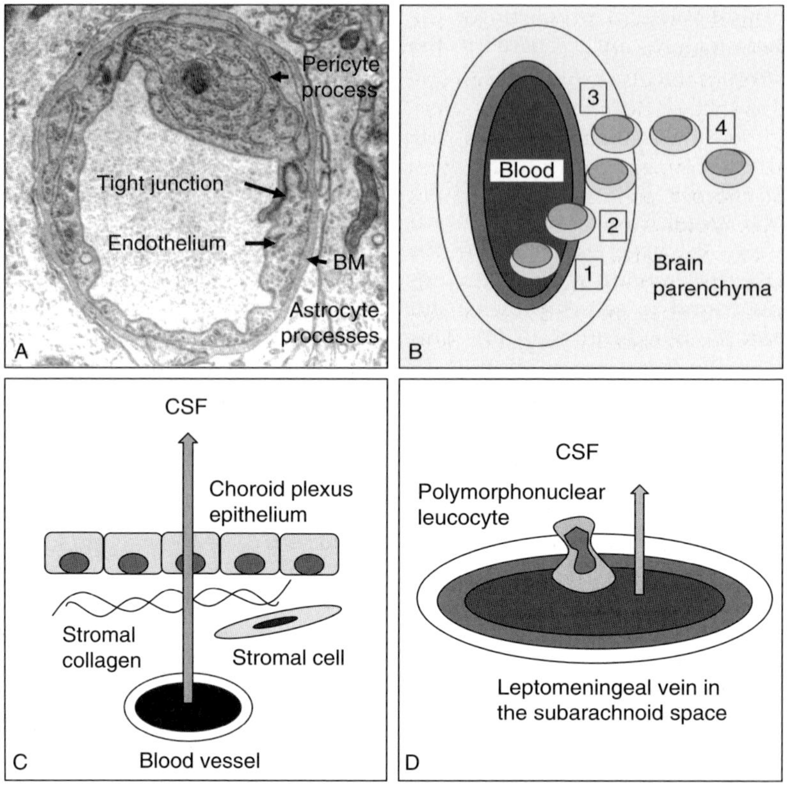

Fig. 2.3. Blood–brain barrier (BBB) and blood–CSF barrier (BCSFB). (A) *BBB for solutes.* An electron micrograph of a capillary in the cerebral cortex showing the site of the BBB for solutes. Tight junctions join the endothelial cells that surround blood in the capillary lumen. Solutes are actively transported through the endothelium into the extracellular space of the CNS. Capillaries are closely invested by astrocyte processes and pericytes; both play a role in the BBB. Capillary endothelial cells are invested by the basement membrane (BM) and this is the beginning of the pathway for the drainage of interstitial fluid out of the CNS. (B) *BBB for inflammatory cells.* Diagram showing a venule within the brain. Lymphocytes with specific integrins on their surface attach to receptors on the venular endothelium [1] and then pass through the endothelium [2] into the perivenular space [3] from where they pierce the perivascular astrocyte basement membrane and pass into the brain parenchyma [4]. (C) *BCSFB in the choroid plexus.* Fluid and solutes pass into the stroma of the choroid plexus and then through the choroid plexus epithelium into the ventricular cavity in the direction of the arrow. The site of the BCSFB is in the choroid plexus epithelium. (D) *Entry of inflammatory cells into the CSF of the SAS.* A PMNL is shown passing from the lumen of a leptomeningeal vein into the CSF in the direction of the arrow. In addition to the venular endothelium, the leucocyte must penetrate the thin layer of leptomeningeal cells that coats the outer surface of the vein.

epithelium where the cells are joined by tight junctions and gap junctions. Proteins and other components of the blood pass into the stroma of the choroid plexus but do not enter the CSF. The composition of CSF differs from the blood as it has very low protein levels and different electrolytes.

Although veins in the SAS are continuous with veins within the brain, they have different characteristics with regard to the migration of inflammatory cells. Whereas PMNLs rarely enter the brain in large numbers, such cells readily migrate from leptomeningeal veins into the CSF of the SAS

(Fig. 2.3d). This difference between venules in the brain and veins in the SAS is further illustrated experimentally. The intracerebral injection of cytokines does not induce entry of leucocytes into the brain but does result in widespread recruitment of inflammatory cells to the choroid plexus, leptomeninges and ventricles (Andersson *et al.*, 1992). It is important to recognize the differences between intra-CNS vessels and those in the leptomeninges, so that the BBB for inflammatory cells is not confused with the BCSFB.

Bacteria and fungi enter the CSF of the SAS either by direct penetration from adjacent infected foci, by haematogenous spread from other sites in the body and possibly by direct penetration through the nasal mucosa (Brown and Gray, 2008). It is unclear how bacteria penetrate the walls of blood vessels to enter the CSF in the SAS, but it is possible that they use the same route as PMNLs (Fig. 2.3d). Nor is it clear how bacteria pass through the choroid plexus into the ventricular CSF. Viruses probably enter the CSF via specific transcellular transport mechanisms. Most bacterial and fungal infections in the brain parenchyma are abscesses. Infected emboli in the blood produce septic infarction and result in bacterial growth and abscess formation. Diffuse infections of the brain parenchyma are uncommon and mainly seen with *Listeria monocytogenes*.

Drainage of CSF

The CSF has a volume in humans of 30 ml in the ventricles and 110 ml in the subarachnoid spaces; it is produced by the choroid plexus at 350 ml/min in humans. Following circulation through the ventricular system, CSF drains from the SAS: (i) via the cribriform plate of the ethmoid bone and nasal lymphatics to regional lymph nodes in the neck; and (ii) through arachnoid granulations and villi into the venous blood (Weller *et al.*, 2009b) (Fig. 2.4).

Experimental studies in rodents and sheep suggest that at least 50% of CSF drains from the SAS via channels that pass alongside olfactory nerves through the cribriform plate of the ethmoid bone to join lymphatics in the nasal mucosa to drain to deep cervical lymph nodes. Drainage of CSF through the cribriform plate has been confirmed in adult humans (Johnston *et al.*, 2004), although the proportion of CSF that drains to lymph nodes in humans is uncertain. The nasal lymphatic route may be the main pathway by which inflammatory cells drain from CSF to regional lymph nodes in animals and in humans (Kaminski *et al.*, 2012).

Arachnoid granulations and villi are invaginations of the arachnoid mater into venous sinuses, most prominent in the superior sagittal sinus and the cavernous sinus. Arachnoid villi in the spine have also been described in association with nerve roots. Each arachnoid granulation or villus consists of a core, a cap of arachnoid cells and a coating of venous endothelial cells (Upton and Weller, 1985). CSF appears to percolate through channels in the core and arachnoid cap to reach the venous endothelium at the apex of the granulation or villus. Final drainage of CSF into blood is thought to occur by bulk flow through macrovacuoles that traverse the endothelial cells from the abluminal to the luminal surface (Tripathi and Tripathi, 1974).

Pathology of CSF

Although tumour cells may invade the surface of the brain, PMNLs and bacteria rarely penetrate the *glia limitans* on the surface of the CNS (Weller, 1999). Arteries and veins in the SAS, on the other hand, may be damaged by infection and inflammation and thrombosis results in infarction of the underlying brain tissue. Hydrocephalus is a major complication following meningitis due to fibrosis and scarring of the leptomeninges and adhesions in the SAS obstructing the drainage of the CSF. Hydrocephalus results in damage to the white matter around dilated ventricles; CSF is infused into the periventricular white matter causing interstitial oedema and tissue destruction (Weller, 1998).

2.4.3 Interstitial fluid

Production and elimination

Interstitial fluid is derived from the blood by the passage of fluid and solutes through the

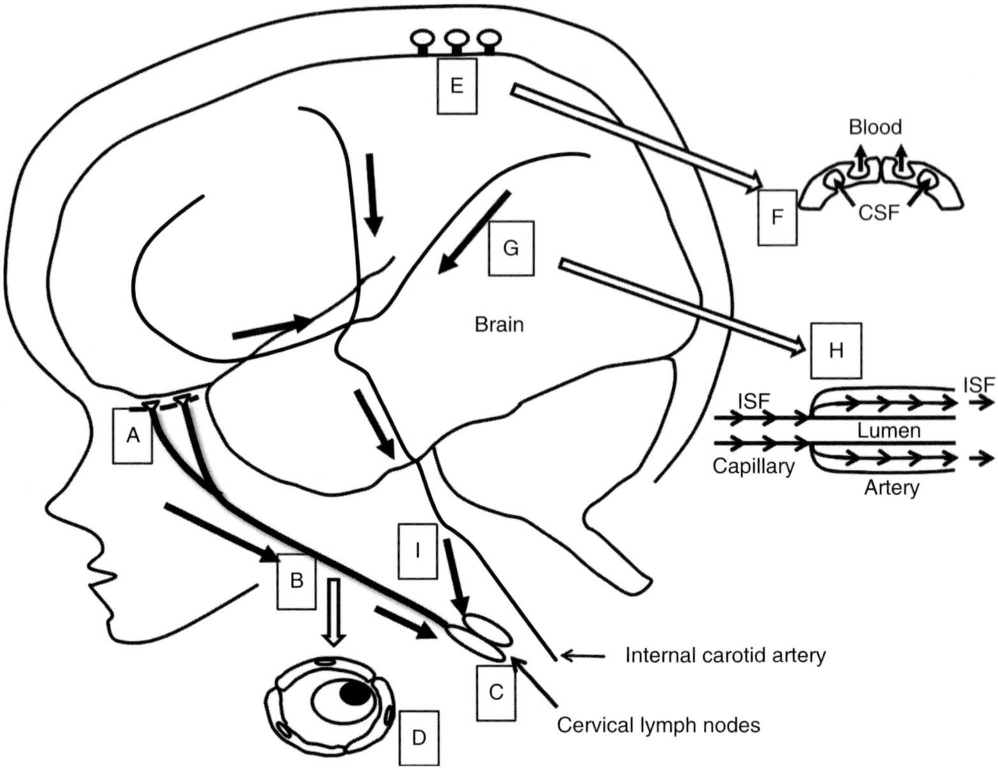

Fig. 2.4. Drainage pathways for CSF from the human brain. (A) CSF drains from the SAS along channels that pass through the cribriform plate of the ethmoid bone alongside branches of the olfactory nerves. (B) From the nasal mucosa underlying the ethmoid bone, CSF drains along nasal lymphatics to deep cervical lymph nodes (C). The nasal and cervical lymphatics (D) are channels that are capable of conducting inflammatory cells from the CSF to cervical lymph nodes. (E) The other major pathway for drainage of intracranial CSF is through arachnoid granulations and villi that protrude into the venous sinuses. (F) CSF reaches the venous endothelium coating the arachnoid granulations and villi by channels in their cores and arachnoid caps. As shown here, CSF appears to be transported into venous blood by bulk flow via large vacuoles that traverse the venous endothelial cells.

Drainage pathways for interstitial fluid from the human brain. (G) Interstitial fluid (ISF) and solutes drain from the brain parenchyma along perivascular pathways in the walls of cerebral capillaries and arteries. (H) Fluid and solutes enter the 100–150 nm wide basement membranes in the walls of capillaries and then pass along the basement membranes between smooth muscle cells in the tunica media of arteries. There is no evidence that inflammatory cells can pass along this narrow drainage pathway. (I) From experimental studies and from observations in humans, it seems that interstitial fluid and solutes from the brain drain along the walls of intracranial arteries to the walls of internal carotid arteries in the neck and thence to cervical lymph nodes. (Modified and reproduced with permission from Laman and Weller, 2012.)

capillary endothelial BBB into the brain and spinal cord. It has a volume of 280 ml in the brain and spinal cord and is eliminated from the CNS at an estimated rate of 0.11–0.29 ml/min/g of brain, which is comparable to the average lymphatic drainage in the rest of the body (Szentistvanyi *et al.*, 1984).

In most organs of the body, except for the CNS and retina, interstitial fluid drains from the tissue by well-recognized lymphatic channels to regional lymph nodes. Furthermore, inflammatory cells such as lymphocytes and dendritic cells also drain by lymphatics to regional lymph nodes. The brain and spinal cord possess no traditional lymphatics; there are no well-defined lymphatic vessels extending from CNS tissue to regional lymph nodes. For many years, it was assumed that interstitial fluid drained into CSF and was eliminated along CSF drainage pathways. However, when solutes such as serum albumin are injected into the brains of experimental animals, they drain along perivascular pathways in the walls of cerebral and carotid arteries to cervical lymph nodes. Only 10–15% of interstitial fluid appears to leak from the perivascular pathways into the CSF (Szentistvanyi *et al.*, 1984): thus, drainage pathways for interstitial fluid appear to be largely independent from the CSF. Intracranial injections of fluorescent tracers in mice have shown that interstitial fluid and solutes drain from the brain along 100–150 nm thick basement membranes in the walls of capillaries and arteries as the perivascular route for the elimination of interstitial fluid and solutes from the brain (Carare *et al.*, 2008) (Fig. 2.4).

Whereas lymphatics from other organs carry inflammatory cells from tissues to the regional lymph nodes, there is no evidence that inflammatory cells drain from the brain along the 100–150 nm thick basement membranes in capillary and artery walls (Carare *et al.*, 2008). The lack of a direct route for the migration of inflammatory cells from the CNS to regional lymph nodes may be an important factor, together with the BBB, in the immunological privilege of CNS tissue.

Pathology of interstitial fluid and its drainage pathways

Two of the major functions ascribed to perivascular drainage of interstitial fluid and solutes from the CNS are: (i) delivery of soluble antigens, but not cells, to regional lymph nodes (Carare *et al.*, 2008); and (ii) maintenance of homeostasis of the extracellular environment in the brain and spinal cord (Weller *et al.*, 2009b).

Although the brain is considered to be an immunologically privileged site, immune-mediated reactions occur in the CNS in response to infections and in autoimmune diseases. In other tissues of the body, T-lymphocyte-mediated immune reactions rely upon the transport of immunologically competent cells from the tissue to regional lymph nodes. This does not seem to occur in the CNS, so it is possible that sensitized lymphocytes migrate from peripheral sites to cervical or lumbar lymph nodes and then respond to antigens draining from the CNS by targeting the brain or spinal cord (Weller *et al.*, 2009b).

As with lymphatic drainage systems in other parts of the body, perivascular drainage of fluid and solutes from the CNS is essential for maintaining homoeostasis of the extracellular environment of neurons and other cells in the brain and spinal cord (Weller *et al.*, 2009b). Theoretical models suggest that the driving force for perivascular drainage of fluid and solutes is derived from pulsations of cerebral arteries (Schley *et al.*, 2006). With advancing age, cerebral arteries stiffen (Weller *et al.*, 2009a), and as the amplitude of pulsations is reduced the efficiency of perivascular drainage may decline. Failure of perivascular drainage is reflected in the accumulation of insoluble amyloid-β (Aβ) both in the brain and in perivascular drainage pathways as cerebral amyloid angiopathy (CAA) in Alzheimer's disease (Weller *et al.*, 2009c). CAA itself further reduces perivascular drainage (Hawkes *et al.*, 2011). Loss of homoeostasis in the brain may be reflected in the rise of soluble Aβ in the brain in Alzheimer's disease (Weller *et al.*, 2009c). CAA has the added complication of intracerebral haemorrhage as smooth muscle cells in the walls of cerebral arteries are replaced by amyloid and the arteries rupture (Auriel and Greenberg, 2012).

Perivascular drainage pathways for interstitial fluid and solutes pass along the walls of leptomeningeal vessels within the SAS. It is probable that inflammation and bacterial infection in the SAS has an effect on interstitial fluid flow, but little is known about it. Problems that arise with the drainage of interstitial fluid in meningitis are almost certainly masked by the inflammation and oedema in the underlying CNS that result from venous and arterial thrombosis and infarction of the underlying brain or spinal cord.

2.5 Conclusions

Meninges coating the brain and spinal cord have diverse structures and functions. The dura mater is the tough, fibrous membrane that covers the human brain and spinal cord, but it is the leptomeninges that show a wide diversity in structure and function. The arachnoid mater surrounding the external aspects of the CNS forms a waterproof layer that contains the CSF. Within the SAS, arachnoid cells form collagen bundles within trabeculae that anchor the parietal arachnoid to the pia mater and subpial collagen. Similarly, arachnoid cells in the cores of the choroid plexus and arachnoid granulations and villi form collagenous structures that stabilize these organs concerned with the production and drainage of CSF. Cytokines and enzymes produced by arachnoid and pial cells contribute to inflammatory reactions in the SAS and to a barrier function between the CSF and the surface of the CNS. Arachnoid cells coating arteries in the SAS may play a key role in separating drainage pathways for interstitial fluid within the walls of the arteries from the surrounding CSF, thus allowing some specificity of drainage pathways for both CSF and interstitial fluid from the CNS.

References

Alcolado, J.C., Moore, I.E. and Weller, R.O. (1986) Calcification in the human choroid plexus, meningiomas and pineal gland. *Neuropathology and Applied Neurobiology* 12, 235–250.

Alcolado, R., Weller, R.O., Parrish, E.P. and Garrod, D. (1988) The cranial arachnoid and pia mater in man: anatomical and ultrastructural observations. *Neuropathology and Applied Neurobiology* 14, 1–17.

Andersson, P.B., Perry, V.H. and Gordon, S. (1992) Intracerebral injection of proinflammatory cytokines or leukocyte chemotaxins induces minimal myelomonocytic cell recruitment to the parenchyma of the central nervous system. *Journal of Experimental Medicine* 176, 255–259.

Auriel, E. and Greenberg, S.M. (2012) The pathophysiology and clinical presentation of cerebral amyloid angiopathy. *Current Atherosclerosis Reports* 14, 343–350.

Blumbergs, P., Reilly, P. and Vink, R. (2008) Trauma. In: Love, S., Louis, D.N. and Ellison, D.W. (eds) *Greenfield's Neuropathology*, 8th edn. Edward Arnold, London, pp. 733–832.

Brown, E. and Gray, F. (2008) Bacterial infections. In: Love, S., Louis, D.N. and Ellison, D.W. (eds) *Greenfield's Neuropathology*, 8th edn. Edward Arnold, London, pp. 1391–1445.

Carare, R.O., Bernardes-Silva, M., Newman, T.A., Page, A.M., Nicoll, J.A.R., Perry, V.H. and Weller, R.O. (2008) Solutes, but not cells, drain from the brain parenchyma along basement membranes of capillaries and arteries. Significance for cerebral amyloid angiopathy and neuroimmunology. *Neuropathology and Applied Neurobiology* 34, 131–144.

Christodoulides, M., Makepeace, B.L., Partridge, K.A., Kaur, D., Fowler, M.I., Weller, R.O. and Heckels, J.E. (2002) Interaction of *Neisseria meningitidis* with human meningeal cells induces the secretion of a distinct group of chemotactic, proinflammatory, and growth-factor cytokines. *Infection and Immunity* 70, 4035–4044.

Engelhardt, B. (2008) Immune cell entry into the central nervous system: involvement of adhesion molecules and chemokines. *Journal of Neurological Science* 274, 23–26.

Fernandez, A.A., *et al.* (2009) Malformations of the craniocervical junction (Chiari type I and syringomyelia: classification, diagnosis and treatment). *BMC Musculoskeletal Disorders* 10 Suppl. 1, S1.

Feurer, D.J. and Weller, R.O. (1991) Barrier functions of the leptomeninges: a study of normal meninges and meningiomas in tissue culture. *Neuropathology and Applied Neurobiology* 17, 391–405.

Ge, S., Song, L. and Pachter, J.S. (2005) Where is the blood–brain barrier ... really? *Journal of Neuroscience Research* 79, 421–427.

Hardy, S.J., Christodoulides, M., Weller, R.O. and Heckels, J.E. (2000) Interactions of *Neisseria meningitidis* with cells of the human meninges. *Molecular Microbiology* 36, 817–829.

Hawkes, C.A., Hartig, W., Kacza, J., Schliebs, R., Weller, R.O., Nicoll, J.A. and Carare, R.O. (2011) Perivascular drainage of solutes is impaired in the ageing mouse brain and in the presence of cerebral amyloid angiopathy. *Acta Neuropathologica* 121, 431–443.

Hutchings, M. and Weller, R.O. (1986) Anatomical relationships of the pia mater to cerebral blood vessels in man. *Journal of Neurosurgery* 65, 316–325.

Ironside, J.W., Moss, T.H., Louis, D.N., Lowe, J.S. and Weller, R.O. (2002) *Diagnostic Pathology of Nervous System Tumours.* Churchill Livingstone, Edinburgh.

Johnston, M., Zakharov, A., Papaiconomou, C., Salmasi, G. and Armstrong, D. (2004) Evidence of connections between cerebrospinal fluid and nasal lymphatic vessels in humans, non-human primates and other mammalian species. *Cerebrospinal Fluid Research* 1, 2–15.

Kaminski, M., Bechmann, I., Pohland, M., Kiwit, J., Nitsch, R. and Glumm, J. (2012) Migration of monocytes after intracerebral injection at entorhinal cortex lesion site. *Journal of Leukocyte Biology* 92, 31–39.

Kaplan, G.P., Hartman, B.K. and Creveling, C.R. (1981) Localization of catechol-*O*-methyltransferase in the leptomeninges, choroid plexus and ciliary epithelium: implications for the separation of central and peripheral catechols. *Brain Research* 204, 353–360.

Kida, S., Pantazis, A. and Weller, R.O. (1993) CSF drains directly from the subarachnoid space into nasal lymphatics in the rat. Anatomy, histology and immunological significance. *Neuropathology and Applied Neurobiology* 19, 480–488.

Krahn, V. (1981) Leukodiapedesis and leukocyte migration in the leptomeninges and in the subarachnoid space. *Journal of Neurology* 226, 43–52.

Laman, J.D. and Weller, R.O. (2012) Editorial: Route by which monocytes leave the brain is revealed. *Journal of Leukocyte Biology* 92, 6–9.

Liu, S., Agalliu, D., Yu, C. and Fisher, M. (2012) The role of pericytes in blood–brain barrier function and stroke. *Current Pharmaceutical Design* 18, 3653–3662.

Louis, D.N., Ohgaki, H., Wiestler, O.D. and Cavenee, W.K. (2007) *WHO Classification of Tumours of the Central Nervous System*, 4th edn. International Agency for Research on Cancer, Lyon.

Nicholas, D.S. and Weller, R.O. (1988) The fine anatomy of the human spinal meninges. A light and scanning electron microscopy study. *Journal of Neurosurgery* 69, 276–282.

O'Rahilly, R. and Muller, F. (1986) The meninges in human development. *Journal of Neuropathology and Experimental Neurolology* 45, 588–608.

Parrish, E.P., Garrod, D.R., Mattey, D.L., Hand, L., Steart, P.V. and Weller, R.O. (1986) Mouse antisera specific for desmosomal adhesion molecules of suprabasal skin cells, meninges, and meningioma. *Proceedings of the National Academy of Sciences USA* 83, 2657–2661.

Pollock, H., Hutchings, M., Weller, R.O. and Zhang, E.T. (1997) Perivascular spaces in the basal ganglia of the human brain: their relationship to lacunes. *Journal of Anatomy* 191, 337–346.

Salzman, K.L., Osborn, A.G., House, P., Jinkins, J.R., Ditchfield, A., Cooper, J.A. and Weller, R.O. (2005) Giant tumefactive perivascular spaces. *American Journal of Neuroradiology* 26, 298–305.

Schley, D., Carare-Nnadi, R., Please, C.P., Perry, V.H. and Weller, R.O. (2006) Mechanisms to explain the reverse perivascular transport of solutes out of the brain. *Journal of Theoretical Biology* 238, 962–974.

Szentistvanyi, I., Patlak, C.S., Ellis, R.A. and Cserr, H.F. (1984) Drainage of interstitial fluid from different regions of rat brain. *American Journal of Physiology* 246, F835–F844.

Tripathi, B.J. and Tripathi, R.C. (1974) Vacuolar transcellular channels as a drainage pathway for cerebrospinal fluid. *Journal of Physiology* 239, 195–206.

Upton, M.L. and Weller, R.O. (1985) The morphology of cerebrospinal fluid drainage pathways in human arachnoid granulations. *Journal of Neurosurgery* 63, 867–875.

Weller, R.O. (1995) Fluid compartments and fluid balance in the central nervous system. In: Williams, P.L. (ed.) *Gray's Anatomy*, 38th edn. Churchill Livingstone, Edinburgh, pp. 1202–1224.

Weller, R.O. (1998) Pathology of cerebrospinal fluid and interstitial fluid of the CNS: significance for Alzheimer disease, prion disorders and multiple sclerosis. *Journal of Neuropathology and Experimental Neurolology* 57, 885–894.

Weller, R.O. (1999) Reaction of intrathecal and epidural spaces to infection and inflammation. In: Yaksh, T.L. (ed.) *Spinal Drug Delivery.* Elsevier, Amsterdam, pp. 297–315.

Weller, R.O. (2005) Microscopic morphology and histology of the human meninges. *Morphologie* 89, 22–34.

Weller, R.O., Boche, D. and Nicoll, J.A. (2009a) Microvasculature changes and cerebral amyloid angiopathy in Alzheimer's disease and their potential impact on therapy. *Acta Neuropathologica* 118, 87–102.

Weller, R.O., Djuanda, E., Yow, H.Y. and Carare, R.O. (2009b) Lymphatic drainage of the brain and the pathophysiology of neurological disease. *Acta Neuropathologica* 117, 1–14.

Weller, R.O., Preston, S.D., Subash, M. and Carare, R.O. (2009c) Cerebral amyloid angiopathy in the aetiology and immunotherapy of Alzheimer disease. *Alzheimers Research and Therapy* 1, 6.

Zhang, E.T., Inman, C.B. and Weller, R.O. (1990) Interrelationships of the pia mater and the perivascular (Virchow–Robin) spaces in the human cerebrum. *Journal of Anatomy* 170, 111–123.

Zhang, E.T., Richards, H.K., Kida, S. and Weller, R.O. (1992) Directional and compartmentalised drainage of interstitial fluid and cerebrospinal fluid from the rat brain. *Acta Neuropathologica* 83, 233–239.

3 Evidence-based Clinical Examination of Meningitis

Sarah Curtis*
Edmonton Clinic Health Academy (ECHA), Edmonton, Canada

3.1 Introduction

Bacterial meningitis still remains a serious threat to global health, despite the success of antibiotic therapy and mass vaccination against organisms causing epidemic disease. Meningitis can and does occur in anyone, but certain children are at increased risk for invasive disease. Neonates and young infants are considered to be relatively immunodeficient with decreased cellular and humoral immunity. Birth to a mother who is positive for *Streptococcus agalactiae* or *Escherichia coli* on prenatal screening, who had prolonged rupture of membranes, chorioamnionitis and/or was unwell or febrile around delivery puts an infant at risk for meningitis after birth. Immunodeficient states such as asplenia, human immunodeficiency virus (HIV) infection and humoral or complement deficiencies also predispose to invasive disease. Anyone with recent exposure to infected individuals or recent travel to areas with endemic disease may also be at risk. Crowded living conditions such as dormitories, camps, army barracks and daycare centres allow easier person-to-person transmission of pathogens. Unimmunized children are at increased risk for meningitis, as are children with advanced or chronic medical illness or poor overall health and nutrition. Otherwise healthy children with another site of bacterial infection such as otitis media, sinusitis or pneumonia are also thought to be at increased risk for meningitis. Penetrating head trauma, central nervous system (CNS) surgery, presence of a ventriculo-peritoneal shunt, cochlear implant devices, recent lumbar puncture (LP) or anatomical defects such as dermal sinus lesions with resultant cerebrospinal fluid (CSF) leaks can result in easy passage of a pathogen into the CNS with subsequent meningitis. A past history of meningitis and population variance of genetic polymorphisms responsible for host defence may also increase the risk of recurrence.

This chapter describes the strength of evidence supporting the use of individual purported clinical features as diagnostic tests for meningitis, as used in the process of weighing an individual patient's risk of having the disease prior to the administration of the more definitive gold standard diagnostic test of CSF analysis. The evidence is described in both children and adults, and recommendations for further research are given.

*scurtis@ualberta.ca

3.2 Anatomical and Physiological Origins of the Clinical Features

During meningeal infection, inflammatory cells spill into the CSF-containing subarachnoid space (SAS), and an increased CSF cell count is a diagnostic hallmark of meningitis. Meningeal inflammation produces the symptoms and signs of the disease. Ensuing damage may be global or focal, resulting from the trade-off between the insult of bacterial invasion and secondary host-driven injury. Pathogens with virulence factors that enable colonization of host mucosal epithelium, invasion and propagation within the bloodstream, penetration of the blood–brain barrier (BBB)/blood–CSF barrier (BCSFB) and proliferation within the CSF can lead to meningitis. Proposed sites of initial invasion into the CSF and the cellular and molecular basis of meningitis caused by diverse organisms are discussed in the following chapters. Potential global outcomes of meningeal inflammation are vasogenic brain oedema, loss of cerebrovascular autoregulation, intracranial hypertension with subsequent focal areas of ischaemia, cytotoxic injury and apoptosis (Weber and Tuomanen, 2007). Vasogenic brain oedema resulting from increased permeability of the BBB/BCSFB and increased intercellular volume can lead to raised intracranial pressure (ICP). Raised ICP can cause altered mental status, headache, irritability, nausea, vomiting, coma, visual changes, papilloedema, bradycardia, hypertension and cerebral herniation. The accumulation of inflammatory cells between the meninges and subsequent inflammation of these membranes, as well as increased CSF volume, causes the pain and limitations in range-of-motion testing of the neck.

Hearing loss, the most common neurological sequelae of meningitis in up to 35% of patients, may be either transient or permanent. Bacteria are believed to either travel with the eighth cranial nerve in the internal auditory canal or reach the cochlea via the cochlear aqueduct from the SAS. Infection leads to loss of hair cells, calcification of perilymphatic channels and damage to the auditory nerve, which results in hearing loss of varying severity.

Clinical neurological manifestations of meningitis may have sudden or gradual onset (Scheld *et al.*, 2002). Both the hippocampus and cerebral cortex are vulnerable to areas of focal ischaemic necrosis during bacterial meningitis. Impairment of learning and memory occur secondary to necrosis of cells in the dentate gyrus of the hippocampus and hippocampal atrophy has been demonstrated in survivors of the disease (Loeffler *et al.*, 2001). Focal ischaemic insults can result in paresis, ataxia, aphasia, visual field defects, cranial nerve palsies, sensory defects and seizures. Bacterial toxins, neurochemical changes and fever are other proposed explanations for seizures in meningitis. Seizures may be generalized or focal and may occur acutely or years after the disease (Pomeroy *et al.*, 1990; Carter *et al.*, 2003).

Subdural effusions may be present in up to 20% of children with meningitis, and in infants these may be evident as a bulging fontanelle on clinical examination. Brain abscesses are rare and usually associated with rare pathogens. Uncommon complications of meningitis include hydrocephalus and spinal cord injury. Systemic features that may also be seen include shock, hypoglycaemia and petechial rash secondary to coagulation cascade abnormalities.

3.3 Purported Key Clinical Examination Features

3.3.1 Meningeal signs

The meningeal signs have been well described and are considered among the most important physical examination features for screening for meningitis. These signs include descriptions of neck stiffness, Kernig's sign, Brudzinski's sign, opisthotonos and Amoss's sign, among others. While meningitis is an important explanation for the presence of meningeal signs in a patient, it is important to remember that other causes such as arthritis, cervical adenitis, retropharyngeal or peritonsillar abscesses, subarachnoid or epidural haemorrhage, and cauda equina tumour, among others, are also possible explanations for the positivity of some or all of these signs.

The mechanistic underpinnings of all these signs can be understood by considering several items. When positive, these signs have both sensory (pain) and motor (movement, resistance to movement or posturing) features. Research on cadavers has demonstrated that flexion of the neck normally produces several millimetres of elevation of the brain stem near the occiput and upward motion of the spinal cord in the lumbar region. Flexion of the hips, with legs extended, pulls on the sciatic nerve, drawing the nerve roots of the spinal cord downward. Flexion of the hips with the knees flexed does not stretch the sciatic nerve. Extension of the hips and flexion of the knees pulls on the femoral nerve. Flexion of the hips and knees relieves stretching of both the sciatic and femoral nerves. The healthy individual should be able to freely undergo reasonable amounts of passive stretching of the spinal canal as described, without resistance or pain. When the meninges of the spinal cord and its nerve roots are diseased (as in meningitis), the physical sequelae may result in both impaired free movement and pain on stretching at any or several points along the length of the irritated cerebrospinal axis. This pain and limitation of motion may be identified by the patient at the neck or lower back (most commonly along the area of the sciatic nerve). However, the pain and stiffness may also be less well described and may be located at multiple sites along the spinal cord. Meningeal signs have been proposed to be difficult to elicit in infants and the elderly (Ziai and Lewin, 2008; Curtis *et al.*, 2010), and it is thus accepted clinical practice that the absence of these signs should not be used to exclude the diagnosis of meningitis in these age groups.

3.3.2 Neck stiffness

Neck stiffness, or nuchal rigidity, is elicited initially by asking the patient to touch their chin to their chest and then turn the head, looking to the extreme right and left. If the patient is unable to do this, the clinician should lean over the supine patient, gather the patient's head in both hands and gently flex the head forward, bringing the chin towards the patient's chest and then secondarily turning the head from right to left. Resistance to smooth flexion of the neck (stiff neck) is characteristic of meningeal irritation.

3.3.3 Kernig–Lasegue sign

In descriptions of meningitis, this sign is more commonly known simply as Kernig's sign, after the Russian neurologist who first described the motor aspects of this sign in 1882. The original description of the sign described a patient sitting on the edge of a bed with legs overhanging. The physician attempted to passively extend the leg at the knee towards 90 degrees. A positive sign was elicited if the legs could not be extended due to contraction of the hamstring muscles maintaining a flexed position. Pain was not a part of the original description by Kernig. J.J. Forst, a pupil of the French physician Charles Lasegue (1816–1883), known for his early descriptions of sciatica, first described the sensory, painful aspect of this sign, in his doctoral thesis in 1881. The sign was considered positive when pain was felt in the area of the sciatic nerve while performing the manoeuvre as described by Kernig. As an acknowledgement of the contributions of both of these physicians (but not of Forst!), the sign is sometimes described as the Kernig–Lasegue sign, and has been somewhat modified. In current medical practice, Kernig's sign is elicited with the patient flat in the supine position. Initially, the hip and knee of one limb are both flexed to 90 degrees. The sign is considered positive if, on passive extension of the leg at the knee joint, resistance or pain is elicited in the lower back, and if the knee will not fully extend as it did when the hip was originally extended in the flat supine position.

3.3.4 Brudzinski's sign

This neck sign was first described by Polish paediatrician Jozef Brudzinski in 1909. This sign is positive when passive flexion of the supine patient's head is painful and is accompanied by flexion of the lower limbs. Flexion of the forearms may also be seen, although this is less well described. Passive head flexion causes stretching on the upper portion of the cerebrospinal axis, which promotes shortening of the lower aspect of the cerebrospinal axis by flexion of the lower extremities at the hips and knees. An accompanying involuntary head retraction may also be felt. A positive sign is bilateral with flexion of both legs at the hips and knees (relieves tension on sciatic and femoral nerves).

3.3.5 Opisthotonos

Opisthotonos (Greek: opistho = behind, and tonos = tone) is the position of supine rigid prolonged hyperextension of the neck and spine, such that *in extremis* only the occiput and lower back or feet touch the bed, secondary to severely aggravated extensor tone. This phenomenon is most commonly thought of as a symptom of spasticity or dystonia and has been noted in other disease states including rabies, tetanus, malaria, encephalitis, asphyxia, cerebral palsy, seizures, psychiatric disorders and medication effects (Hooda *et al.*, 1995; Ceulemans *et al.*, 2008; Haden *et al.*, 2009; Chauhan and Pickens, 2011).

3.3.6 Tripoding or Amoss's sign

The term 'tripod position' may be more commonly known in the context of obstructive airway diseases such as epiglottitis, retropharyngeal abscesses or chronic obstructive pulmonary disease. Impending airway obstruction promotes the tripod position in which the patient leans forward, supporting the upper body with outstretched hands on the flat surface between his knees anterior to the frontal plane. This position optimizes use of the accessory muscles of the neck and helps to elevate the anterior wall of the chest (Bhatt *et al.*, 2009). In meningitis, the position is the reflective opposite. American pathologist Harold Lindsay Amoss (1886–1956) first described the tripod sign as a protective position in the context of the pain of meningeal irritation. In order to relieve pressure on the irritated spinal canal, the patient tries to sit up by supporting himself with his hands outstretched directly behind him on the bed. The back is arched in lordosis with neck extended and knees and hips flexed when irritation is extreme (Suvarna and Keskar, 2009). While infrequently noted in the literature, several case records do exist (Nichols, 1994; Oostenbrink *et al.*, 2001).

3.3.7 Bulging fontanelle

The bones of the skull join together at suture lines, which progressively mineralize and fuse together over late infancy. In early infancy, the fibrous membrane-covered soft spot where two sutures join together forms a small space called a fontanelle. The word fontanelle comes from the Latin 'fonticulus' and the French word 'fontaine', meaning a little fountain or spring. Ideally, the infant's fontanelle should be examined while the infant is upright and calm. Fontanelles should feel firm and just slightly concaved to the touch. When bulging, fontanelles feel full, tense and convex. The most likely explanation for a bulging fontanelle in meningitis is expansion of the SAS, secondary to obstruction of CSF absorption by congested arachnoid granulations in the sagittal sinus. Alternative explanations include increased intravascular volume, hydrocephalus and subdural effusions; however, radiographic evidence for these explanations is not forthcoming (Rothman and Lee, 1998; Kiesler and Ricer, 2003; Wellons *et al.*, 2013).

3.4 Relevance of the Clinical Examination

Until relatively recently, the clinical examination was the main or only means of arriving at a clinical diagnosis. The past century has seen a rapid increase in the availability and sophistication of laboratory and sometimes even bedside testing, to aid the clinician in achieving a timely and accurate diagnosis. However, despite these advances, in the majority of clinical situations, the history and physical exam still play vital roles and are the mainstay of the clinician (Ende and Fosnocht, 2002). The bedside clinical assessment, the history and physical examination, can be viewed as a collection of rapidly administered diagnostic tests, which either together – or sometimes in isolation – will shed light on the aetiology and severity of the patient's medical complaint. Each finding from the medical history and physical examination is a test result that bears weight on the direction of clinical decision-making. It is these individual bedside clinical 'test results', prioritized within the process of data gathering, that lead the clinician to the correct choice of next steps, of either further more definitive testing or arrival at a diagnosis with subsequent treatment and management. Ranking these clinical 'pre-tests' in order of decreasing magnitude of diagnostic accuracy will help clinicians to selectively choose the most efficient examinations on which to focus, for a given condition. Continued clinical use of tests with minimal or no diagnostic weight is inefficient and does not help with the diagnostic process (King *et al.*, 2005). Therefore, identification of the key and most useful items of the physical examination is of extreme relevance to the clinician, patient and healthcare system (Straus, 2006).

Unfortunately, most diseases do not present with a singular identifying feature but rather a constellation of symptoms. Many similar symptoms are common to quite disparate diseases and overlap of symptomatology makes accurate diagnosis challenging. Missed disease is devastating, with significant mortality and lifetime morbidity. Reviews of paediatric malpractice claims in the USA reveal that missed meningitis is one of the top three medical litigations and the medical entity with the highest associated mortality. The most common medical misadventure noted in these claims is that of error in accurate diagnosis (Selbst *et al.*, 2005; Carroll and Buddenbaum, 2007). Accurate diagnosis appears to be most difficult in patients at both extremes of the age spectrum and in those with developmental delays, due to the understandable challenges in assessing these vulnerable populations.

Despite centuries of painstaking descriptions of the clinical features of ill individuals, we still have very little certainty about how to clinically recognize or rule out severe disease in ill individuals. The exactitude of our clinical examination has not been examined scientifically in most cases, with very few methodologically rigorous studies available to support the clinical assessments used historically. Thus, clinicians are uncertain about the faith they can place in the accuracy and reliability of the clinical examination. While ancillary laboratory and imaging tests are a key aspect of clinical appraisal, these tests also have varying degrees of accuracy and reliability, they may be expensive or burdensomely invasive and moreover, for many medical conditions, are not yet available. The challenge for the clinician is to correctly identify the sickest individuals contained within a large group of patients with apparently undifferentiated features. Improved recognition of the physical features that best differentiate truly unwell individuals from those who have more minor illnesses will result in more efficient and improved care.

3.5 How Useful Are Clinical Tests for Clinical Care?

A useful bedside examination test is one that will alter the clinician's initial estimates of the pre-test probability of disease and should help to determine if further testing, treatment or management is required in an individual patient. Tests are of greatest use when a diagnostic dilemma is present. For example, when considering the likelihood of meningitis, a well-appearing, playful, happy, 4-year-old with fever and upper respiratory tract infection clearly does not require definitive CSF testing to determine that meningitis is not present. Similarly, a 70-year-old presenting to the emergency department with a fever, headache, vomiting, neck stiffness and altered level of consciousness does not immediately require the results from CSF testing to prompt the administration of broad-spectrum antibiotic treatment for meningitis. A diagnostic dilemma in next-step decision-making is not present in either initial clinical scenario, although the latter patient will, when stable, require CSF testing to confirm the diagnosis and determine details surrounding treatment selection and duration. While without CSF testing we cannot be 100% sure that meningitis is absent or present, respectively, in each case, we can weigh up, based on the clinical presentations, that the likelihood of disease is low enough and high enough, respectively, that further diagnostic testing and treatment is unnecessary in the first case but warranted in the second. Unfortunately, the clinical presentations of many patients fall in between these extremes, into a region of diagnostic uncertainty, and it is here that careful application of the various diagnostic tests of the clinical examination may be most useful (Fig. 3.1).

The gold standard diagnostic test for meningitis is laboratory examination of the CSF through the performance of LP. However, performance of this particular anxiety-provoking, painful, invasive, time-consuming and expensive diagnostic test in each individual who presents to a clinician with undifferentiated symptom constellations is not always feasible or desirable. Selective identification of those patients most likely to benefit from the information derived from LP, through discriminating application of the most accurate screening 'pre-tests' of the clinical examination, is the most efficient approach. The usefulness of each of these tests of the clinical examination is directly related to how accurately they identify the target disorder of meningitis and thus, as a proxy, for how each test compares with the gold standard test for disease.

3.6 Reliability of the Clinical Examination

When thinking about tests used to assist in the process of diagnosis, information about how accurately a test identifies or excludes a condition (the diagnostic accuracy estimate) is of utmost importance. However, it is also important to feel confident that administration of that same test on other occasions under similar conditions will yield the same result. If not, then it is not a very reliable instrument. For example, information about how to perform or interpret clinical examination tests such as Kernig's or Brudzinski's sign, while somewhat standardized through bedside teaching in medical schools or descriptions in medical textbooks, is susceptible to human error or variations in style, ability or understanding of that test. Reliability, or the consistency of a tool, can be assessed by examining the agreement between two or more measures of the same thing. The most well-known measures of reliability are inter-rater and test–retest reliability. Inter-rater reliability, estimated by calculation of the kappa statistic, is assessed by examining the agreement of the results of

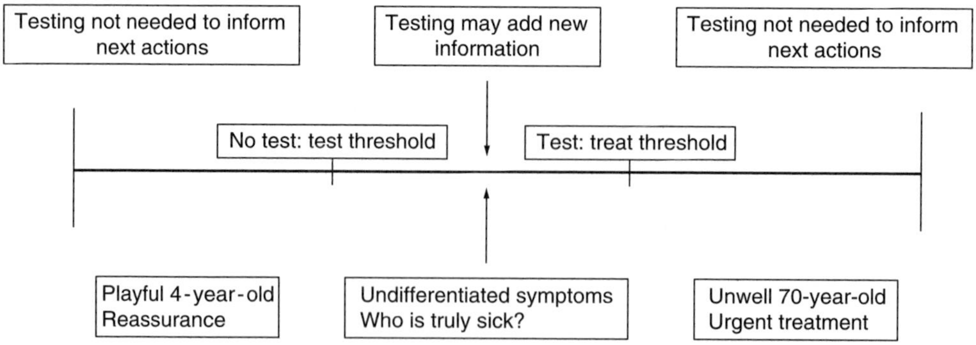

Fig. 3.1. Decision-making: how information provided by a test may influence next steps. (Adapted from Hayden and Brown, 1999; Meates-Dennis, 2004; Brown *et al.*, 2004.)

the test as applied by two or more raters. Test–retest reliability is a comparison of the scores obtained by the same rater on two or more separate occasions. To date, review of the literature for adult and paediatric meningitis does not reveal any information surrounding the reliability of the clinical tests performed to diagnose this disease entity. None of the studies of diagnostic accuracy described in this chapter include parallel estimates of the reliability of the clinical features examined within those studies. Without certainty as to whether the tests (signs and symptoms) are uniformly understood or applied in a consistent manner, interpretation of the accuracy of the data may be challenging. Without precision evaluations of inter-rater reliability throughout each prospective study, it is difficult to assess the extent and thus influence of this variability. While this may in fact reflect the reality of clinical practice, a general interpretation can be kept in mind. However, in future research of this topic, performance of inter-rater reliability should be assessed in parallel with diagnostic accuracy studies and would be useful to further inform clinicians of the performance metrics of the clinical tests applied. Ideally, each prospective study would benefit from pre-study demonstration of each sign and symptom as well as standardized, clearly written definitions maintained as a part of each study proforma.

3.7 Diagnostic Accuracy of the Clinical Examination

Historically, the incorporation of particular systems-based clinical examination features into the clinician's toolkit was a didactic one, with the identification and sharing of knowledge through clinical bedside teaching or descriptive case reports. Clinical features of meningitis have been frequently described in case reports and textbooks. However, the evidence behind the diagnostic accuracy and reliability of these often undifferentiated features has only recently begun to be examined in a rigorous manner.

Diagnostic accuracy is a statistical measure of how well a test identifies or excludes a condition. Diagnostic tests rarely confirm or exclude the diagnosis with certainty but rather support the clinician's estimate that a disease is likely or unlikely in an individual patient. A good diagnostic test should be able to differentiate between patients who have the condition of interest (target condition) and those who do not. A useful diagnostic test will be used to modify a clinician's initial estimation of disease probability (pre-test probability). Pre-test probabilities of disease (ranging from 0 to 100%) may be derived from knowledge of disease prevalence in the local population or from clinical experience.

The goal of any test application is to provide information that can inform a revised estimate of the probability of disease (post-test probability of disease). This post-test probability is useful to clinicians and patients to discuss at the bedside, because this information may help to shed light on the likelihood of disease and whether further tests or treatment are needed. If the clinical signs and symptoms are reassuring, the patient's post-test probability of disease may be the same or even lower than pre-test estimates and the patient may not require any further assistance. However, if post-test probabilities of disease are raised because of the new information acquired from physical tests, then the clinician and patient will need to decide whether the increase is large enough to warrant further definitive testing or treatments.

Throughout the clinical assessment, the clinician is constantly querying the probability of disease in a given patient. Each question on history and each physical exam manoeuvre can sequentially update the opinion about pre-test probability of disease, to generate a modified post-test probability of disease. Logically, after conducting one test, the modified disease estimate or post-test probability of disease becomes the new pre-test probability of disease, prior to examining the information revealed by the next clinical test. This is a reasonable approach, providing that the tests are independent of one another mechanistically. When many tests are performed in series as described, the cumulative nature of the weight borne by the information derived from each individual test can result in powerful overall estimates of disease likelihood even if each individual test weight is small (Gill *et al.*, 2005).

3.7.1 Statistical tests of diagnostic accuracy

Many statistical tests of diagnostic accuracy exist, including sensitivity, specificity and positive and negative predictive values. Likelihood ratios (LRs) may be the most useful statistical estimates of test accuracy for the clinician and have several advantages over other statistical measures. LR estimates help the clinician incorporate and adapt test properties such as sensitivity and specificity to individual patients and can be calculated from the knowledge of both test accuracy measures. LRs can be used to describe test accuracy for tests that have a wide range of outcomes (continuous results) and can be calculated for several levels of the test result. Importantly, they are less likely to change with the prevalence of the disorder and, unlike other measures, their use is considered 'transferable' and comparable between differing populations, regardless of disease prevalence. In addition, they can be used to combine the results of several independent diagnostic tests and, most importantly, they can be used easily to calculate the post-test probability for a target disease. It is the generation of this probability that is of most importance to the patient and clinician in deciding on the next course of action.

The LR is defined as the ratio between the probability of observing the test result (positive or negative) in patients with disease and the probability of observing the same test result (positive or negative) in patients without the disease. The LR is the ratio of two proportions and is a ratio that describes either positive test results (LR+) or negative test results (LR–). Intuitively, the larger the positive LR, the larger the likelihood of disease; the smaller the negative LR, the lesser the likelihood of disease. By convention, LRs > 10 significantly increase the probability of disease while LRs that are very low (< 0.1) significantly decrease the chance that the individual has the target disorder (Hayden and Brown, 1999). As with any test statistic, an accompanying confidence interval (CI) should be calculated for each diagnostic test accuracy estimate, in order to best interpret and reflect the statistical significance of each accuracy measure. Easy conversion from pre-test to post-test probability can be achieved using the LR value and a simple nomogram (Fagen, 1975; Hayden and Brown, 1999).

3.7.2 How is the diagnostic accuracy data of clinical features (or any other test) derived?

In the ideal clinical scenario, a clinician would be able to access an array of highly accurate diagnostic tests to assist in differentiating well and unwell patients. However, in reality, relatively few such tests exist, despite the importance of diagnosis to the clinician's function. Before coming into clinical use, any test (laboratory or other) should be subjected to assessments of diagnostic rigour to ensure that the purported diagnostic accuracy of the test is realistic. The methods by which the diagnostic accuracy of a given test has been derived are therefore an important consideration, as poor methodologies can significantly misrepresent estimates of test accuracy.

Diagnostic tests should initially be evaluated in a clinically relevant population, by prospectively comparing the results of the index test under evaluation with the results of the reference or gold standard on the same patient population. In the clinical context of meningitis, the index tests are a standardized and prospective evaluation of each individual sign or symptom of disease in each patient under clinical suspicion of disease. The gold standard test (CSF analysis via LP) should be performed on each patient in the population, and blinding of the clinical outcome assessor to the results of the subsequently performed gold standard is paramount to minimize ascertainment bias. This will result in a study that can provide data derived from two groups of a cohort, one of which contains individuals with the target disease and the other containing individuals without. The researchers can then compare the performance of the index test in each group and provide LRs to reflect the strength of the test's ability to identify sick individuals. Primary studies that do not provide data about test performance in two or more comparison groups measured against the gold standard are more susceptible to bias and cannot provide all of the data points required to appropriately assess test accuracy.

Methodological consistency among the numerous reports of the clinical examination for meningitis is not high, and the vast majority of these reports are retrospective in nature. Unfortunately, retrospective studies, while easier to perform than prospective studies via review of charts, are subject to high amounts of bias, largely reporting bias. Clinical features may or may not have been noted in the chart due to other chance factors, such as the particular level of knowledge, focus, efficiency or time available for accurate charting by the individual physician. Retrospective studies also have large degrees of heterogeneity with respect to clinical presentations reviewed (selection bias), patient characteristics such as age and general level of health, country of origin and baseline prevalence of disease among other features, leading to considerable limitations in meaningful data synthesis. Most of these studies lack a comparison group and, most importantly, these studies also have large variations in the gold standard definition. Even though CSF analysis is the gold standard for diagnosis of meningitis, laboratory definitions are variable and the effect of these variations is uncertain (Curtis *et al.*, 2010).

3.7.3 Summary of adult evidence surrounding diagnostic accuracy of clinical features

The medical literature regarding clinical features of meningitis in adults is voluminous. Previously, Attia *et al.* (1999) published a comprehensive meta-analysis that summarized the data from 14 retrospectively designed studies. Unfortunately, the data were of limited use due to the retrospective study designs, lack of control groups and large heterogeneity with respect to key clinical features. To date, only three methodologically appropriate studies of the diagnostic accuracy of clinical features of meningitis in adults have been forthcoming (Uchihara and Tsukagoshi, 1991; Thomas *et al.*, 2002; Waghdhare *et al.*, 2010). Key findings from these studies are listed in Table 3.1. Each study reviewed various features of both the clinical examination and the clinical history. These studies provide useful numerical descriptors of the weight of diagnostic accuracy of each individual clinical feature studied through provision of data that allow calculation of LRs. From these rigorous studies, it would seem that relatively few (if any) signs or symptoms, which have long been used to clinically discriminate adult patients with meningitis from those without the disease, are in fact useful.

It would also seem that there is a lack of evidence to support use of these clinical features to distinguish between meningitis of differing aetiologies (Waghdhare *et al.*, 2010) (Table 3.2). Similarly, review of a series of papers from several cohorts of individuals with meningitis also sheds light on whether different bacteria are likely to cause significantly different features in presentation. While only retrospective and proportional data are presented, the proportions of clinical features displayed across groups of individuals with confirmed pneumococcal, meningococcal and *Listeria* meningitis do not appear to be strikingly different from each other (Weisfelt *et al.*, 2006a; Heckenberg *et al.*, 2008; Amaya-Villar *et al.*, 2010).

Weisfelt *et al.* (2006b) also examined whether any clinical features are more prevalent in elderly patients (>60 years) as compared with younger patients (17–59 years). Again, within the limitations of retrospectively gathered data, it was noted that the classic triad of fever, neck stiffness and altered mental status (Glasgow Coma Score <14) was present more often in older adults than younger adults (149/257 (58%) versus 156/439 (36%); $P = 0.01$), a larger proportion of

Table 3.1. Accuracy of clinical features adults: single studies: prospective data with control group. LR+, positive likelihood ratio; LR–, negative likelihood ratio; GCS, Glasgow Coma Scale; Hx, history.

Study and clinical feature	No. of patients (%)	Sensitivity % (95% CI)	Specificity % (95% CI)	LR+ (95% CI)	LR– (95% CI)
Waghdhare *et al.*, 2010	**190**	–	–	–	–
Nuchal rigidity	66 (34)	39.4 (29.7, 49.7)	70.3 (59.8, 79.5)	1.33 (0.89, 1.98)	0.86 (0.7, 1.06)
Kernig	21 (11)	14.1 (7.95, 22.6)	92.3 (84.8, 96.9)	1.84 (0.77, 4.35)	0.93 (0.84, 1.03)
Brudzinski	17 (9)	11.1 (5.68, 19)	93.4 (86.2, 97.5)	1.69 (0.65, 4.37)	0.95 (0.87, 1.04)
Jolt accentuation	7 (4)	6.06 (2.26, 12.7)	98.9 (94, 100)	5.52 (0.67, 44.9)	0.95 (0.89, 1.00)
Thomas *et al.*, 2002	**297**	–	–	–	–
Nuchal rigidity	93 (31)	30	68	0.94 (0.64, 1.39)	1.02 (0.87, 1.22)
Kernig	11 (4)	5	95	0.97 (0.27, 3.55)	1.0 (0.94, 1.07)
Brudzinski	11 (4)	5	95	0.97 (0.26, 3.53)	0.97 (0.94, 1.07)
Temp. > 38°C	146 (49)	42.5 (32.2, 53.4)	48.4 (41.8, 55.0)	0.82 (0.62, 1.09)	1.2 (0.94, 1.5)
GCS < 13	24 (8)	10 (5.2, 18.5)	92.6 (88.4, 95.4)	1.36 (0.6, 3.0)	0.97 (0.89, 1.06)
Hx headache	237 (84)	92 (83, 96)	18.8 (14.1, 24.7)	1.13 (1.03, 1.245)	0.43 (0.19, 0.96)
Hx fever	199 (67)	77 (68, 84)	33 (27, 39)	1.15 (1.005, 1.33)	0.68 (0.46, 1.025)
Hx photophobia	148 (50)	57.3 (46, 68)	49 (42, 58)	1.13 (0.88, 1.43)	0.87 (0.65, 1.17)
Hx vomiting	167 (56)	70.1 (59.2, 79.2)	47 (40.4, 53.6)	1.32 (1.09, 1.60)	0.636 (0.439, 0.922)
Hx stiff neck	135 (45)	48 (37, 58)	55 (49, 62)	1.07 (0.82, 1.41)	0.94 (0.74, 1.9)
Hx focal motor deficit	25 (8)	6.4 (2.8, 14)	90.5 (85.7, 94.0)	0.67 (0.262, 1.73)	1.03 (0.96, 1.11)
Hx focal sensory deficit	19 (6)	2.6 (0.7, 9.1)	95 (91, 97)	0.493 (0.112, 2.173)	1.029 (0.979, 1.08)
Hx seizure	19	8.9 (4.4, 17.2)	94.4 (90.5, 97.0)	1.67 (0.68, 4.09)	0.96 (0.89, 1.04)
Uchihara and Tsukagoshi, 1991	**54**	–	–	–	–
Jolt accentuation	33 (61)	97.1	60	2.43 (1.41, 4.16)	0.05 (0.01, 0.35)

older individuals had altered mental status (216/256 (84%) versus 261/438 (60%); $P <$ 0.001) and focal neurological abnormalities were more likely in older individuals. However, data leading to calculation of LRs were not available from these studies and thus applicability of these features for clinical assessment of individual patients is uncertain.

While these descriptions may be somewhat useful for the adult patient, it is worth considering that only three rigorous but heterogeneous studies have been performed to date, resulting in information gleaned from relatively small sample sizes overall. Ideally in the future, further more homogeneously designed studies appropriate for meta-analysis might provide more firm conclusions on the usefulness of these clinical examination features.

Applying the information to adults

Two adults living where the known prevalence of meningitis is 15%, present to the local hospital with histories of headache and vomiting. Assuming that these clinical features are independent of each other (using the data in Table 3.1), the combination of the clinical features of fever (LR+ 1.15), headache (LR+ 1.13) and vomiting (LR+ 1.32) (combined

Table 3.2. Diagnostic accuracy of physical signs from a single study with control group using prospective data, in different aetiological types of meningitis. LR+, positive likelihood ratio; LR–, negative likelihood ratio. (Adapted from Waghdhare *et al.*, 2010.)

Clinical feature	No. of patients	LR+ (95% CI)	LR– (95% CI)
Aseptic meningitis	62	–	–
Nuchal rigidity	18	0.97 (0.59, 1.62)	1.01 (0.82, 1.24)
Kernig	4	0.83 (0.25, 2.74)	1.01 (0.92, 1.11)
Brudzinski	3	0.73 (0.19, 2.82)	1.02 (0.94, 1.11)
Jolt accentuation	1	1.47 (0.09, 23.0)	0.99 (0.95, 1.03)
Tuberculous meningitis	30	–	–
Nuchal rigidity	17	1.91 (1.22, 2.98)	0.61 (0.40, 0.94)
Kernig	7	3.03 (1.25, 7.95)	0.83 (0.67, 1.02)
Brudzinski	7	3.54 (1.29, 9.71)	0.82 (0.66, 1.01)
Jolt accentuation	3	9.1 (0.98, 84.2)	0.91 (0.67, 1.02)
Bacterial meningitis	7	–	–
Nuchal rigidity	4	1.93 (0.94, 3.94)	0.60 (0.25, 1.45)
Kernig	3	5.57 (1.83, 17)	0.61 (0.32, 1.18)
Brudzinski	1	2.17 (0.30, 15.6)	0.91 (0.67, 1.25)
Jolt accentuation	2	26.00 (0.26, 2.53)	0.72 (0.45, 1.15)

LR+ of 3.60) raises these adults' likelihood of disease a small amount, from what was already assumed as the pre-test probability of meningitis of 15% to a post-test probability of ~20% (Fig. 3.2). If the first patient has a normal clinical examination but the second adult has a positive jolt accentuation test (LR+ 2.43), the combined LR becomes 4.98 and the post-test probability is raised to 40% in the second adult. Thus, for both adults, the detection of these signs raises the risk of meningitis, but for the second adult the risk is doubled. Ideally, given the high pre-test and post-test probability of disease and the devastation of missed disease, both patients would receive definitive diagnostic testing and antimicrobial treatment.

However, consider the same patients presenting in a highly malarious region where very large volumes of patients present with very similar initial symptoms. The challenge clinically, particularly in resource-limited settings, is how to appropriately triage patients towards the appropriate diagnostic tests and treatments. While the presence of a positive jolt accentuation test may raise the suspicion of meningitis in an adult by twofold – even by fivefold (Waghdhare *et al.*, 2010) – further studies to confirm its use as a distinguishing feature for meningitis are still warranted, as the evidence is scanty. When considering the usefulness of other clinical examination features (Table 3.1), as supported by evidence from the very few available derivation studies, no other clinical examination feature proves to have useful weight for its use as an identifying test for meningitis in adults.

While clinical examination features may not look promising as identifying tests from the current evidence, further well-designed studies should be performed to confirm or refute the paucity of evidence that does exist, so that clinical and educational emphasis can be tailored appropriately. Furthermore, construction of logistic regression models of varying combinations of features, in an attempt to obtain sets of predictor variables with an optimal balance of sensitivities and specificities, may still prove useful.

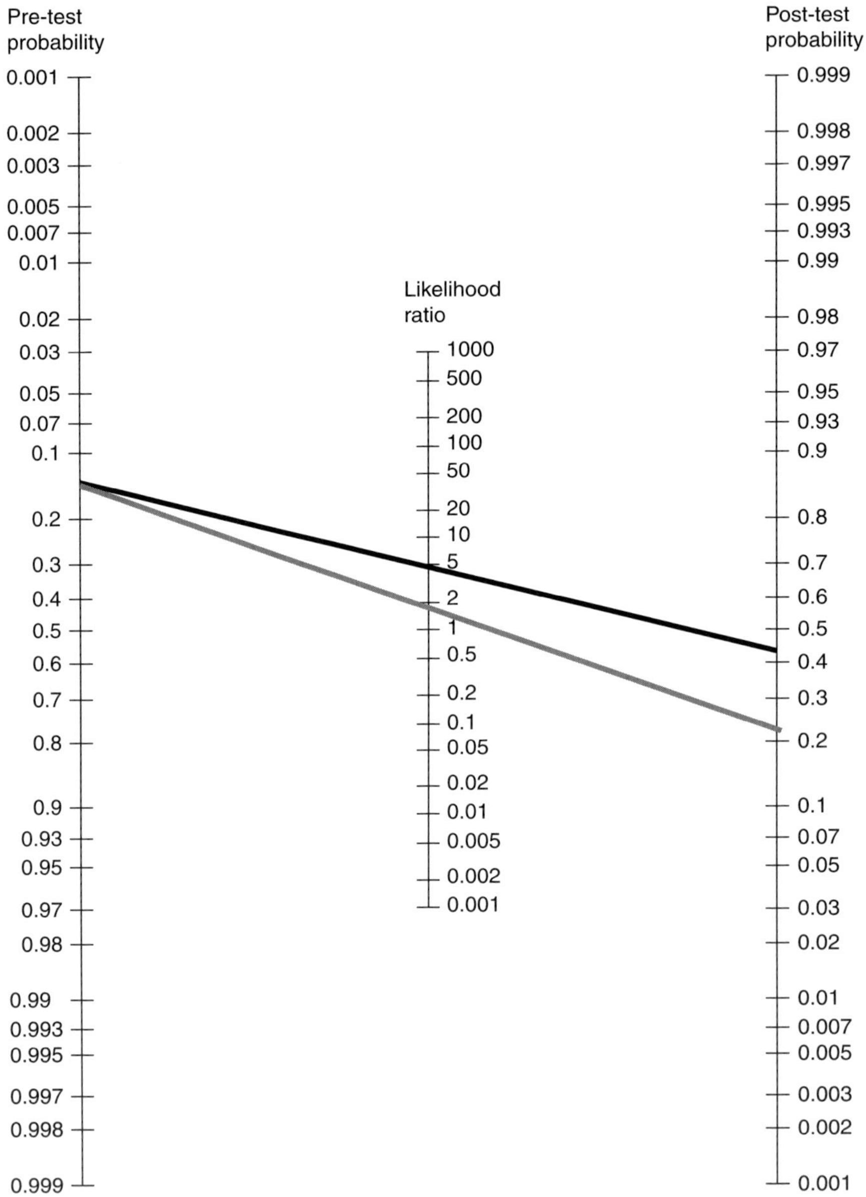

Fig. 3.2. Fagan nomogram for adult meningitis. To use the nomogram, draw a straight line from the patient's pre-test probability of disease through the likelihood ratio for the test result to the post-test probability of disease. (Adapted from Fagen, 1975.)

3.7.4 Summary of paediatric evidence surrounding diagnostic accuracy of clinical features

In contrast to the adult literature, methodologically appropriate studies of the diagnostic accuracy of clinical features of meningitis in children, from an equally voluminous literature, are more forthcoming. A large systematic review of the clinical features suggestive of meningitis in children provides an overview of the strength of evidence supporting the accuracy of numerous clinical features in paediatric meningitis (Curtis *et al.*, 2010). Each of the ten studies included in this review had collected data on clinical features proforma and prospectively in two groups of ill children – those with CSF-confirmed meningitis and those without meningitis (CSF negative). Within each study, clinicians assessed the clinical features in each patient prior to LP and so were appropriately blinded to the final diagnosis of disease. While study quality was generally rated well, the review was somewhat limited by common contributions to meta-analysis heterogeneity such as study settings, patient age, co-morbidities, inclusion criteria, gold standard and index-test definitions. Ideally, index-test definitions in each study would have been more rigorous and transparent to ensure reproducibility and more confidence in interpretation. Additionally, as paediatric physiology changes rapidly across the age spectrum, the essential stratifications of data across clinically relevant paediatric subgroups are important but were unfortunately largely unavailable in the primary studies.

The review findings (Table 3.3) list features in decreasing magnitude of LR. Only six out of 18 symptoms and 15 out of 48 signs were suitable for meta-analysis. Notable features derived from medical histories included: a caregiver's report of a bulging fontanelle (LR+ 8.0), of neck stiffness (LR+ 7.7), of seizures (outside the febrile convulsion range) (LR+ 4.4) or of reduced feeds (LR+ 2.0). Thus, the presence of these features on history appears to raise the likelihood of meningitis, but to varying degrees. Notable features derived from a clinician's physical examination of a child included the presence of petechiae (LR+ 37.0), jaundice (LR+ 5.9), being toxic or moribund (LR+ 5.8), meningeal signs (LR+ 4.5), neck stiffness (LR+ 4.0), bulging fontanelle (LR+ 3.5), Kernig's sign (LR+ 3.5), tone up (LR+ 3.2), fever >40°C (LR+ 2.9) or Brudzinski's sign (LR+ 2.5). Thus, the presence of any of these features independently raises the likelihood of meningitis in the paediatric patient. Several other clinical features have LRs between 1.3 and 2.5 (Table 3.3). The absence of meningeal signs (LR+ 0.41) or of an abnormal cry (LR+ 0.30) were the most useful findings for lowering the likelihood of meningitis. Strikingly, the absence of fever does not rule out meningitis (LR+ 0.70).

Since publication of this systematic review, three new prospective studies are of note and would be of benefit to include in an updated meta-analysis in the future. Bilavsky *et al.* (2012) prospectively assessed the diagnostic accuracy of three physical examination features, namely Kernig's sign, Brudzinski's sign and nuchal rigidity in CSF-confirmed paediatric meningitis. Eighty-six patients, aged 3 months to 17 years (median 25.5 months) were examined. *Streptococcus pneumoniae* (57.5%) and *Neisseria meningitidis* (42.5%) were the causative organisms isolated from the study population. Kernig's sign had the highest LR (10.3 (95% CI 2.57, 41.1)) and the diagnostic accuracy was not altered significantly, whether used alone or in combination with Brudzinski's sign and/or nuchal rigidity. Brudzinski's sign and nuchal rigidity were less useful tests with lower discriminating abilities (LR+ 2.34 and 1.39, respectively). Bilavsky *et al.* (2012) also reported that the accuracy of these three tests did not vary with changes in severity of disease or with causative organism.

Laman *et al.* (2012) prospectively assessed 554 children aged 8 months to 10 years of age (median 24 months) in whom meningitis was clinically suspected and LP was performed. A standardized clinical report form was completed and clinicians screened for clinical findings including neck stiffness, Kernig's sign, Brudzinski's sign, bulging fontanelle, number of seizures, coma and impaired consciousness. These index tests and the gold standard CSF test were well described in the

Table 3.3. Accuracy of clinical features children: summary of prospective data with control group. LR+, positive likelihood ratio; LR–, negative likelihood ratio; NOS, no other symsptoms. (Adapted from Curtis *et al.*, 2010.)

Symptom/Sign	No. of patients	Summary sensitivity %	Summary specificity %	Summary LR+ (95% CI)	Summary LR– (95% CI)
Bulging fontanelle	284	14	98	8.0 (2.4, 26)	0.88 (0.79,0.98)
Neck stiffness or bulging fontanelle	341	20	98	7.7 (3.2,19)	0.82 (0.73,0.93)
History of seizures outside febrile convulsions age range	965	32	93	4.4 (3.0,6.4)	0.73 (0.64,0.85)
Reduced feeds	1890	52	70	2.0 (1.2, 3.4)	0.66 (0.54, 0.81)
Lethargy or drowsy	925	29	78	1.3 (1.0, 1.7)	0.91 (0.82, 1.0)
Irritable	284	82	34	1.3 (1.1, 1.5)	0.52 (0.28, 0.97)
Petechiae	341	6	100	37 (2.0, 680)	0.94 (0.88, 0.99)
Jaundice	2059	6	99	5.9 (1.8, 19)	0.95 (0.89, 1.0)
Toxic or moribund	172	49	92	5.8 (3.0, 11)	0.56 (0.42, 0.73)
Meningeal signs[a]	2399	64	89	4.5 (2.4, 8.3)	0.41 (0.30, 0.57)
Neck stiffness	3118	51	89	4.0 (2.6, 6.3)	0.56 (0.43, 0.72)
Bulging fontanelle	2247	36	90	3.5 (2.0, 6.0)	0.74 (0.61, 0.89)
Kernig	172	53	85	3.5 (2.1, 5.7)	0.56 (0.41, 0.75)
Tone up	284	59	82	3.2 (2.2, 4.5)	0.50 (0.36, 0.70)
Fever >40°C	433	19	93	2.9 (1.6, 5.5)	0.81 (0.55, 1.2)
Brudzinski	172	66	74	2.5 (1.8, 3.6)	0.46 (0.31, 0.68)
Staring eyes	640	42	82	2.4 (1.8, 3.2)	0.70 (0.60, 0.82)
Can't or won't feed	284	61	70	2.1 (1.5, 2.8)	0.56 (0.39, 0.79)
Complex Sz[b]	1400	27	82	2.0 (1.2, 3.4)	0.86 (0.70, 1.1)
Lethargic or drowsy (sign)	376	40	79	1.9 (1.3, 2.9)	0.58 (0.20, 1.7)
Unconscious or coma	3313	23	86	1.8 (1.2, 2.7)	0.94 (0.85, 1.1)
Abnormal cry	284	84	52	1.8 (1.5, 2.1)	0.30 (0.16, 0.57)
Restless/irritable/ agitated	758	37	79	1.6 (1.2, 2.1)	0.77 (0.50, 1.2)
Multiple seizures	522	64	57	1.5 (1.1, 2.1)	0.62 (0.36, 1.3)
Seizures non-specific	1095	54	63	1.4 (1.2, 1.7)	0.75 (0.48, 1.2)
Change mental status[c]	1815	72	47	1.4 (1.2, 1.7)	0.54 (0.34, 0.87)
Fever NOS	885	–	–	1.2 (0.98, 1.4)	0.7 (0.53, 0.92)

[a]Stiffness or rigidity or meningeal irritation or Brudzinski or Kernig.
[b]Focal or multiple or >15 min duration or complex.
[c]Lethargic/agitated/impaired consciousness.

report. Fifteen per cent of these children had proven ($n=47$) or probable ($n=36$) meningitis. Causative organisms included 22 with *Haemophilus influenzae* type B, 22 with *S. pneumoniae*, two with *Cryptococcus gattii* and one with *Staphylococcus aureus*. The most useful of the physical screening tests was neck stiffness and bulging fontanelle (LR+ 7.6–7.7). The presence of deep coma doubled the chances of meningitis (LR+ 2.1). Neck stiffness was the only sign whose absence may have contributed to lowering the suspicion for meningitis (LR– 0.3). In general, the findings reflected the direction and magnitudes of the systematic review. Of interest, the presence of malarial parasites on peripheral smear (LR+ 0.04) was associated with a dramatically reduced likelihood of acute bacterial meningitis (ABM) in this population, a finding that is quite unique among studies. Laman *et al.* (2012) have emphasized the importance of the development and validation of ABM predictive models that are specific to the influences of local epidemiology.

Mwaniki *et al.* (2011) prospectively assessed 2411 young infants with suspected meningitis. The goal was to identify clinical indicators of ABM in young infants and compare the performance of these indicators with the World Health Organization guidelines. The methodological approach was rigorous with documented specific pre-study training for clinical staff in the recognition of the clinical signs of meningitis. Data were gathered and analysed in two clinical age-based subgroups of 7 days and 7–59 days. *S. pneumoniae*, *S. agalactiae* and *H. influenzae* were the most common species identified. Meningitis was diagnosed more often at 7–59 days than in the first week of life (4.8% versus 3.0%, $P < 0.001$). Blood cultures were positive in 71% of cases and 28% had an obviously turbid CSF.

For infants in the first week of life, the most useful indicators appeared to be history of fever (LR+ 2.16), history of seizure (LR+ 2.03), irritability (LR+ 3.83), bulging fontanelle (LR+ 8.46) and axillary temperature >39°C (LR+ 3.57). A lack of a history of fever was somewhat suggestive of decreased likelihood of meningitis (LR– 0.41). For infants aged 7–59 days, these same features were similarly useful, with absence of fever more strongly lowering the likelihood of meningitis (LR– 0.29). In this group, neck stiffness had a LR of 4.90. A simple scoring system based on these features was designed by the research team and this system was validated in a subsequent population of similar infants. Overall, one case of meningitis would be identified for every 21 (95% CI, 15, 35) infants undergoing LP or presumptive treatment based on the signs in this scoring system, compared with 28 (95% CI, 19, 61) using the WHO recommended signs.

Applying the information to children

A 6-month-old infant presents to a busy medical clinic in Canada with symptoms of poor feeding and irritability. The medical trainee takes a thorough medical history and describes the history of poor feeding (LR+ 2.0) and irritability (LR+ 1.3) to the senior clinician (Table 3.3). While considering a broad differential diagnosis in this ill infant, the clinician reflects that, from the limited history, the likelihood of meningitis is probably only slightly higher (3%) than the known North American population prevalence of ~1%. The infant has received the first two routine vaccinations and so is partially protected and also benefits somewhat from herd immunity, as vaccine uptake in the locale is very strong. Furthermore, the physician stays abreast of local microbiology reports and is not aware of local epidemics or outbreaks of meningitis-causing organisms. On the other hand, the clinician weighs that such non-specific symptoms in a child could be the result of a serious bacterial illness and that such considerations should be conservative in young children. She seeks further information through physical examination. On examination, the infant is noted to have an abnormal cry (LR+ 1.8), a bulging fontanelle (LR+ 3.5) and neck stiffness (LR+ 4.0). As each piece of information is elicited from the examination, the post-test probability is raised from 1–3% to ~40% (Fig. 3.3). LP is carefully performed, CSF is sent for analysis and broad-spectrum antimicrobial therapy is swiftly initiated.

Although the evidence describing the weight of clinical examination features for paediatric meningitis is more substantial than that for adult meningitis, further well-designed studies are still warranted in children. Some features have been examined only in single studies and/or in small numbers of patients. Furthermore, evidence derived from studies with robust patient numbers in relevant paediatric age or stage subgroups has not yet been forthcoming and could be of considerable clinical relevance. Several

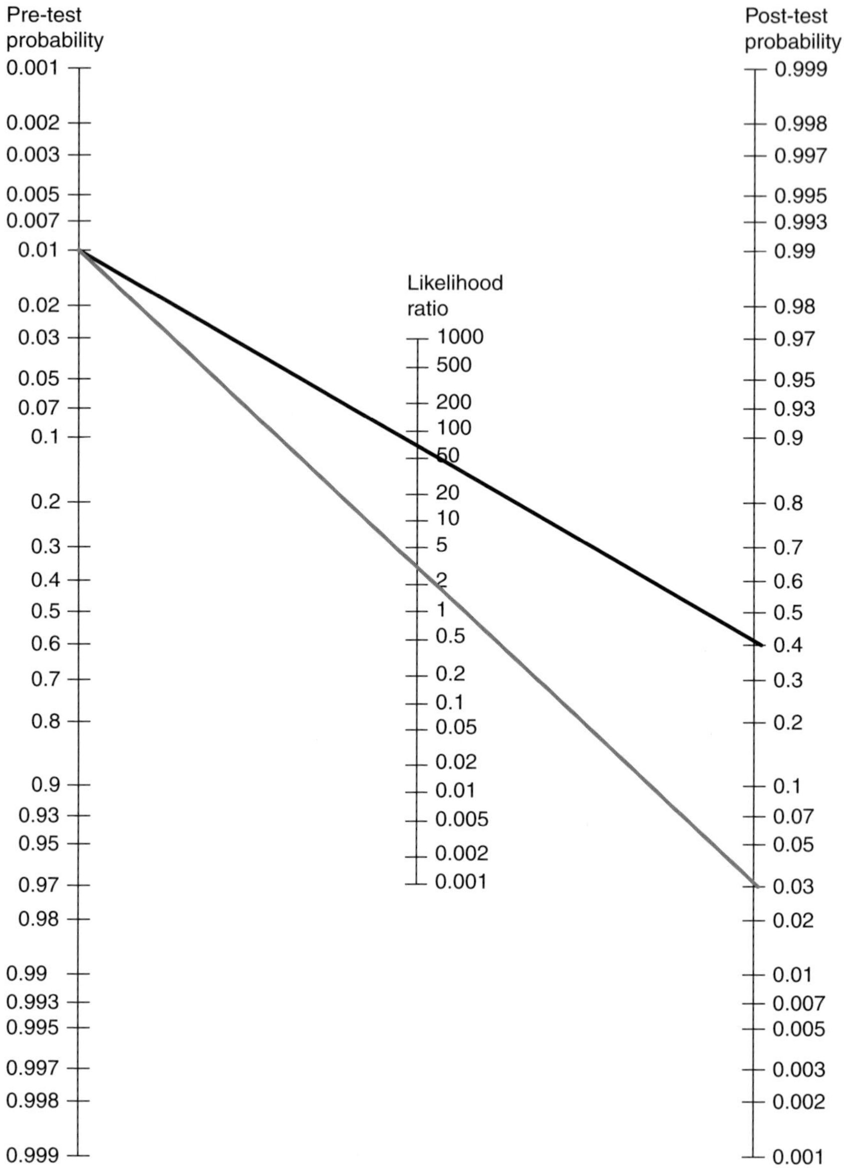

Fig. 3.3. Fagan nomogram for child meningitis. To use the nomogram, draw a straight line from the patient's pre-test probability of disease through the likelihood ratio (LR) for the test result to the post-test probability of disease. (Adapted from Fagen, 1975.)

clinical features are of some use to raise suspicion of meningitis with many positive LRs ranging from 2 to 8 (Table 3.3). While the weight of these LRs may not seem strong when considering common definitions, many assert that these values can still be of use, particularly when used in series as described above. As in adults, construction of logistical regression models of varying combinations of paediatric features, in an attempt to obtain sets of paediatric age subgroup-specific predictor variables with an optimal balance of sensitivities and specificities, may also prove useful.

3.8 Conclusions

Clinical features thought to be predictive of meningitis in adults have been tentatively identified but have not been appropriately studied for drawing confident conclusions surrounding accuracy or reliability of these features for clinical use. For children, identifying features have been more rigorously studied and several clinical features appear to be useful. Further methodologically rigorous studies in both populations are warranted. Given the severe sequelae of this disease and prevailing clinical uncertainty about the directive weight of clinical features, any individual under suspicion of disease, particularly those who are difficult to assess clinically, should undergo definitive testing or treatment.

References

Amaya-Villar, R., Garcia-Cabrera, E., Sulleiro-Igual, E., Fernandez-Viladrich, P., Fontanals-Aymerich, D., Catalan-Alonso, P., Rodrigo-Gonzalo de, L.C., Coloma-Conde, A., Grill-Diaz, F., Guerrero-Espejo, A., Pachon, J. and Prats-Pastor, G. (2010) Three-year multicenter surveillance of community-acquired *Listeria monocytogenes* meningitis in adults. *BMC Infectious Diseases* 10, 324.

Attia, J., Hatala, R., Cook, D.J. and Wong, J.G. (1999) The rational clinical examination. Does this adult patient have acute meningitis? *Journal of the American Medical Association* 282, 175–181.

Bhatt, S.P., Guleria, R., Luqman-Arafath, T.K., Gupta, A.K., Mohan, A., Nanda, S. and Stoltzfus, J.C. (2009) Effect of tripod position on objective parameters of respiratory function in stable chronic obstructive pulmonary disease. *Indian Journal of Chest Diseases and Allied Sciences* 51, 83–85.

Bilavsky, E., Leibovitz, E., Elkon-Tamir, E., Fruchtman, Y., Ifergan, G. and Greenberg, D. (2012) The diagnostic accuracy of the 'classic meningeal signs' in children with suspected bacterial meningitis. *European Journal of Emergency Medicine* doi: 10.1097/MEJ.0b013e3283585f20. Epub ahead of print.

Brown, J.C., Klassen, T. and Wiebe, N.M. (2004) Croup. In: Moyer, V.A., Elliot, E.J., Gilbert, R., Klassen, T., Logan, S., Mellis, C., Henderson-Smart, D. and Williams, K. (eds) *Evidence-based Paediatrics*. BMJ Books, London, pp. 305–318.

Carroll, A.E. and Buddenbaum, J.L. (2007) Malpractice claims involving pediatricians: epidemiology and etiology. *Pediatrics* 120, 10–17.

Carter, J.A., Neville, B.G. and Newton, C.R. (2003) Neuro-cognitive impairment following acquired central nervous system infections in childhood: a systematic review. *Brain Research & Brain Research Reviews* 43, 57–69.

Ceulemans, B., van Rhijn, J., Kenis, S., Krols, R., Laridon, A. and Van Havenbergh, T. (2008) Opisthotonus and intrathecal treatment with baclofen (ITB) in children. *European Journal of Pediatrics* 167, 641–645.

Chauhan, V.V. and Pickens, A.T. (2011) Opisthotonus in neurosyphilis: a case report. *Journal of Emergency Medicine* 41, 613–615.

Curtis, S., Stobart, K., Vandermeer, B., Simel, D.L. and Klassen, T. (2010) Clinical features suggestive of meningitis in children: a systematic review of prospective data. *Pediatrics* 126, 952–960.

Ende, J. and Fosnocht, K.M. (2002) Clinical examination: still a tool for our times? *Transactions of the American Clinical and Climatological Association* 113, 137–150.

Fagen, T.J. (1975) Nomogram for Baye's theorem. *New England Journal of Medicine* 293, 257.

Gill, C.J., Sabin, L. and Schmid, C.H. (2005) Why clinicians are natural bayesians. *British Medical Journal* 330, 1080–1083.

Haden, S.V., McShane, M.A. and Holt, C.M. (2009) Opsoclonus myoclonus: a non-epileptic movement disorder that may present as status epilepticus. *Archives of Disease in Childhood* 94, 897–899.

Hayden, S.R. and Brown, M.D. (1999) Likelihood ratio: a powerful tool for incorporating the results of a diagnostic test into clinical decision making. *Annals of Emergency Medicine* 33, 575–580.

Heckenberg, S.G., de Gans, J., Brouwer, M.C., Weisfelt, M., Piet, J.R., Spanjaard, L., van der Ende, A. and van de Beek, D. (2008) Clinical features, outcome, and meningococcal genotype in 258 adults with meningococcal meningitis: a prospective cohort study. *Medicine (Baltimore)* 87, 185–192.

Hooda, S., Kiran, S., Thapa, D. and Chhabra, B. (1995) Opisthotonus and thiopental. *Anesthesia and Analgesia* 81, 1309–1310.

Kiesler, J. and Ricer, R. (2003) The abnormal fontanel. *American Family Physician* 67, 2547–2552.

King, D.B., Dickinson, J.A., Boulton, M.-R. and Toumpas, C. (2005) Clinical skills textbooks fail evidence-based examination. *Evidence Based Medicine* 10, 131–132.

Laman, M., Manning, L., Greenhill, A.R., Mare, T., Michael, A., Shem, S., Vince, J., Lagani, W., Hwaiwhanje, I., Siba, P.M., Mueller, I. and Davis, T.M. (2012) Predictors of acute bacterial meningitis in children from a malaria-endemic area of Papua New Guinea. *American Journal of Tropical Medicine and Hygiene* 86, 240–245.

Loeffler, J.M., Ringer, R., Hablutzel, M., Tauber, M.G. and Leib, S.L. (2001) The free radical scavenger alpha-phenyl-tert-butyl nitrone aggravates hippocampal apoptosis and learning deficits in experimental pneumococcal meningitis. *Journal of Infectious Diseases* 183, 247–252.

Meates-Dennis, M. (2004) Bronchiolitis. In: Moyer, V.A., Elliot, E.J., Gilbert, R., Klassen, T., Logan, S., Mellis, C., Henderson-Smart, D. and Williams, K. (eds) *Evidence-based Paediatrics.* BMJ Books, London, pp. 319–330.

Mwaniki, M.K., Talbert, A.W., Njuguna, P., English, M., Were, E., Lowe, B.S., Newton, C.R. and Berkley, J.A. (2011) Clinical indicators of bacterial meningitis among neonates and young infants in rural Kenya. *BMC Infectious Diseases* 11, 301.

Nichols, M.M. (1994) The tripod sign and knee kissing in polio. *Hospital Practice (Off Ed)* 29, 12.

Oostenbrink, R., Moons, K.G., Theunissen, C.C., Derksen-Lubsen, G., Grobbee, D.E. and Moll, H.A. (2001) Signs of meningeal irritation at the emergency department: how often bacterial meningitis? *Pediatric Emergency Care* 17, 161–164.

Pomeroy, S.L., Holmes, S.J., Dodge, P.R. and Feigin, R.D. (1990) Seizures and other neurologic sequelae of bacterial meningitis in children. *New England Journal of Medicine* 323, 1651–1657.

Rothman, S.M. and Lee, B.C. (1998) What bulges under a bulging fontanel? *Archives of Pediatrics and Adolescent Medicine* 152, 100–101.

Scheld, W.M., Koedel, U., Nathan, B. and Pfister, H.W. (2002) Pathophysiology of bacterial meningitis: mechanism(s) of neuronal injury. *Journal of Infectious Diseases* 186 Suppl. 2, S225–S233.

Selbst, S.M., Friedman, M.J. and Singh, S.B. (2005) Epidemiology and etiology of malpractice lawsuits involving children in US emergency departments and urgent care centers. *Pediatric Emergency Care* 21, 165–169.

Straus, S.E. (2006) Bridging the gaps in evidence based diagnosis. *British Medical Journal* 333, 405–406.

Suvarna, J.C. and Keskar, V.S. (2009) Tripod sign. *Journal of Postgraduate Medicine* 55, 211–213.

Thomas, K.E., Hasbun, R., Jekel, J. and Quagliarello, V.J. (2002) The diagnostic accuracy of Kernig's sign, Brudzinski's sign, and nuchal rigidity in adults with suspected meningitis. *Clinical Infectious Diseases* 35, 46–52.

Uchihara, T. and Tsukagoshi, H. (1991) Jolt accentuation of headache: the most sensitive sign of CSF pleocytosis. *Headache* 31, 167–171.

Waghdhare, S., Kalantri, A., Joshi, R. and Kalantri, S. (2010) Accuracy of physical signs for detecting meningitis: a hospital-based diagnostic accuracy study. *Clinical Neurology and Neurosurgery* 112, 752–757.

Weber, J.R. and Tuomanen, E.I. (2007) Cellular damage in bacterial meningitis: an interplay of bacterial and host driven toxicity. *Journal of Neuroimmunology* 184, 45–52.

Weisfelt, M., van de Beek, D., Spanjaard, L., Reitsma, J.B. and de Gans, J. (2006a) Clinical features, complications, and outcome in adults with pneumococcal meningitis: a prospective case series. *Lancet Neurology* 5, 123–129.

Weisfelt, M., van de Beek, D., Spanjaard, L., Reitsma, J.B. and de Gans, J. (2006b) Community-acquired bacterial meningitis in older people. *Journal of the American Geriatrics Society* 54, 1500–1507.

Wellons, J.C., Holubkov, R., Browd, S.R., Riva-Cambrin, J., Whitehead, W., Kestle, J. and Kulkarni, A.V. (2013) The assessment of bulging fontanel and splitting of sutures in premature infants: an interrater reliability study by the Hydrocephalus Clinical Research Network. *Journal of Neurosurgery: Pediatrics* 11, 12–14.

Ziai, W.C. and Lewin, J.J. (2008) Update in the diagnosis and management of central nervous system infections. *Neurologic Clinics* 26, 427–468.

4 Viral Meningitis

David N. Irani*
University of Michigan Medical School, Ann Arbor, USA

4.1 Introduction

Viral infections of the human central nervous system (CNS) encompass both acute and chronic conditions caused by over 100 different pathogens (Johnson, 1998). As a group, these diseases exert complex effects on the CNS, and multiple host, viral and environmental factors influence the pathogenesis of individual disorders. In terms of frequency, cases of viral meningitis exceed the total number of meningitis episodes reported each year caused by all other aetiologies combined, and some estimates suggest that unreported cases of viral meningitis exceed reported ones by tenfold. This disorder results from dissemination of viruses to the meningeal coverings and subarachnoid spaces of the CNS. This chapter will review the important clinical features, epidemiology, diagnostic approaches, pathophysiology and management strategies for patients with viral meningitis. Particular emphasis will be placed on the diseases caused by enteroviruses (EVs), which as a group account for the vast majority of all human viral meningitis cases.

4.2 Definitions

The term aseptic meningitis describes a clinical syndrome characterized by meningeal inflammation not caused by an identifiable bacterial pathogen in the cerebrospinal fluid (CSF) (Wallgren, 1951). It also distinguishes a group of disorders that do not typically cause notable parenchymal involvement of the brain (encephalitis) or spinal cord (myelitis). Implicit to the definition of aseptic meningitis is a somewhat more benign clinical course compared with either bacterial meningitis or the hybrid syndromes of meningoencephalitis or encephalomyelitis. As might be anticipated, however, sufficient clinical overlap exists among the infectious causes of aseptic meningitis, meningoencephalitis and encephalomyelitis to require that all potential aetiological agents be considered in an individual patient. It is also worth remembering that aseptic meningitis can occur in the setting of underlying systemic disorders such as connective tissue diseases or via cancer metastasis to the meninges, and it can appear as a reaction that follows certain drug

*davidira@med.umich.edu

administrations. This necessitates a thorough search for non-infectious aetiologies as well (Irani, 2008). The aseptic meningitis syndrome will be reviewed here, with particular emphasis on viral causes of this disorder.

4.3 Clinical Features

Clinical features that develop in patients with viral meningitis can vary widely with the age and underlying immune status of the host, while disease severity can range from an asymptomatic CSF pleocytosis to an illness causing an alarming degree of neurological impairment. Despite this heterogeneity, however, most adult patients with aseptic meningitis present with fever accompanied by complaints of headache, neck stiffness, malaise, anorexia and vomiting. The disorder is more heterogeneous in paediatric populations; CNS involvement in neonates may or may not be evidenced by overt signs of meningeal inflammation (nuchal rigidity, bulging of the anterior fontanelle). Furthermore, neonatal EV infections can show prominent systemic involvement in the form of hepatic necrosis, myocarditis and even necrotizing enterocolitis (Rotbart, 2000). Indeed, such multi-organ failure may closely resemble overwhelming bacterial sepsis. The CNS disease caused by EVs in older newborns commonly progresses to a more overt encephalitic picture with the appearance of seizures and focal neurological deficits. Death in this setting, however, is still more likely to occur as the result of hepatic or cardiac failure (Abzug *et al.*, 1993; Rotbart, 2000). The morbidity and mortality that accompany perinatal EV infections can be as high as 70% and 10%, respectively (Modlin, 1986; Abzug *et al.*, 1993; Abzug, 1995; Rotbart, 2000).

In older infants and children, EV meningitis is rarely fatal but may still be complicated by significant short-term morbidity and a prolonged convalescence. These patients present with the abrupt onset of fever to 38–40°C; temperature curves are often biphasic with the first peak accompanying systemic constitutional symptoms and the second one appearing with the onset of meningeal signs (Wilfert *et al.*, 1983; Rotbart, 2000). If old enough to report them, affected children complain of headache, photophobia and myalgias, and many also experience vomiting, diarrhoea, cough, sore throat and rash (Wilfert *et al.*, 1983; Rotbart, 2000). Some EV serotypes also produce distinctive clinical stigmata – during a large EV-71 outbreak in Taiwan, young patients developed a characteristic hand, foot and mouth disease with vesicular lesions erupting over these body regions (Ho *et al.*, 1999). Febrile seizures may accompany EV meningitis in children without other evidence of parenchymal CNS involvement, and the syndrome of inappropriate antidiuretic hormone (SIADH) secretion can occasionally be seen (Chemtob *et al.*, 1985). Such infections are often symptomatic for more than a week, thereby causing significant economic impact on their care providers (Pichichero *et al.*, 1998). Full recovery eventually ensues in the vast majority of patients, and despite lingering suspicions otherwise, there is no convincing evidence that EV meningitis leads to any subsequent neurodevelopmental abnormalities (Rorabaugh *et al.*, 1992). One exception to this rule occurs in young patients with congenital hypo- or agammaglobulinaemia; defects in the antibody-dependent mechanisms critical for EV clearance from the CNS lead to a chronic meningitis or meningoencephalitis that can be fatal (McKinney *et al.*, 1987). Paediatric survivors of chronic EV infections can develop superimposed rheumatological disorders, commonly in the form of dermatomyositis, hypothesized to result from lingering extracerebral tissue infection (McKinney *et al.*, 1987).

Older infants and children are also susceptible to other forms of viral meningitis beyond those caused by EVs, albeit at much lower rates. The mosquito-borne flaviviruses and bunyaviruses (especially St Louis encephalitis virus (SLEV) and La Crosse virus), mumps virus (either with or without an accompanying parotitis) and various members of the herpesvirus family (herpes simplex virus (HSV)-1 and -2, varicella-zoster virus (VZV) and human herpesvirus type 6 (HHV-6)) all can cause meningitis in this age group. In most cases, a distinguishing clinical feature that identifies a particular pathogen is not observed, and a specific diagnosis rests heavily on epidemiological and laboratory data. Occasionally, a highly distinctive rash (VZV) or the occurrence of parotitis (mumps) can render a specific diagnosis clear. While cases of encephalitis caused by all of these pathogens can produce adverse outcomes, the aseptic meningitis they induce is typically self-limited and followed by full recovery in the majority of patients (Rotbart, 2000).

Adults with EV meningitis may have symptoms that persist for several weeks, although the overall severity of these illnesses tends to be somewhat lower than in children (Rotbart, 1997; Rotbart *et al.*, 1998). Other forms of viral meningitis in adults are, for the most part, similarly benign. Primary genital infections caused by HSV-2 are accompanied by meningitis in more than a third of women and 11% of men (Corey *et al.*, 1983), although many cases of both HSV-1 and HSV-2 meningitis occur without any history of recent genital lesions (Hartford *et al.*, 1975; Schlesinger *et al.*, 1995). These two pathogens must also be kept in mind in adults with recurrent episodes of aseptic meningitis; so-called Molleret's meningitis has been linked using polymerase chain reaction (PCR) with HSV, particularly HSV-2, in the absence of signs or symptoms of concurrent genital infection (Tedder *et al.*, 1994). In the clinical setting of aseptic meningitis accompanied by acute weakness of the extremities occurring in the summer or autumn months, West Nile virus (WNV) has become the modern-day paralytic poliomyelitis and is the most common infectious cause of acute flaccid paralysis in the western hemisphere (Davis *et al.*, 2006). This diagnosis must be considered in any patient with a CSF pleocytosis and clinical or electrophysiological findings consistent with lower motor neuron involvement.

4.4 Epidemiology

Because more than 90% of all viral meningitis cases are caused by EVs, patterns associated with the occurrence of this syndrome at a population level are driven largely by the epidemiology of these pathogens. Overall, EVs occur worldwide (Melnick, 1996), although only a handful of specific serotypes predominate in particular parts of the world in any given year (Strikas *et al.*, 1986). Humans are their only natural reservoir, and the viruses are transmitted primarily by faecal–oral contamination and less commonly in respiratory secretions (Melnick, 1996). As such, EVs exhibit a summer-to-autumn seasonality in temperate climates and a high year-round incidence in tropical and subtropical areas (ostensibly due to sparse clothing and lower hygiene standards among children in these environments) (Fig. 4.1). Indeed, while EVs are still the most common cause of viral meningitis in adults (Rotbart *et al.*, 1998), the majority of cases occur in children under the age of 5 years (Modlin, 1986; Abzug *et al.*, 1993; Melnick, 1996; Rotbart, 2000). In the USA, the 15 or so most common serotypes that cause disease cycle with varying periodicity, probably reflecting the birth of new susceptible hosts (i.e. non-immune children) within a given community (Strikas *et al.*, 1986). Occasional outbreaks in adults are caused by those serotypes not present within a community for some time, again because a pool of susceptible hosts without pre-existing immunity needs a longer time to develop (Kinnunen *et al.*, 1987). Among the many EV serotypes that cycle from year to year, certain ones are more strongly associated with the development of aseptic meningitis than others.

Many non-EV cases of viral meningitis also demonstrate seasonality, even as much less common causes of this syndrome. For vector-borne pathogens such as SLEV, WNV and La Crosse virus, the resultant disease occurs predominantly during the summer and autumn months in geographical regions where infected mosquitoes are abundant. Often only a small proportion (< 5%) of these arthropod-borne infections actually produce symptoms, and even when they do, febrile illness may or may not be accompanied by signs of meningitis. SLEV was first identified in the midwestern USA, but it is now recognized to cause disease throughout Central and North America. Symptomatic infections caused by this pathogen are more meningitic in children but tend to be more encephalitic in older patients (Tsai *et al.*,

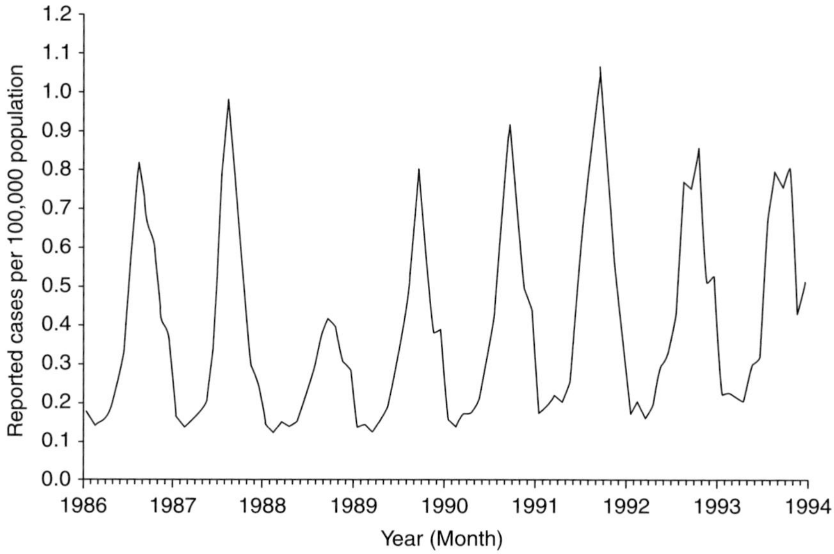

Fig. 4.1. The seasonal occurrence of aseptic meningitis in the USA from 1986 to 1994, as reported to the Centers for Disease Control and Prevention. The striking peak of cases during the summer and early autumn months in each year reflects the predominance of EV as the main aetiologic agent of this disorder (Centers for Disease Control and Prevention, 1994).

1988). Paradoxically, exposure to infected vectors among all age groups can occur indoors as often as outdoors, and open windows are a known predisposing factor (Tsai *et al.*, 1988). For WNV, neuroinvasive disease occurs in only 1–2% of all infections, but nearly half of these cases (more than 20,000 since 1999) are manifest primarily as aseptic meningitis clustering from March through to October (Davis *et al.*, 2006). Each year since 1999 has brought clusters of WNV cases to different regions of the USA, Canada and Mexico. La Crosse virus is endemic in forested regions of the USA, especially around the Great Lakes, and mostly causes aseptic meningitis in children (Rotbart, 2000; Irani, 2008).

Mumps virus is transmitted via respiratory secretions, and clinical infections predominate in the winter and early spring months when person-to-person transmissions are most common. With the widespread use of the attenuated live-virus vaccine, however, mumps has gone from being one of the most common identifiable causes of meningitis to being only rarely diagnosed in the USA today (Centers for Disease Control and Prevention, 1989). When it occurs, symptomatic mumps infection is twice as frequent in males as it is in females, and neurological involvement is three times more common in the male population (Rotbart, 2000; Irani, 2008). These unusual gender differences in the pathogenesis of mumps infection have never been adequately explained.

4.5 Differential Diagnosis

Patients who develop the syndrome of acute aseptic meningitis may or may not actually have an underlying infectious illness. Of primary importance is the exclusion of partially treated bacterial meningitis that can occur in the setting of preceding antibiotic exposure and that requires further antibiotic therapy. Other bacteria such as *Mycoplasma*, spirochaetes (*Borrelia*, *Treponema* and *Leptospira*), *Mycobacteria* and *Brucella*, along with various fungi, can occasionally present as acute aseptic meningitis. Non-infectious aetiologies are rare, but include certain drugs (especially non-steroidal anti-inflammatory drugs (NSAIDs) and intravenous immunoglobulin (IVIg)), vaccines, systemic illnesses including connective-tissue disorders (notably systemic lupus erythematosus), vasculitides (such as Kawasaki disease), granulomatous conditions (mostly sarcoidosis), neoplasms that have spread to the meninges and, rarely, migraine. The broad differential diagnosis of the acute aseptic meningitis syndrome as it segregates based on the relative frequency of each disorder among the general population is outlined in Table 4.1.

4.6 Pathophysiology and Pathogenesis

Viruses that cause meningitis spread to the CNS via extracerebral routes. For EVs, it is likely that the initial inoculum is swallowed and passes into the lower intestinal tract where it infects enterocytes (Rotbart, 1997, 1999). The virus then traverses the intestinal wall and moves into gut-associated lymphoid tissue such as Peyer's patches where primary replication occurs. A viraemia ensues, and multiple tissues (liver, lungs, heart, CNS) can be seeded (Rotbart, 1997, 1999). Even if the meninges do not become infected at this stage, further replication at these extracerebral sites can produce a second viraemia that then causes neurological involvement (Rotbart, 1997, 1999). The pathogenesis of routine EV infections within the CNS is not very well understood because pathological data are scarce and fatal cases invariably reflect a more severe encephalitic syndrome rather than more typical meningitis. Still, a single case of a child who died of coxsackievirus B5 myocarditis and who also had meningitis has been reported; here, prominent inflammation of the choroid plexus and ependymal lining of the ventricles was described (Price *et al.*, 1970). Fibrotic changes in the basal leptomeninges were also seen, but there was limited direct parenchymal involvement by the pathogen (Price *et al.*, 1970).

For the vector-borne viruses, local subcutaneous replication after virus inoculation leads to regional lymph node spread, viraemia and dissemination to the CNS via a haematogenous route (Johnson, 1998). In some cases, prominent infection of olfactory

Table 4.1. Causes of the aseptic meningitis syndrome segregated based on their relative frequency in the general population.

Common	Uncommon	Rare
Viruses	Viruses	Viruses
Enteroviruses, arboviruses[a,b], HSV-2	Mumps, lymphocytic choriomeningitis virus, human immunodeficiency virus, HHV-6	HSV-1, VZV, cytomegalovirus, Epstein–Barr virus, measles, influenza viruses A and B, parvovirus B19
Bacteria	Bacteria	
Borrelia burgdorferi[b]	*Mycobacterium tuberculosis*	
Partially-treated bacterial meningitis (common agents)	*Leptospira* spp.[b]	
Mycoplasma pneumoniae		
Parameningeal bacterial infection (sinusitis, otitis, mastoiditis)		
	Other	Other
	Fungi[b]	*Brucella* spp., fungi, autoimmune diseases (Lupus, Sjögren's), drugs (NSAIDs, IVIg), malignancy, vasculitis (Kawasaki)

[a]Arthropod-borne viruses (including alphaviruses, flaviviruses, bunyaviruses and reoviruses).
[b]Incidence varies significantly with geographical region.

neurons suggests that CNS entry can occasionally be achieved via inhalation and passage across the cribriform plate (Monath *et al.*, 1983). Mumps is contracted via respiratory secretions and the virus replicates initially in the upper respiratory epithelium. Local invasion causes the prototypical parotitis, but viraemia and CNS spread can occur in the absence of overt parotid involvement (Kilham, 1949). The passage of infected mononuclear cells across the choroid plexus into the CSF is believed to result in meningoencephalitis (Wolinsky *et al.*, 1976). With lymphocytic choriomeningitis virus (LCMV), an arenavirus previously known to be a major cause of aseptic meningitis, human transmissions occur via inhalation or ingestion of contaminated rodent urine and faeces (Peters *et al.*, 1996). Spread to the CNS follows replication in the lungs and hilar lymph nodes, probably via the bloodstream (Peters *et al.*, 1996). Aseptic meningitis due to infections caused by the herpesviruses can occur with either primary or reactivated infection; both haematogenous and intraneuronal routes of CNS dissemination are described (Roizman, 1996).

Animal models have been used for a number of years to study the pathogenesis of viral meningitis. Although human EVs can be inoculated into primates, LCMV infection of mice has served as the premier animal model of viral meningitis and has been the foundation of seminal contributions to the fields of both virology and immunology. Direct intracerebral inoculation of LCMV into adult immunocompetent mice results in the development of an acute, uniformly fatal choriomeningitis over the next 6–8 days (Kang and McGavern, 2008). In this setting, virus localizes to the choroid plexus, ependyma and meningeal coverings of the brain, with little found in the CNS parenchyma itself. Because LCMV is a non-cytopathic virus, the damage induced by infection resulting in death of the host is not a direct result of the pathogen itself but rather is caused by the host immune response. Detailed neuropathological studies have shown extensive inflammatory cell infiltration of the meningeal and ventricular regions of the brain, closely corresponding to the site of viral localization (Mims, 1960; Schwendemann *et al.*, 1983). A brisk virus-specific CD8+ T-cell response is mounted in the periphery of infected animals within a few days of virus challenge (Lynch *et al.*, 1989); these T-cells then accumulate in the CSF (Zinkernagel and Doherty, 1973; Ceredig *et al.*, 1987), and numerous studies have demonstrated that they are essential for the development of lethal choriomeningitis (Baenziger *et al.*, 1986; Leist *et al.*, 1987; Fung-Leung *et al.*, 1991; Oldstone *et al.*, 1999). Beyond viral pathogenesis, the LCMV infection model has been used to study the molecular mechanisms of CD8+ T-cell trafficking to the CNS and CD8+ T-cell effector function within the brain (Kang and McGavern, 2008). From a historical perspective, the central immunological principle of major histocompatibility restriction was first demonstrated by Zinkernagel and Doherty (1973) in the LCMV infection model – a finding for which they were subsequently awarded the Nobel Prize.

4.7 Common Aetiological Agents

4.7.1 Enteroviruses

The EVs constitute more than 60 viral serotypes within the picornavirus family; they are subdivided into the polioviruses, the coxsackieviruses, the echoviruses and the newer 'numbered' EVs. Although genetic variability in the coding region of the capsid protein produces the many serotypes, all EV virions consist of a small icosahedral capsid that surrounds a single strand of positive-sense RNA (Melnick, 1996). Most picornaviruses use cell-surface molecules belonging to the immunoglobulin superfamily to bind to cells; canyon-like features on the surfaces of virus particles allow them to destabilize and initiate the uncoating process, whereby the viral genome is directly released into the target cell cytoplasm (Rossmann *et al.*, 2002). A single polyprotein is then translated directly from this RNA strand, and its rapid cleavage produces individual products that regulate viral RNA transcription and others that create new capsids (Melnick, 1996). Viral replication rapidly shuts down host cell protein synthesis, and the cell becomes a factory for new viral production. Finally, direct lysis causes the release of infectious virions that spread quickly to adjacent cells. Current therapeutic strategies against EVs largely have focused on the development of low molecular weight substances or soluble receptor analogues that bind to the viral capsid and inhibit its uptake by target cells (Fechner *et al.*, 2011).

4.7.2 Flaviviruses

SLEV and WNV are two of 69 known flaviviruses. These pathogens are also small, enveloped viruses containing a spherical ribonucleoprotein core that surrounds a single-stranded, positive-sense RNA genome. A membrane and an envelope protein are present in the outer lipid envelope of the virion; variability in the latter distinguishes the many viral subtypes, and epitopes therein are the main targets of host immunity. Although virions are inactivated by high temperature, ultraviolet light, gamma irradiation and various disinfectants, virus-containing aerosols are stable at room temperature for up to 6 h, making this route of transmission conceivable in certain settings (Monath and Heinz, 1996). Cells infected *in vitro* demonstrate reduced macromolecular synthesis late in the replication process, around the time when cytopathic effects appear. Only some of these viruses are neurotropic *in vivo*, while others infect visceral organs and cause fatal haemorrhagic fevers. Mechanisms of neuroinvasion remain poorly understood; haematogenous dissemination to the olfactory bulb as well as retrograde axonal transport up peripheral nerve tracts have both been proposed (Hollidge *et al.*, 2010).

4.7.3 Mumps

Mumps virus is a paramyxovirus that exists as a single serotype. Its virions are larger enveloped structures that contain a ribonucleoprotein core with a single strand of negative-sense RNA. Proteins associated with the core assist with genomic replication and maintenance of the core structure. Two surface glycoproteins mediate neuraminidase, haemagglutination and fusion functions that allow virus adsorption to host cells and penetration of the genome into the cytoplasm. Mumps RNA replication occurs via the production of a positive-strand intermediate, which serves as both the template for negative-sense RNA replication as well as mRNA for protein translation (Wolinsky, 1996). After infection via respiratory droplets, the virus replicates in the upper respiratory epithelium. Local invasion of the parotid gland is common at this point but is not required for more widespread dissemination. Based on findings reported in a hamster model, infection of circulating mononuclear cells is probably responsible for CNS dissemination and meningitis (Wolinsky *et al.*, 1976).

4.7.4 Herpesviruses

Herpesviruses are large, enveloped viruses with an icosadeltahedral capsid that surrounds a complex, double-stranded DNA genome. Eight of the nearly 100 known herpesviruses cause observable disease in humans, either as primary infections or by means of reactivation. Virus assembly takes place in the nucleus, and the replication of progeny virus invariably destroys the infected target cell. While some human herpesviruses (HSV-1, HSV-2) infect a wide range of host cells *in vivo*, others (Epstein-Barr virus (EBV), HHV-6) are much more restricted in their cellular targets (Roizman, 1996). Latency is another property of herpesviruses that influences the type of disease these pathogens can produce, and the nervous system is a common site of this event. As such, neurological involvement may or may not be accompanied by signs of systemic infection. Invasion of the CNS from the periphery can occur either by haematogenous dissemination or via retrograde axonal transport (Roizman, 1996).

4.7.5 Non-viral pathogens

More fastidious bacteria as well as various fungi usually cause chronic meningitis, but CNS involvement by these pathogens can occasionally present as an acute illness. A specific microbiological diagnosis can be difficult in this setting owing to a lack of reliable culture methods and/or the very slow growth of these organisms. PCR assays applicable to CSF are being investigated for some of these pathogens (*Mycobacterium tuberculosis, Borrelia burgdorferi*), but none has achieved routine clinical use at present. However, many patients with these infections will have extracerebral foci of involvement at the same time as their meningitis, and a search for systemic involvement is often warranted. Even if such a diagnostic approach does not confirm one of these infections, it can sometimes uncover a previously undocumented malignancy or granulomatous disease that could explain the CNS symptoms.

4.7.6 Non-infectious aetiologies

Aseptic meningitis can occur in 2–4% of patients with systemic lupus erythematosus, usually as part of the ongoing disease evolution but rarely as an initial manifestation of the disorder (Johnson and Richardson, 1968). Leptomeningeal metastasis has been estimated to occur in up to 5% of all patients with cancer, and, unlike those with solid tumours, patients with leukaemias or lymphomas can develop neoplastic meningitis without any evidence of systemic disease, during periods of remission and even rarely at the time of clinical presentation (Chamberlain *et al.*, 2005). An occasional patient taking NSAIDs may develop aseptic meningitis without any other underlying explanatory cause, and a handful of individuals have developed this syndrome in the setting of pre-existing IVIg infusions. Here, most symptoms occur within 24 h of completing an infusion, may recur with reinfusion and always recover spontaneously in less than a week after their onset (Hamrock, 2006).

4.8 Diagnostic Approach

A diagnosis of aseptic meningitis begins with the identification of a CSF pleocytosis (either mononuclear or polymorphonuclear cell predominant) in a patient with the appropriate clinical features. Bacterial smears and cultures of the CSF are uniformly negative. Variability from patient to patient in the total CSF cell count (usually 100–1000 cells/mm^3), protein concentration (usually normal to mildly elevated) and glucose level (usually normal to slightly depressed) is the norm, even during confirmed outbreaks caused by a single viral serotype (Rotbart, 2000; Greenberg, 2009). Much effort has gone into the development of predictive algorithms to analyse routine CSF parameters in the setting of acute meningitis, but they retain little practical significance for use at the bedside. Indeed, the difficulty distinguishing between aseptic and partially treated bacterial meningitis on clinical and routine laboratory grounds alone means that most patients should be treated for the latter disorder, until an alternative cause is uncovered or the patient demonstrates significant clinical improvement.

For EV meningitis, a specific diagnosis traditionally has depended on recovery of virus from the CSF using cell culture techniques. Studies conducted in the pre-PCR era for all patients with aseptic meningitis identified a specific viral pathogen in 55–70% of cases, and they consistently confirmed that EVs were the predominant virus isolated using various culture methodologies (Table 4.2). Still, the mean interval to a positive viral culture can range from 3.7 to 8.2 days (Rotbart, 1999), often well after a final CSF bacterial culture result has been available and clinical outcome has been determined, making the practical clinical significance of these techniques unclear. Application of PCR methods to the analysis of CSF samples has resulted in higher rates of EV isolation in much shorter periods of time; more than two-thirds of what turn out to be culture-negative specimens are positive for an EV using these techniques, with turnaround times of less than 1 day (Sawyer *et al.*, 1994). This means that EVs now account for 85–90% of all cases

Table 4.2. Viral causes of aseptic meningitis as reported in selected case series.

		Viruses identified (%)								
Years	Cases	P	NPE	Arbo	Mumps	HSV	LCMV	Other[a]	None	References
1941–1946	374				15.3		11.2	No	73.5	Rasmussen (1946)
1947–1952	480				13.3	5.3	9.7	No	74.8	Adair *et al.* (1953)
1953–1958	430	8.8	29.8	0.7	15.8	1.4	8.8	No	29.0	Meyer *et al.* (1960)
1955–1958	407	7.0	41.0		8.0			No	46.0	Lepow *et al.* (1962)
1958–1959	368	2.0	57.0		9.0	1.0		Yes	31.0	Lennette *et al.* (1962)
1958–1963	374	4.8	38.5	0.8	7.5	0.5	1.9	Yes	43.5	Buescher *et al.* (1968)
1972–1979	2382	0.5	24.0	1.4	1.2	2.7	0.5	Yes	68.3	Deibel *et al.* (1974, 1975, 1977); Deibel and Flanagan (1979); Flanagan and Deibel (1981)
1986–1990	274	0.007	61.3					Yes	38.4	Berlin *et al.* (1993)

P, polioviruses; NPE, non-polio enteroviruses; Arbo, arthropod-borne viruses.
[a]Rare cases of adenovirus, measles virus, EBV, influenza A virus, cytomegalovirus, VZV, rubella virus, influenza B virus, parainfluenza type 3 virus, respiratory syncytial virus.

of aseptic meningitis where an aetiological agent is identified (Rotbart, 2000). On the other hand, EVs have been found by PCR in only about one-half of CSF samples tested in large retrospective cohorts (Lee *et al.*, 2006; Michos *et al.*, 2007), raising some question about whether hospital laboratories should routinely use EV PCR for the evaluation of aseptic meningitis and at what frequency the assay should be performed. In one series, patients with positive CSF EV PCR results had shorter durations of antibiotic coverage and hospitalization compared with patients with negative results or for whom the PCR assay was not performed (Michos *et al.*, 2007). Prospective studies are needed to determine the optimal cost–benefit strategy for diagnostic testing in patients with aseptic meningitis.

4.9 Management

Management of patients with acute aseptic meningitis is largely supportive in nature. Appropriate interventions include aggressive fluid, electrolyte and pain management, as well as close observation for potential neurological and neuroendocrine sequelae (seizures, brain oedema, SIADH secretion). Antiviral therapies active against many of the causative agents underlying viral meningitis either do not exist (arthropod-borne viruses, mumps virus, LCMV) or have not been convincingly shown to accelerate recovery in clinical trials (herpesviruses) (Landry *et al.*, 2009). This latter point must not, however, be confused with the established benefit of acyclovir in patients with herpes simplex encephalitis. Two therapies recently used against EVs are immune serum globulin (ISG) and pleconaril, the latter being a newly developed anti-picornaviral agent. Both have relatively limited data behind their use: ISG has been given therapeutically in neonates and prophylactically in immunocompromised hosts, while pleconaril has been studied in only a few placebo-controlled trials. In neonates with systemic EV infection, one study showed that ISG treatment produced lower serum viral titres, but it was too small to demonstrate any clinical benefit to this approach (Abzug *et al.*, 1995). In agammaglobulinaemic adults given regular doses of ISG, the incidence of chronic EV meningoencephalitis appears to have fallen, and the course of such infections in these patients may be attenuated (Webster *et al.*, 1993). The therapeutic benefit of such treatment in established cases of chronic EV meningoencephalitis has also been anecdotally reported (Rotbart, 2000).

Pleconaril binds to the viral capsid, presumably blocking EV attachment to cellular receptors and inhibiting the viral uncoating process. The drug has broad-spectrum anti-EV activity *in vitro* and high oral bioavailability *in vivo* (Rotbart, 2000). Unfortunately, despite promising initial results, the drug was recently found to have no detectable clinical or virological benefit in infants with EV meningitis compared with placebo (Abzug *et al.*, 2003). In two randomized studies with more 600 combined patients, pleconaril only modestly shortened the course of the illness in a subgroup of adults with EV meningitis who experienced more severe symptoms and who were treated early in disease (Desmond *et al.*, 2006). Applications for federal approval of the drug have not yet been accepted based on these data, and it remains unclear what future the drug has in these diseases.

4.10 Conclusions

Aseptic meningitis is frequently caused by the spread of a viral pathogen to the meninges and subarachnoid space, and this syndrome remains the most common manifestation of CNS viral infection. EV infections of the CNS underlie most cases of viral meningitis, although it can have other viral, non-viral infectious and non-infectious aetiologies as well. Patients with acute aseptic meningitis typically have a favourable long-term clinical outcome. Therapies for these disorders are still in their infancy, but as pathogenesis studies in animal models unravel disease mechanisms, novel treatment interventions are expected to follow. In this regard, it seems conceivable that both the pathogens themselves as well as the host responses elicited by these infections may be future drug targets.

References

Abzug, M.J. (1995) Perinatal enterovirus infections. In: Rotbart, H.A. (ed.) *Human Enterovirus Infections.* ASM Press, Washingon, DC, pp. 221–238.

Abzug, M.J., Levin, M.J. and Rotbart, H.A. (1993) Profile of enterovirus disease in the first two weeks of life. *Pediatric Infectious Disease Journal* 12, 820–824.

Abzug, M.J., Kevserling, H.L., Lee, M.L., Levin, M.J. and Rotbart, H.A. (1995) Neonatal enterovirus infection: virology, serology, and effects of intravenous immune globulin. *Clinical Infectious Diseases* 20, 1201–1206.

Abzug, M.J., *et al.* (2003) Double blind placebo-controlled trial of pleconaril in infants with enteroviral meningitis. *Pediatric Infectious Disease Journal* 22, 335–341.

Adair, C.V., Gauld, R.L. and Smadel, J.E. (1953) Aseptic meningitis, a disease of diverse etiology: clinical and etiologic studies on 854 cases. *Annals of Internal Medicine* 39, 675–704.

Baenziger, J., Hengartner, H., Zinkernagel, R.M. and Cole, A. (1986) Induction or prevention of immunopathological disease by cloned cytotoxic T cell lines specific for lymphocytic choriomeningitis virus. *European Journal of Immunology* 16, 387–393.

Berlin, L.E., Rorabaugh, M.L., Heldrich, F., Roberts, K., Doran, T. and Modlin, J.F. (1993) Aseptic meningitis in infants <2 years of age: diagnosis and etiology. *Journal of Infectious Diseases* 168, 888–892.

Buescher, E.L., Artenstein, M.S. and Olson, L.C. (1968) Central nervous system infections of viral etiology: the changing pattern. *Research Publications – Association for Research in Nervous and Mental Disease* 44, 147–163.

Centers for Disease Control and Prevention (1989) Mumps: United States, 1985–1988. *Morbidity and Mortality Weekly Report* 38, 101–105.

Centers for Disease Control and Prevention (1994) Summary of notifiable diseases, United States, 1993. *Morbidity and Mortality Weekly Report* 42, 1–73.

Ceredig, R., Allan, J.E., Tabi, Z., Lynch, F. and Doherty, P.C. (1987) Phenotypic analysis of the inflammatory exudate in murine lymphocytic choriomeningitis. *Journal of Experimental Medicine* 165, 1539–1551.

Chamberlain, M.C., Nolan, C. and Abrey, L.E. (2005) Leukemic and lymphomatous meningitis: incidence, prognosis, and treatment. *Journal of Neuro-Oncology* 75, 71–83.

Chemtob, S., Reece, E.R. and Mills, E.L. (1985) Syndrome of inappropriate secretion of antidiuretic hormone in enteroviral meningitis. *American Journal of Diseases of Children* 139, 292–294.

Corey, L., Adams, H.G., Brown, Z.A. and Holmes, K.K. (1983) Genital herpes simplex virus infections: clinical manifestations, course, and complications. *Annals of Internal Medicine* 98, 958–972.

Davis, L.E., DeBiasi, R., Goade, D.E., Haaland, K.Y., Harrington, J.A., Harnar, J.B., Pergam, S.A., King, M.K., DeMasters, B.K. and Tyler, K.L. (2006) West Nile virus neuroinvasive disease. *Annals of Neurology* 60, 286–300.

Deibel, R. and Flanagan, T.D. (1979) Central nervous system infections: etiologic and epidemiologic observations in New York State, 1976–1977. *New York State Journal of Medicine* 79, 689–695.

Deibel, R., Barron, A., Millian, S. and Smith, V. (1974) Central nervous system infections in New York State: etiologic and epidemiologic observations, 1972. *New York State Journal of Medicine* 74, 1929–1935.

Deibel, R., Flanagan, T.D. and Smith, V. (1975) Central nervous system infections in New York State: etiologic and epidemiologic observations, 1974. *New York State Journal of Medicine* 75, 2337–2342.

Deibel, R., Flanagan, T.D. and Smith, V. (1977) Central nervous system infections in New York State: etiologic and epidemiologic observations, 1975. *New York State Journal of Medicine* 77, 1398–1404.

Desmond, R.A., Accortt, N.A., Talley, L., Villano, S.A., Soong, S.J. and Whitley, R.J. (2006) Enteroviral meningitis: natural history and outcome of pleconaril therapy. *Antimicrobial Agents and Chemotherapy* 50, 2409–2414.

Fechner, H., Pinkert, S., Geisler, A., Poller, W. and Kurreck, J. (2011) Pharmacological and biological antiviral therapeutics for coxsackievirus infections. *Molecules* 16, 8475–8503.

Flanagan, T.D. and Deibel, R. (1981) Central nervous system infections: etiologic and epidemiologic observations in New York State, 1978–1979. *New York State Journal of Medicine* 81, 346–353.

Fung-Leung, W.P., Kundig, T.M., Zinkernagel, R.M. and Mak, T.W. (1991) Immune response against lymphocytic choriomeningitis virus infection in mice without CD8 expression. *Journal of Experimental Medicine* 174, 1425–1429.

Greenberg, B.M. (2009) Viral infections. In: Irani, D.N. (ed.) *Cerebrospinal Fluid in Clinical Practice.* Saunders Elsevier, Philadelphia, PA, pp. 177–189.

Hamrock, D.J. (2006) Adverse events associated with intravenous immunoglobulin therapy. *International Immunopharmacology* 6, 535–542.

Hartford, C.G., Wellinghoff, W. and Weinstein, R.A. (1975) Isolation of herpes simplex virus from the cerebrospinal fluid in viral meningitis. *Neurology (Minneapolis)* 25, 198–200.

Ho, M., Chen, E.-R., Hsu, K.-H., Twu, S.J., Chen, K.T., Tsai, S.F., Wang, J.R. and Shih, S.R. (1999) An epidemic of enterovirus 71 infection in Taiwan. *New England Journal of Medicine* 341, 929–935.

Hollidge, B.S., Gonzalez-Scarano, F. and Soldan, S.S. (2010) Arboviral encephalitides: transmission, emergence, and pathogenesis. *Journal of Neuroimmune Pharmacology* 5, 428–442.

Irani, D.N. (2008) Aseptic meningitis and viral myelitis. *Neurologic Clinics* 26, 635–655.

Johnson, R.T. (1998) *Viral Infections of the Nervous System,* 2nd edn. Lippincott-Raven Publishers, Philadelphia, PA.

Johnson, R.T. and Richardson, E.P. (1968) The neurological manifestations of systemic lupus erythematosus. *Medicine* 47, 337–369.

Kang, S.S. and McGavern, D.B. (2008) Lymphocytic choriomeningitis infection of the central nervous system. *Frontiers in Bioscience* 13, 4529–4543.

Kilham, L. (1949) Mumps meningoencephalitis with and without parotitis. *American Journal of Diseases of Children* 78, 324–333.

Kinnunen, E., Hovi, T., Stenvik, M., Hellstrom, O., Porras, J., Kleemola, M. and Kantanen, M.C. (1987) Localized outbreak of enteroviral meningitis in adults. *Acta Neurologica Scandinavica* 75, 346–351.

Landry, M.L., Greenwold, J. and Vikram, H.R. (2009) Herpes simplex type-2 meningitis: presentation and lack of standardized therapy. *American Journal of Medicine* 122, 688–691.

Lee, B.E., *et al.* (2006) Pediatric Investigators Collaborative Network on Infections in Canada (PICNIC) study of aseptic meningitis. *BMC Infectious Diseases* 6, 68–75.

Leist, T.P., Cobbold, S.P., Waldmann, H., Aguet, M. and Zinkernagel, R.M. (1987) Functional analysis of the T lymphocyte subsets in antiviral host defense. *Journal of Immunology* 138, 2278–2281.

Lennette, E.H., Magoffin, R.L. and Knouf, E.G. (1962) Viral central nervous system disease: an etiologic study conducted at the Los Angeles County General Hospital. *Journal of the American Medical Association* 179, 687–695.

Lepow, M.L., Coyne, N., Thompson, L.B., Carver, D.H. and Robbins, F.C. (1962) A clinical, epidemiologic and laboratory study of aseptic meningitis during the four-year period, 1955–1958: II. The clinical disease and its sequelae. *New England Journal of Medicine* 266, 1188–1193.

Lynch, F., Doherty, P.C. and Ceredig, R. (1989) Phenotypic and functional analysis of the cellular response in regional lymphoid tissue during acute virus infection. *Journal of Immunology* 142, 3592–3598.

McKinney, R.E., Katz, S.L. and Wilfert, C.M. (1987) Chronic enteroviral meningoencephalitis in agammaglobulinemic patients. *Reviews of Infectious Diseases* 9, 334–356.

Melnick, J.L. (1996) Enteroviruses: polioviruses, coxsackieviruses, echoviruses, and newer enteroviruses. In: Fields, B.N., Knipe, D.M. and Howley, P.M. (eds) *Fields Virology*, 3rd edn. Lippincott-Raven Press, New York, pp. 655–712.

Meyer, H.M. Jr, Johnson, R.T., Crawford, I.P., Dascomb, H.E. and Rogers, N.G. (1960) Central nervous syndromes of "viral" etiology. *American Journal of Medicine* 29, 334–347.

Michos, A.G., Syriopoulou, V.P., Hadjichristodoulou, C., Daikos, G.L., Lagona, E., Douridas, P., Mostrou, G. and Theodoridou, M. (2007) Aseptic meningitis in children: analysis of 506 cases. *PLoS ONE* 2, e674.

Mims, C.A. (1960) Intracerebral injections and the growth of viruses in the mouse brain. *British Journal of Experimental Pathology* 41, 52–59.

Modlin, J.F. (1986) Perinatal echovirus infection: insights from a literature review of 61 cases of serious infection and 16 outbreaks in nurseries. *Reviews of Infectious Disease* 8, 918–926.

Monath, T.P. and Heinz, F.X. (1996) Flaviviruses. In: Fields, B.N., Knipe, D.M. and Howley, P.M. (eds) *Fields Virology,* 3rd edn. Lippincott-Raven Press, New York, pp. 961–1034.

Monath, T.P., Cropp, C.B. and Harrison, A.K. (1983) Mode of entry of a neurotropic arbovirus into the central nervous system: reinvestigation of an old controversy. *Laboratory Investigation* 48, 399–410.

Oldstone, M.B., von Herrath, M., Lewicki, H., Hudrisier, D., Whitton, J.L. and Gairin, J.E. (1999) Use of a high-affinity peptide that aborts MHC-restricted cytotoxic T lymphocyte activity against multiple viruses *in vitro* and virus-induced immunopathologic disease *in vivo*. *Virology* 256, 246–257.

Peters, C.J., Buchmeier, M., Rollin, P.E. and Ksiazek, T.G. (1996) Arenaviruses. In: Fields, B.N., Knipe, D.M. and Howley, P.M. (eds) *Fields Virology*, 3rd edn. Lippincott-Raven Press, New York, pp. 1521–1551.

Pichichero, M.E., McLinn, S., Rotbart, H.A., Menegus, M.A., Cascino, M. and Reidenberg, B.E. (1998) Clinical and economic impact of enterovirus illness in private pediatric practice. *Pediatrics* 102, 1126–1134.

Price, R.A., Garcia, J.H. and Rightsel, W.A. (1970) Choriomeningitis and myocarditis in an adolescent with isolation of Coxsackie B5 virus. *American Journal of Clinical Pathology* 53, 825–831.

Rasmussen, A.F. Jr (1946) The laboratory diagnosis of lymphocytic choriomeningitis and mumps. In: *Rocky Mountain Conference on Infantile Paralysis*, University of Colorado School of Medicine and Hospitals, Denver, Colorado, pp. 87–97.

Roizman B. (1996) *Herpesviridae*. In: Fields, B.N., Knipe, D.M. and Howley, P.M. (eds) *Fields Virology*, 3rd edn. Lippincott-Raven Press, New York, pp. 2221–2230.

Rorabaugh, M.L., Berlin, L.E., Rosenberg, L., Rossman, M., Allen, M. and Modlin, J.F. (1992) Absence of neurodevelopmental sequelae from aseptic meningitis. *Pediatric Research* 30, 177–180.

Rossmann, M.G., He, Y. and Kuhn, R.J. (2002) Picornavirus–receptor interactions. *Trends in Microbiology* 10, 324–331.

Rotbart, H.A. (1997) Viral meningitis and the aseptic meningitis syndrome. In: Scheld, W.M., Whitley, R.J. and Durack, D.T. (eds) *Infections of the Central Nervous System*, 2nd edn. Lippincott-Raven Publishers, Philadelphia, PA, pp. 23–46.

Rotbart, H.A. (1999) Enteroviruses. In: Murray, P.R., Baron, E.J., Pfaller, M.A., Tenover, F.C. and Yolken, R.H. (eds) *Manual of Clinical Microbiology.* ASM Press, Washington, DC, pp. 990–998.

Rotbart, H.A. (2000) Viral meningitis. *Seminars in Neurology* 20, 277–292.

Rotbart, H.A., Brennan, P.J., Fife, K.H., Romero, J.R., Griffin, J.A., McKinlay, M.A. and Hayden, F.G. (1998) Enterovirus meningitis in adults. *Clinical Infectious Diseases* 27, 896–898.

Sawyer, M.H., Holland, D. and Aintablian, N. (1994) Diagnosis of enteroviral central nervous system infection by polymerase chain reaction during a large community outbreak. *Pediatric Infectious Disease Journal* 3, 177–182.

Schlesinger, Y., Tebes, P., Gaudreault-Keener, M., Buller, R.S. and Storch, G.A. (1995) Herpes simplex virus type 2 meningitis in the absence of genital lesions: improved recognition with use of the polymerase chain reaction. *Clinical Infectious Diseases* 20, 842–848.

Schwendemann, G., Lohler, J. and Lehmann-Grube, F. (1983) Evidence for cytotoxic T-lymphocyte-target cell interaction in brains of mice infected intracerebrally with lymphocytic choriomeningitis virus. *Acta Neuropathologica* 61, 183–195.

Strikas, R.A., Anderson, L.J. and Parker, R.A. (1986) Temporal and geographic patterns of isolates of nonpolio enterovirus in the United States, 1970–1983. *Journal of Infectious Diseases* 153, 346–351.

Tedder, D.G., Ashley, R., Tyler, K.L. and Levin, M.J. (1994) Herpes simplex virus infection as a cause of benign recurrent lymphocytic meningitis. *Annals of Internal Medicine* 121, 334–338.

Tsai, T.F., Canfield, M.A., Reed, C.M., Flannery, V.L., Sullivan, K.H., Reeve, G.R., Bailey, R.E. and Poland, J.D. (1988) Epidemiological aspects of a St. Louis encephalitis outbreak in Harris County, Texas, 1986. *Journal of Infectious Diseases* 157, 351–356.

Wallgren A. (1951) Die atiologie der enzephalomeningitis bei kindern, besonders des syndromes der akuten abakteriellen (aseptichen) meningitis. *Acta Paediatrica Scandinavica* 40, 541–565.

Webster, A.D., Rotbart, H.A., Warner, T., Rudge, P. and Hyman, N. (1993) Diagnosis of enterovirus brain disease in hypogammaglobulinemic patients by polymerase chain reaction. *Clinical Infectious Diseases* 17, 657–661.

Wilfert, C.M., Lehrman, S.N. and Katz, S.L. (1983) Enteroviruses and meningitis. *Pediatric Infectious Diseases* 2, 333–341.

Wolinsky, J.S. (1996) Mumps virus. In: Fields, B.N., Knipe, D.M. and Howley, P.M. (eds) *Fields Virology*, 3rd edn. Lippincott-Raven Press, New York, pp. 1243–1266.

Wolinsky, J.S., Klassen, T. and Baringer, J.R. (1976) Persistence of neuroadapted mumps virus in brains of newborn hamsters after intraperitoneal inoculation. *Journal of Infectious Diseases* 133, 260–267.

Zinkernagel, R.M. and Doherty, P.C. (1973) Cytotoxic thymus-derived lymphocytes in cerebrospinal fluid of mice with lymphocytic choriomeningitis. *Journal of Experimental Medicine* 138, 1266–1269.

5 Pathogenesis of Cerebrospinal Meningitis Caused by *Neisseria meningitidis*

Mathieu Coureuil,[1] Florence Miller,[1] Olivier Join-Lambert,[1,2] Hervé Lécuyer,[1,2] Sandrine Bourdoulous,[1,3,4] Stefano Marullo[1,3,4] and Xavier Nassif[1,2*]

[1]*Université Paris Descartes, Paris, France;* [2]*Assistance Publique – Hôpitaux de Paris, Hôpital Necker Enfants Malades, Paris, France;* [3]*Institut Cochin, Paris, France;* [4]*CNRS, Paris, France*

5.1 Introduction

Neisseria meningitidis (meningococcus) is a Gram-negative coccus restricted to humans that is responsible for two major diseases, cerebrospinal meningitis and/or septicaemia. The latter can lead to a *purpura fulminans,* an often fatal condition due to the associated septic shock. Paradoxically, *N. meningitidis* is a common inhabitant of the human nasopharynx, and as such is a normal saprophytic organism that is transmitted from person to person by direct contact. Only in a small proportion of colonized subjects do bacteria invade the bloodstream where they are responsible for septicaemia and/or meningitis after crossing the blood–brain barrier (BBB). The mechanisms responsible for nasopharyngeal colonization and crossing of the nasopharyngeal mucosa remain largely unexplained.

Human genetic polymorphism is likely to be important in determining outcome, particularly regarding the risk of developing *purpura fulminans* (Brouwer *et al.,* 2009). In addition, not all meningococci have the same pathogenic potential. Indeed, analysis of results from multi-locus sequence typing has demonstrated the existence of distinct phylogenetic groups (clonal complexes). Some of them are more likely to be isolated from patients than from asymptomatic carriers (Maiden *et al.,* 1998), corresponding to the so-called 'hypervirulent' or 'hyperinvasive' lineages. Recently, the presence of a prophage has been correlated with the invasiveness of strains belonging to hyperinvasive lineages (Bille *et al.,* 2008). This element, inserted into the bacterial chromosome, can be induced to produce a filamentous phage.

Only a limited number of bacterial species are capable of invading the meninges, suggesting that specific virulence factors are required for bacteria to enter the subarachnoid space (SAS). Among the extracellular bacteria, *N. meningitidis* is the pathogen that most

*xavier.nassif@inserm.fr

consistently invades the meninges following bacteraemia. Approximately 63% of bacteraemia cases due to *N. meningitidis* are associated with meningitis (INVS, 2009).

Due to the lack of reliable animal models, most hypotheses regarding the pathogenesis of meningococcal infections are derived from post-mortem studies of patients who died from meningococcal meningitis or *purpura fulminans* or from biopsies of skin purpuric lesions (Pron *et al.*, 1997; Faust *et al.*, 2001; Harrison *et al.*, 2002; Dupin *et al.*, 2012). In the brain, data obtained from a patient who died of fulminant meningococcaemia, when bacteria were invading the cerebrospinal fluid (CSF), revealed that *N. meningitidis* adheres on to endothelial cells and forms small colonies on the endoluminal surface of the microvasculature. Bacteria are also found inside cells and in intercellular spaces (Pron *et al.*, 1997). These data suggest that *N. meningitidis* crosses the BBB through a direct interaction between bacteria and endothelial cells. Thus, *in vivo* observations suggest that meningeal invasion by *N. meningitidis* relies on the ability of the bacteria to: (i) survive and/or grow in the bloodstream; and (ii) interact and to signal to endothelial cells throughout the body.

From these *in vivo* data, it can be speculated that the clinical forms of meningococcal disease mostly reflect the levels of bacteraemia. When a low or moderate number of meningococci circulate in the bloodstream, the bacteria interacting with peripheral capillaries cause only few localized purpuric lesions, although the interaction with brain endothelial cells is sufficient to lead to meningeal invasion. In this case, meningitis is the prominent clinical sign of the disease. In contrast, in cases of high bacteraemia, peripheral endothelial cells are probably massively colonized by meningococci, leading to a significant increase of vascular permeability, which can be associated with extensive thrombosis and purpura. In this case, bacteria also invade meningeal spaces, but the clinical presentation includes septic shock and *purpura fulminans* lesions. This review will concentrate on the two main obstacles that *N. meningitidis* has to overcome before reaching the meninges: the bloodstream and the BBB.

5.2 *Neisseria meningitidis* in the Blood

Meningeal invasion by *N. meningitidis* is directly correlated with bacteraemia, which is believed to favour invasion by directly increasing the likelihood of the interaction between bacteria and components of the BBB. Therefore, the bacterial attributes involved in growth and/or survival in the extracellular fluids play an essential role in meningococcal meningitis.

Studies aimed at identifying factors responsible for bacterial survival, multiplication or adaptation in the bloodstream were based on the screening of transposon mutagenesis libraries using either an infant rat model (Sun *et al.*, 2000) or survival in complemented serum (Geoffroy *et al.*, 2003) as readouts. More recently, a transcriptomic analysis of bacteria grown in human whole blood was reported (Echenique-Rivera *et al.*, 2011). These studies demonstrated the major role of virulence factors commonly observed in most extracellular pathogens. In addition to iron chelation systems that are essential for pathogenic bacteria to obtain the necessary ferric iron *in vivo* (Stojiljkovic *et al.*, 1995), the polysaccharide capsule (Cap) and the lipopolysaccharide (LPS; strictly a lipo-oligosaccharide) participate in the prevention of bacterial killing by host innate immune system effectors such as complement. A new virulence factor, the 28 kDa surface-exposed lipoprotein factor H-binding protein (fHbp), was identified recently (Seib *et al.*, 2009). fHbp binds to human factor H in the bloodstream of infected individuals and enables *N. meningitidis* to effectively evade host immune responses by preventing complement-mediated bacterial cell lysis. Based on sequence diversity, fHbp proteins are classified into three variants and two subfamilies (Masignani *et al.*, 2003; Fletcher *et al.*, 2004). More recently, a modular structural organization has been described for fHbp, whereby a combination of five distinct variable segments defines six unique modular groups (Beernink and Granoff, 2009). This protein is expressed by all *N. meningitidis* strains studied to date, although the level of expression varies among strains (high, intermediate and low expressers). Antibodies directed against fHbp are bactericidal and this protein is currently a promising vaccine candidate.

Less is known about how other components of the innate immune system, such as polymorphonuclear neutrophils (PMNs), confer protection against meningococcal disease. These phagocytic cells elaborate multiple mechanisms effective at killing microorganisms, such as the production of antimicrobial peptides, degradative enzymes and reactive oxygen species (ROS) derived from the oxidative burst. Recently, it has been shown that a mechanism by which *N. meningitidis* escapes killing by PMNs to survive in the bloodstream is due to its ability to uptake L-glutamate and to convert it to glutathione; by maintaining intracellular redox potential, this key molecule protects the bacterium from ROS such as hydrogen peroxide (Tala *et al.*, 2011).

It should be pointed out that meningococcal infections are very often discovered at the stage of cerebrospinal meningitis, thus suggesting that the bloodstream phase can be totally asymptomatic until the bacteria cross the BBB and infect the CSF. As for all Gram-negative bacteria, LPS is the major inducer of the pro-inflammatory response via activation of Toll-like receptor (TLR) 4. This response is believed to be beneficial. However, it can become detrimental for the infected host when excessive stimulation occurs (Beutler and Rietschel, 2003). Meningococcal sepsis is generally seen as the prototypical endotoxin-mediated disease. The chemical composition of the lipid A determines how well it is recognized by TLR4. *N. meningitidis* has been reported to produce lipid A with six acyl chains, the optimal number for TLR4 recognition. Recent data have shown that, in a significant percentage of invasive meningococcal isolates, the lipid A was penta-acylated. This modification is the consequence of a mutation in the *lpX1* gene. The corresponding strains were dramatically less efficient in inducing cytokine production. Furthermore, patients infected by these strains presented less frequently with petechial rash and platelet counts were higher, consistent with reduced cytokine induction and less activation of tissue factor-mediated coagulopathy (Fransen *et al.*, 2009). Because penta-acylation of lipid A aids bacterial evasion of the innate immune system, this might explain why the blood phase could remain asymptomatic. However, such a mutation was observed in only 9% of the isolates obtained in meningococcal invasive diseases. It is therefore likely that *N. meningitidis* possesses other mechanisms to reduce activation of the host innate immune system.

5.3 The Interaction of *N. meningitidis* with Endothelial Cells

The tropism of bacteria for microvasculature endothelial cells that constitute the BBB and blood–cerebrospinal fluid barrier (BCSFB) (see Weller, Chapter 2, this volume) is a major pathophysiological issue in meningococcal infections. Various bacterial surface components have been described that enable meningococcal interactions with human cells. These include type IV pili (Tfp, Pil) and outer-membrane (OM) proteins such as Opa or Opc proteins (Virji, 2009). However, in Cap^+ bacteria, type IV pili are the main bacterial attributes capable of promoting adhesion, because Pil^-Cap^+ bacteria adhere poorly to any cell type. Early work performed with Pil^+Cap^+ meningococci showed that interactions with human cells can be divided into two phases. The first phase is adhesion of single diplococci but in a rather inefficient manner. The second phase corresponds to bacterial division on to the apical surface of the cells. Therefore, the high number of bacteria that interact with cells is a consequence of local bacterial division of the few meningococci that have initially succeeded at adherence. Type IV pili are required for both phases. They promote the initial interaction of diplococci with the endothelial cells, and then generate bacteria–bacteria interactions that lead to spreading of the bacteria on the apical surface of the cells.

5.3.1 Type IV pili and pilus biogenesis

Type IV pili are polymeric filaments found on many Gram-negative bacteria (Wolfgang *et al.*, 2000). These structures correspond to the multimeric assembly of a pilin subunit. Functional Tfp are dynamic structures: pilin subunits are constantly assembled into fibres from a platform in the inner membrane. The fibre is then extruded through the OM via the secretin PilQ (Wolfgang *et al.*, 2000). A remarkable property of Tfp is their ability to retract into the bacterium, via the action of the force-generating ATPase PilT (Merz *et al.*, 2000; Skerker and Berg, 2001). Retraction is a consequence of the disassembly of pilin subunits that are then stored in the cytoplasmic membrane (Morand *et al.*, 2004). Tfp retraction is essential for bacterial (twitching) motility, competence for DNA transformation and pilus-associated signalling to host cells (Lee *et al.*, 2005).

The *pilE* gene, encoding the major neisserial pilus subunit, pilin, is subject to antigenic variation following recombination with silent loci (*pilS*). Pilin is synthesized as a pre-protein. A short leader sequence (5–6 residues) is cleaved by the pre-pilin peptidase PilD (Lory and Strom, 1997), which also methylates the N-terminal phenylalanine of the mature protein product. Pilins are packed through internal hydrophobic interactions between conserved N-terminal α-helices, leaving hypervariable C-terminal globular regions exposed (Parge *et al.*, 1995). PilE undergoes several post-translational modifications of serine residues including glycosylation at position 63, whereas the residue at position 68 was reported to be modified by the addition of phosphate, phosphoethanolamine or phosphorylcholine (Forest *et al.*, 1999; Hegge *et al.*, 2004). The structure of the added sugar is different, depending on the strain (Virji, 1997; Chamot-Rooke *et al.*, 2007).

In addition to PilE, pili also contain the less abundant proteins PilX, PilV and ComP. These are called minor pilins (Winther-Larsen *et al.*, 2001; Helaine *et al.*, 2005) as they structurally resemble PilE and are likely to be assembled within the filaments in a similar way (Craig and Li, 2008). Importantly, each minor pilin modulates Tfp-linked properties (Brown *et al.*, 2010). PilX is crucial for the formation of bacterial aggregates and indirectly controls the adhesion to human cells by promoting bacteria–bacteria interactions (Helaine *et al.*, 2005, 2007), and ComP is essential for competence for DNA transformation (Wolfgang *et al.*, 1999), while PilV affects several pilus-linked properties such as signalling to endothelial cells (Brown *et al.*, 2010).

The PilC proteins play a crucial but still enigmatic role (Jonsson *et al.*, 1991; Nassif *et al.*, 1994; Rudel *et al.*, 1995a,b). Two alleles were originally discovered (Jonsson *et al.*, 1991). Expression of both variants is subject to phase variation as a result of frameshift in homopolymeric 'G' tracts located in the open reading frames (Jonsson *et al.*, 1991). PilC-null strains show impaired pilus expression and lack the ability for transformation competence. Abolition of *pilT* in a PilC-null background restores piliation, confirming the hypothesis that PilC acts as an antagonist of PilT by preventing PilT-mediated retraction (Wolfgang *et al.*, 1998; Morand *et al.*, 2004).

5.3.2 Mechanism of meningococcal adhesion to host cells

The molecular mechanism responsible for the first step of *N. meningitidis* adhesion, i.e. the initial attachment of individual diplococci to the cells, requires both bacterial attributes and accommodating flow shear stresses. *In vivo*, blood flow generates mechanical forces that vary depending on the vessels. *N. meningitidis* can only adhere to endothelial cells in the presence of a very low shear stress, which is present only in capillaries and microvessels (Mairey *et al.*, 2006). This highlights how efficiently *N. meningitidis* colonizes capillaries in the brain and the skin. Bacterial adhesion is dependent on the PilC1 and PilC2 protein, depending on the cell type (Rudel *et al.*, 1992; Nassif *et al.*, 1994; Morand *et al.*, 2001, 2009). One report suggested that the PilC proteins could carry a cell-binding domain (Rudel *et al.*, 1995b) and this hypothesis was based on the inhibition of adhesion using purified PilC molecules. However, non-adhesive, non-piliated isolates of a serogroup B strain with high PilC expression have been described, as well as piliated adhesive isolates with barely detectable PilC expression (Virji *et al.*, 1995). In addition, another PilC$^+$/PilE$^-$ strain, in which PilC location has been demonstrated in the OM, is unable to interact with eukaryotic cells (X. Nassif, 2013, unpublished observations), thus raising doubts over the role of PilC as an adhesion molecule. It is therefore likely that the cell-binding domain on the type IV pili remains to be identified.

After initial attachment, meningococci resist high blood velocities to multiply, and to form microcolonies on the apical surface of endothelial cells. This is dependent on both bacterial aggregation and bacterial signalling to the endothelial cells. A strain lacking the minor pilin pilV is defective in signalling to cells and cannot resist shear stress *in vitro* (Mikaty *et al.*, 2009). Inter-bacterial interaction is also essential to form aggregates and to multiply on the cell surface. A strain that expresses the hypo-aggregative pilin variant PilE-SA is unable to form large colonies on the surface of human cells (Nassif *et al.*, 1993; Marceau *et al.*, 1995). Measurements using optical tweezers showed that retraction of a single Tfp generates forces up to 110 pN, in a transient manner for each fibre. Bundles of Tfp, which result from the association of eight to ten pili, act as coordinated retractable units. Thus, bundles can generate retraction forces in the nanonewton range (Biais *et al.*, 2008). These forces allow the transition of the Tfp into a new conformation, which is longer and narrower than the usual structure (Biais *et al.*, 2010). This transition reveals some new epitopes like the SM1 epitope (residues 49–53 of mature pilin: EYYLN), previously reported to be buried in the fibre. Brissac *et al.* (2012) have recently shown that, upon adhesion to endothelial cells, the SM1 epitope is revealed and this correlates with Tfp-induced signalling to the cell. Interestingly, PilX is required for this transition. It was previously shown that the minor pilin PilX is essential to promote inter-bacterial interactions and that *pilX* mutants are unable to form aggregates. It is now clear that the *pilX* mutant is defective for both aggregation and signalling to the cell, thus making it unable to multiply on top of the endothelial cell layer. During infection, meningococci also modulate their aggregative properties, without influencing adhesion and signalling, by adding a phosphoglycerol molecule on pilins. This modification enhances the ability of the bacteria to detach from the adherent aggregates and to disseminate (Chamot-Rooke *et al.*, 2011).

5.3.3 Consequence of the type IV pilus-mediated interaction and involvement of the host cell β2-adrenergic receptor

Adhesion and signalling are independent but both depend on Tfp. A strain defective in PilC1 that possesses non-adherent Tfp is still able to induce cellular signalling (Merz *et al.*, 1999; Brissac *et al.*, 2012): conversely, the inhibition of meningococcus-induced signalling by the use of drugs or strains defective in signalling does not impair bacterial initial adhesion (Mikaty *et al.*, 2009; Coureuil *et al.*, 2010). To date, the cellular receptor responsible for pilus-mediated adhesion remains unknown. CD46 was proposed as the host cell receptor for both *Neisseria gonorrhoeae* and *N. meningitidis* Tfp (Kallstrom *et al.*, 1997). However, this finding has been strongly contested and has not been confirmed by subsequent studies (Kirchner *et al.*, 2005). Laminin has also been described as a potential receptor for the meningococcal PilQ secretin and the PorA protein (Orihuela *et al.*, 2009). However, considering that PilQ is expressed in Pil$^-$ mutants and that Pil$^-$Cap$^-$ strains are unable to interact with endothelial cells, its role remains unclear. The I-domain-containing integrins were described as essential for *N. gonorrhoeae* adhesion to primary urethral epithelial cells (Edwards and Apicella, 2005), but similar data have not been reported for *N. meningitidis* interactions with endothelial cells.

However, recruitment of the β2-adrenergic receptor at the site of bacterial cell interaction has been shown and was described as an important signalling receptor for *N. meningitidis* (Coureuil *et al.*, 2010; Lecuyer *et al.*, 2012). The expression of both the β2-adrenergic receptor and the receptor-interacting β-arrestins proteins is sufficient to promote a *N. meningitidis*-induced cell response in an incompetent cell line, such as HEK293 cells (Coureuil *et al.*, 2010). The β2-adrenergic receptor is a G-protein-coupled receptor (GPCR) that signals via the heterotrimeric Gαs protein and β-arrestins. This adrenaline receptor is also important in vascular homeostasis and vascular disease. PilE and PilV directly interact with the extracellular N-terminal domain of the β2-adrenergic receptor to transmit the signal (Coureuil *et al.*, 2010). This interaction is believed to modify the conformation of the receptor, resulting in the activation of β-arrestin-mediated signalling without activating the heterotrimeric Gαs protein and the downstream adenyl cyclase/cAMP pathway, a property referred to as 'biased activation' (Drake *et al.*, 2008; Coureuil *et al.*, 2010). β-Arrestins are scaffolding proteins involved in many cellular processes such as receptor internalization, MAP kinase activation and actin polymerization (DeWire *et al.*, 2007). It is likely that accumulated β-arrestins underneath microcolonies play a major role in the sequestration of these signalling molecules.

In summary, following initial adhesion, *N. meningitidis* recruits and activates the β2-adrenergic receptor and the β-arrestins. This is the first stage of meningococcal-induced cellular signalling (Fig. 5.1).

5.3.4 *N. meningitidis*-induced signalling in endothelial cells

Activation of the β2-adrenergic receptor by *N. meningitidis* and the accumulation of β-arrestins leads to the formation of a 'raft-like' membrane domain enriched in cholesterol and phosphatidylinositol 4,5-bisphosphate (PIP2) (Mikaty *et al.*, 2009). Production of PIP2 is critical during meningococcal-induced signalling (Doulet *et al.*, 2006; S. Bourdoulous, 2013, unpublished observations). Nevertheless, how PIP2 is produced at the site of bacterial adhesion is unknown. Two pathways might be involved downstream of the β2-adrenergic receptor and β-arrestins

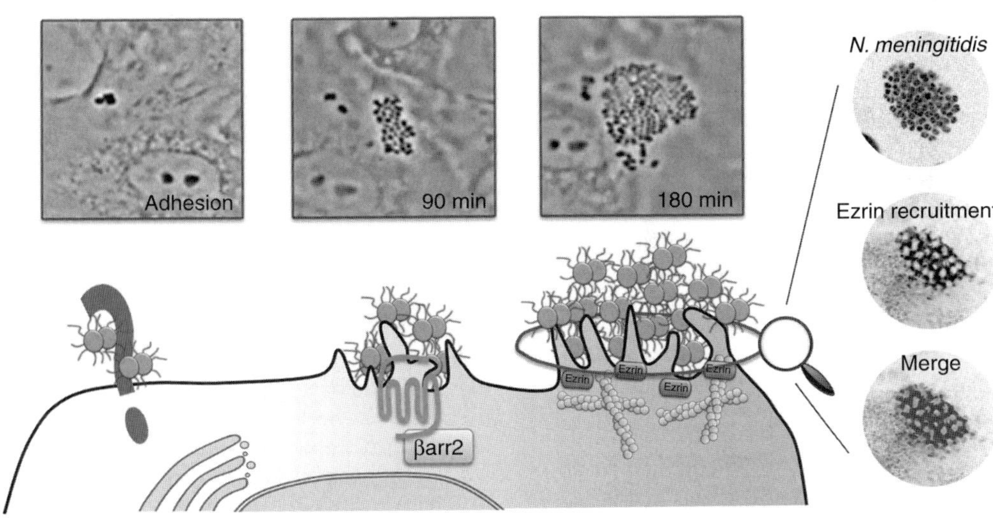

Fig. 5.1. Interaction of *N. meningitidis* with endothelial cells. *N. meningitidis* adhere to microvascular endothelial cells through an interaction between type IV pili and an unknown adhesion receptor. Following initial bacterial adhesion, type IV pili mediate the recruitment and the activation of the β2-adrenoceptor and β-arrestins, thus leading to the organization of a specific cytoplasmic molecular complex, referred to as a 'cortical plaque'. The formation of cortical plaques results from the local accumulation of ezrin and ezrin-binding proteins and actin-binding proteins. The resulting microvilli aid meningococci in resisting shear stress in the bloodstream. The three panels on the top are light microscope images of bacteria (black dots) at the time of adhesion and at 90 and 180 min after adhesion. The three panels on the right are confocal microscope images of ezrin recruitment detected by immunolabelling (negative of images).

(β2AR-βarrs) pathway: (i) the recruitment of phosphoinositide 5-kinase (PIP5K), which catalyses the formation of PIP2 from phosphatidylinositol phosphate (PIP) (Oude Weernink *et al.*, 2007); and (ii) the recruitment of PTEN (phosphatidylinositol 3,4,5-trisphosphate 3-phosphatase and dual-specificity protein phosphatase), via the β-arrestins, which catalyses the production of PIP2 from phosphatidylinositol (3,4,5)-triphosphate (PIP3) (Lima-Fernandes *et al.*, 2011). The local production of PIP2 is necessary for the recruitment of ezrin (Fievet *et al.*, 2004). Once activated by the β2AR-βarrs pathway (Cant and Pitcher, 2005), phosphorylated ezrin can sequester transmembrane receptors, organize actin filament and link the cortical actin network to the membrane (Doulet *et al.*, 2006; Coureuil *et al.*, 2010; Fehon *et al.*, 2010), thus leading to the subsequent formation of a cortical plaque. This is accompanied by a robust local stimulation of actin polymerization leading to the elongation of membrane protrusions around bacteria (Merz *et al.*, 1999; Eugene *et al.*, 2002). Interestingly, the formation of such protrusions was also observed *in vivo* on brain endothelial cells by transmission electron microscopy analysis of brain sections from a child who died of fulminant meningococcaemia (Pujol *et al.*, 1997). The pathophysiological role of these projections is believed to be associated with both an increase of the cell membrane surface to favour adhesion of the bacteria, and the shielding of growing microcolonies against shear stress in the bloodstream (Mairey *et al.*, 2006).

Actin polymerization

Actin polymerization and the formation of membrane protrusions rely on the activation of the small GTPases of the Rho family, i.e. CDC42, Rac1 and RhoA (Eugene *et al.*, 2002; Lambotin *et al.*, 2005). GTPases control diverse cellular function such as polarity, migration, endocytosis and cell-cycle progression. GTPases are recruited following meningococcal adhesion and promote the recruitment of the polarity complex PAR6/PAR3/PKCζ that relocalizes the cortactin-Arp2/3 complex at the site of bacterial adhesion. Cortactin (or cortical actin-binding protein) is a perinuclear cytoplasmic protein that is involved in reorganization of the actin cytoskeleton. Cortactin interacts directly with the Arp2/3 complex (i.e. an actin nucleation complex) to promote actin branching and polymerization (Uruno *et al.*, 2001; Coureuil *et al.*, 2009). In addition to its recruitment, cortactin has to be activated. This activation is controlled by the tyrosine kinase Src, which is sequestered in the cortical plaque. Interestingly, Src recruitment is independent of the CDC42-PAR6/PKCζ pathway. After infection, Src is recruited by direct interaction with the β-arrestins (Coureuil *et al.*, 2010) and regulated by the ERBB2 tyrosine kinase receptor, which subsequently regulates cortactin phosphorylation (Hoffmann *et al.*, 2001). The ERBB2 tyrosine kinase receptor belongs to the family of epidermal growth factor (EGF) receptors. The interaction of *N. meningitidis* with human endothelial cells leads to ERBB2 activation in the cortical plaque, most likely via homodimerization. This is an example of a secondary signalling event, activated by accumulation of a cellular receptor at the site of bacterial adhesion that contributes to the formation of the cortical plaque.

Opening of the paracellular route

Another consequence of the recruitment of the polarity complex PAR6/PAR3/PKCζ is the opening of inter-endothelial cell junctions, allowing the transmigration of bacteria via the paracellular route (Coureuil *et al.*, 2009). Indeed, it has been shown that *N. meningitidis* recruits junctional proteins underneath the colony into the cortical plaque. The CDC42-PAR3/PAR6/PKCζ pathway is usually involved in organization of the cellular junctions (i.e. adherens and tight junctions). Here, ectopic activation of the polarity complex PAR3/PAR6/PKCζ leads to abnormal recruitment of adherens junction proteins (such as VE-cadherin, p120-catenin) that are then sequestrated underneath bacterial colonies through their interaction with β-arrestins. Importantly, cellular junction proteins are recruited from the existing pool of proteins present at the cell–cell contact. As a consequence, these molecules are depleted at the intercellular junctions causing endothelium leakage. Adhesion of *N. meningitidis* also promotes the cleavage of occludin (a component of the cellular junction) by the metalloproteinase MMP-8 (Schubert-Unkmeir *et al.*, 2010), further altering the intercellular junctions.

5.4 Consequences of *N. meningitidis*–Endothelial Cell Interactions on Meningeal Invasion

Following the interaction of bacteria with endothelial cells, there are at least four strategies for a meningeal pathogen to cross brain endothelial cell monolayers: (i) transcellular transport by passive or adhesion-induced transcytosis; (ii) paracellular passage through open tight junctions; (iii) disruption of the endothelial barrier due to a direct cytotoxic effect; and (iv) leucocyte-facilitated transport by infected phagocytes.

Extracellular pathogens, such as *N. meningitidis*, do not use leucocytes as vehicles to cross the BCSFB. A breakdown of the blood–CNS barrier due to apoptosis or bacterial cytotoxity is unlikely because tissue lesions, such as haemorrhages in the SAS, are uncommon during bacterial meningitis. Therefore, the entry of blood-borne pathogens, including meningococci, most probably respects the architecture of the blood–CNS barrier (Koedel *et al.*, 2002). Accordingly, adhesion of *N. meningitidis* to endothelial cells can induce an intracellular signalling pathway leading to disruption of intercellular tight junctions or, alternatively, bacteria may induce their own transcytosis through the cell monolayer. *In vitro*, transcytosis of bacteria through human brain microvascular endothelial cells (HBMECs) has been demonstrated for *Streptococcus pneumoniae*, *Escherichia coli* and *Streptococcus agalactiae*, and through human umbilical vein endothelial cells for *Haemophilus influenzae* (see Klein *et al.*, Chapter 6, Hill and Christodoulides, Chapter 7, Kim, Chapter 8 and Nizet and Doran, Chapter 9, this volume). Although *N. meningitidis* can readily be internalized *in vitro* within vacuoles in HBMECs (Nikulin *et al.*, 2006), the fact that *N. meningitidis* can open gaps in a monolayer of brain endothelial cells as a consequence of the delocalization of junctional components suggests that *N. meningitidis* cross the BBB/BCSFB using the paracellular route. Interestingly, a recent study of skin biopsies indicated that *N. meningitidis* is likely to open the paracellular route *in vivo* (Dupin *et al.*, 2012). Entry of meningococci into the CSF-filled SAS induces a compartmentalized inflammatory response centred on the leptomeninges. The molecular nature of the host innate immune response to invading meningeal pathogens, including meningococci, is described in the chapter by Christodoulides (Chapter 17, this volume).

5.5 Conclusions

Recent exciting findings have considerably expanded our understanding of the cellular events involved in meningococcal interactions with endothelial cells, thus leading to several hypotheses to explain the pathogenesis of meningeal invasion and the development of *purpura fulminans*. However, in spite of these recent findings, much remains to be discovered about the complex molecular networks involved. Among the major issues is identifying the receptor for meningococcal adhesion, which would constitute a significant breakthrough in the field, and developing suitable animal models that would confirm the *in vitro* observations.

Acknowledgements

The laboratory of X.N. is supported by INSERM, Université Paris Descartes, a grant from 'La Fondation pour la Recherche Médicale' and ANR grant no. ANR-AAP-2009-06-26. M.C. is supported by an ANR grant # ANR-11-JSV3-0002 and a grant from 'Mairie de Paris - Programme EMERGENCE'.

References

Beernink, P.T. and Granoff, D.M. (2009) The modular architecture of meningococcal factor H-binding protein. *Microbiology* 155, 2873–2883.

Beutler, B. and Rietschel, E.T. (2003) Innate immune sensing and its roots: the story of endotoxin. *Nature Reviews Immunology* 3, 169–176.

Biais, N., Ladoux, B., Higashi, D., So, M. and Sheetz, M. (2008) Cooperative retraction of bundled type IV pili enables nanonewton force generation. *PLOS Biology* 6, 907–913.

Biais, N., Higashi, D.L., Brujic, J., So, M. and Sheetz, M.P. (2010) Force-dependent polymorphism in type IV pili reveals hidden epitopes. *Proceedings of the National Academy of Sciences USA* 107, 11358–11363.

Bille, E., Ure, R., Gray, S.J., Kaczmarski, E.B., McCarthy, N.D., Nassif, X., Maiden, M.C. and Tinsley, C.R. (2008) Association of a bacteriophage with meningococcal disease in young adults. *PLoS One* 3, e3885.

Brissac, T., Mikaty, G., Dumenil, G., Coureuil, M. and Nassif, X. (2012) The meningococcal minor pilin PilX is responsible for Type IV pilus conformational changes associated with signaling to endothelial cells. *Infection and Immunity* 80, 3297–3306.

Brouwer, M.C., de Gans, J., Heckenberg, S.G., Zwinderman, A.H., van der Poll, T. and van de Beek, D. (2009) Host genetic susceptibility to pneumococcal and meningococcal disease: a systematic review and meta-analysis. *Lancet Infectious Diseases* 9, 31–44.

Brown, D.R., Helaine, S., Carbonnelle, E. and Pelicic, V. (2010) Systematic functional analysis reveals that a set of seven genes is involved in fine-tuning of the multiple functions mediated by Type IV pili in *Neisseria meningitidis. Infection and Immunity* 78, 3053–3063.

Cant, S.H. and Pitcher, J.A. (2005) G protein-coupled receptor kinase 2-mediated phosphorylation of ezrin is required for G protein-coupled receptor-dependent reorganization of the actin cytoskeleton. *Molecular Biology of the Cell* 16, 3088–3099.

Chamot-Rooke, J., Rousseau, B., Lanternier, F., Mikaty, G., Mairey, E., Malosse, C., Bouchoux, G., Pelicic, V., Camoin, L., Nassif, X. and Dumenil, G. (2007) Alternative *Neisseria* spp. type IV pilin glycosylation with a glyceramido acetamido trideoxyhexose residue. *Proceedings of the National Academy of Sciences USA* 104, 14783–14788.

Chamot-Rooke, J., *et al.* (2011) Posttranslational modification of pili upon cell contact triggers *N. meningitidis* dissemination. *Science* 331, 778–782.

Coureuil, M., Mikaty, G., Miller, F., Lecuyer, H., Bernard, C., Bourdoulous, S., Dumenil, G., Mege, R.M., Weksler, B.B., Romero, I.A., Couraud, P.O. and Nassif, X. (2009) Meningococcal Type IV pili recruit the polarity complex to cross the brain endothelium. *Science* 325, 83–87.

Coureuil, M., Lecuyer, H., Scott, M.G., Boularan, C., Enslen, H., Soyer, M., Mikaty, G., Bourdoulous, S., Nassif, X. and Marullo, S. (2010) Meningococcus hijacks a β2-adrenoceptor/β-arrestin pathway to cross brain microvasculature endothelium. *Cell* 143, 1149–1160.

Craig, L. and Li, J. (2008) Type IV pili: paradoxes in form and function. *Current Opinion in Structural Biology* 18, 267–277.

DeWire, S.M., Ahn, S., Lefkowitz, R.J. and Shenoy, S.K. (2007) β-Arrestins and cell signaling. *Annual Review of Physiology* 69, 483–510.

Doulet, N., Donnadieu, E., Laran-Chich, M.P., Niedergang, F., Nassif, X., Couraud, P.O. and Bourdoulous, S. (2006) *Neisseria meningitidis* infection of human endothelial cells interferes with leukocyte transmigration by preventing the formation of endothelial docking structures. *Journal of Cell Biology* 173, 627–637.

Drake, M.T., Violin, J.D., Whalen, E.J., Wisler, J.W., Shenoy, S.K. and Lefkowitz, R.J. (2008) β-Arrestin-biased agonism at the β-2-adrenergic receptor. *Journal of Biological Chemistry* 283, 5669–5676.

Dupin, N., Lecuyer, H., Carlotti, A., Poyart, C., Coureuil, M., Chanal, J., Schmitt, A., Vacher-Lavenu, M.C., Taha, M.K., Nassif, X. and Morand, P.C. (2012) Chronic meningococcemia cutaneous lesions involve meningococcal perivascular invasion through the remodeling of endothelial barriers. *Clinical Infectious Diseases* 54, 1162–1165.

Echenique-Rivera, H., Muzzi, A., Del Tordello, E., Seib, K.L., Francois, P., Rappuoli, R., Pizza, M. and Serruto, D. (2011) Transcriptome analysis of *Neisseria meningitidis* in human whole blood and mutagenesis studies identify virulence factors involved in blood survival. *PLoS Pathogens* 7, e1002027.

Edwards, J.L. and Apicella, M.A. (2005) I-domain-containing integrins serve as pilus receptors for *Neisseria gonorrhoeae* adherence to human epithelial cells. *Cellular Microbiology* 7, 1197–1211.

Eugene, E., Hoffmann, I., Pujol, C., Couraud, P.O., Bourdoulous, S. and Nassif, X. (2002) Microvilli-like structures are associated with the internalization of virulent capsulated *Neisseria meningitidis* into vascular endothelial cells. *Journal of Cell Science* 115, 1231–1241.

Faust, S.N., Levin, M., Harrison, O.B., Goldin, R.D., Lockhart, M.S., Kondaveeti, S., Laszik, Z., Esmon, C.T. and Heyderman, R.S. (2001) Dysfunction of endothelial protein C activation in severe meningococcal sepsis. *New England Journal of Medicine* 345, 408–416.

Fehon, R.G., McClatchey, A.I. and Bretscher, A. (2010) Organizing the cell cortex: the role of ERM proteins. *Nature Reviews Molecular Cell Biology* 11, 276–287.

Fievet, B.T., Gautreau, A., Roy, C., Del Maestro, L., Mangeat, P., Louvard, D. and Arpin, M. (2004) Phosphoinositide binding and phosphorylation act sequentially in the activation mechanism of ezrin. *Journal of Cell Biology* 164, 653–659.

Fletcher, L.D., *et al.* (2004) Vaccine potential of the *Neisseria meningitidis* 2086 lipoprotein. *Infection and Immunity* 72, 2088–2100.

Forest, K.T., Dunham, S.A., Koomey, M. and Tainer, J.A. (1999) Crystallographic structure reveals phosphorylated pilin from *Neisseria*: phosphoserine sites modify type IV pilus surface chemistry and fibre morphology. *Molecular Microbiology* 31, 743–752.

Fransen, F., Heckenberg, S.G.B., Hamstra, H.J., Feller, M., Boog, C.J.P., van Putten, J.P.M., van de Beek, D., van der Ende, A. and van der Ley, P. (2009) Naturally occurring lipid A mutants in *Neisseria meningitidis* from patients with invasive meningococcal disease are associated with reduced coagulopathy. *PLoS Pathogens* 5, e1000396.

Geoffroy, M.C., Floquet, S., Metais, A., Nassif, X. and Pelicic, V. (2003) Large-scale analysis of the meningococcus genome by gene disruption: resistance to complement-mediated lysis. *Genome Research* 13, 391–398.

Harrison, O.B., Robertson, B.D., Faust, S.N., Jepson, M.A., Goldin, R.D., Levin, M. and Heyderman, R.S. (2002) Analysis of pathogen–host cell interactions in purpura fulminans: expression of capsule, type IV pili, and PorA by *Neisseria meningitidis in vivo*. *Infection and Immunity* 70, 5193–5201.

Hegge, F.T., *et al.* (2004) Unique modifications with phosphocholine and phosphoethanolamine define alternate antigenic forms of *Neisseria gonorrhoeae* type IV pili. *Proceedings of the National Academy of Sciences USA* 101, 10798–10803.

Helaine, S., Carbonnelle, E., Prouvensier, L., Beretti, J.L., Nassif, X. and Pelicic, V. (2005) PilX, a pilus-associated protein essential for bacterial aggregation, is a key to pilus-facilitated attachment of *Neisseria meningitidis* to human cells. *Molecular Microbiology* 55, 65–77.

Helaine, S., Dyer, D.H., Nassif, X., Pelicic, V. and Forest, K.T. (2007) 3D structure/function analysis of PilX reveals how minor pilins can modulate the virulence properties of type IV pili. *Proceedings of the National Academy of Sciences USA* 104, 15888–15893.

Hoffmann, I., Eugene, E., Nassif, X., Couraud, P.O. and Bourdoulous, S. (2001) Activation of ErbB2 receptor tyrosine kinase supports invasion of endothelial cells by *Neisseria meningitidis*. *Journal of Cell Biology* 155, 133–143.

INVS (2009) Réseau EPIBAC. Surveillance des infections invasives à *Haemophilus influenzae, Listeria monocytogenes, Neisseria meningitidis, Streptococcus pneumoniae, Streptococcus agalactiae* (B) et *Streptococcus pyogenes* (A) en France métropolitaine. Institut National de Veille Sanitaire (InVs), Paris.

Jonsson, A.B., Nyberg, G. and Normark, S. (1991) Phase variation of gonococcal pili by frameshift mutation in PilC, a novel gene for pilus assembly. *EMBO Journal* 10, 477–488.

Kallstrom, H., Liszewski, M.K., Atkinson, J.P. and Jonsson, A.B. (1997) Membrane cofactor protein (MCP or CD46) is a cellular pilus receptor for pathogenic *Neisseria*. *Molecular Microbiology* 25, 639–647.

Kirchner, M., Heuer, D. and Meyer, T.F. (2005) CD46-independent binding of neisserial type IV pili and the major pilus adhesin, PilC, to human epithelial cells. *Infection and Immunity* 73, 3072–3082.

Koedel, U., Scheld, W.M. and Pfister, H.W. (2002) Pathogenesis and pathophysiology of pneumococcal meningitis. *Lancet Infectious Diseases* 2, 721–736.

Lambotin, M., Hoffmann, I., Laran-Chich, M.P., Nassif, X., Couraud, P.O. and Bourdoulous, S. (2005) Invasion of endothelial cells by *Neisseria meningitidis* requires cortactin recruitment by a phosphoinositide-3-kinase/Rac1 signalling pathway triggered by the lipo-oligosaccharide. *Journal of Cell Science* 118, 3805–3816.

Lecuyer, H., Nassif, X. and Coureuil, M. (2012) Two strikingly different signaling pathways are induced by meningococcal Type IV pili on endothelial and epithelial cells. *Infection and Immunity* 80, 175–186.

Lee, S.W., Higashi, D.L., Snyder, A., Merz, A.J., Potter, L. and So, M. (2005) PilT is required for PI(3,4,5)P3-mediated crosstalk between

Neisseria gonorrhoeae and epithelial cells. *Cellular Microbiology* 7, 1271–1284.

Lima-Fernandes, E., *et al.* (2011) Distinct functional outputs of PTEN signalling are controlled by dynamic association with β-arrestins. *EMBO Journal* 30, 2557–2568.

Lory, S. and Strom, M.S. (1997) Structure–function relationship of type-IV prepilin peptidase of *Pseudomonas aeruginosa* – a review. *Gene* 192, 117–121.

Maiden, M.C.J., *et al.* (1998) Multilocus sequence typing: A portable approach to the identification of clones within populations of pathogenic microorganisms. *Proceedings of the National Academy of Sciences USA* 95, 3140–3145.

Mairey, E., Genovesio, A., Donnadieu, E., Bernard, C., Jaubert, F., Pinard, E., Seylaz, J., Olivo-Marin, J.C., Nassif, X. and Dumenil, G. (2006) Cerebral microcirculation shear stress levels determine *Neisseria meningitidis* attachment sites along the blood-brain barrier. *Journal of Experimental Medicine* 203, 1939–1950.

Marceau, M., Beretti, J.L. and Nassif, X. (1995) High adhesiveness of encapsulated *Neisseria meningitidis* to epithelial cells is associated with the formation of bundles of pili. *Molecular Microbiology* 17, 855–863.

Masignani, V., *et al.* (2003) Vaccination against *Neisseria meningitidis* using three variants of the lipoprotein GNA1870. *Journal of Experimental Medicine* 197, 789–799.

Merz, A.J., Enns, C.A. and So, M. (1999) Type IV pili of pathogenic *Neisseriae* elicit cortical plaque formation in epithelial cells. *Molecular Microbiology* 32, 1316–1332.

Merz, A.J., So, M. and Sheetz, M.P. (2000) Pilus retraction powers bacterial twitching motility. *Nature* 407, 98–102.

Mikaty, G., Soyer, M., Mairey, E., Henry, N., Dyer, D., Forest, K.T., Morand, P., Guadagnini, S., Prevost, M.C., Nassif, X. and Dumenil, G. (2009) Extracellular bacterial pathogen induces host cell surface reorganization to resist shear stress. *PLoS Pathogens* 5, e1000314.

Morand, P.C., Tattevin, P., Eugene, E., Beretti, J.L. and Nassif, X. (2001) The adhesive property of the type IV pilus-associated component PilC1 of pathogenic *Neisseria* is supported by the conformational structure of the N-terminal part of the molecule. *Molecular Microbiology* 40, 846–856.

Morand, P.C., Bille, E., Morelle, S., Eugene, E., Beretti, J.L., Wolfgang, M., Meyer, T.F., Koomey, M. and Nassif, X. (2004) Type IV pilus retraction in pathogenic *Neisseria* is regulated by the PilC proteins. *EMBO Journal* 23, 2009–2017.

Morand, P.C., Drab, M., Rajalingam, K., Nassif, X. and Meyer, T.F. (2009) *Neisseria meningitidis* differentially controls host cell motility through PilC1 and PilC2 components of Type IV pili. *Plos One* 4, e6834.

Nassif, X., Lowy, J., Stenberg, P., Ogaora, P., Ganji, A. and So, M. (1993) Antigenic variation of pilin regulates adhesion of *Neisseria meningitidis* to human epithelial cells. *Molecular Microbiology* 8, 719–725.

Nassif, X., Beretti, J.L., Lowy, J., Stenberg, P., Ogaora, P., Pfeifer, J., Normark, S. and So, M. (1994) Roles of Pilin and Pilc in adhesion of *Neisseria meningitidis* to human epithelial and endothelial cells. *Proceedings of the National Academy of Sciences USA* 91, 3769–3773.

Nikulin, J., Panzner, U., Frosch, M. and Schubert-Unkmeir, A. (2006) Intracellular survival and replication of *Neisseria meningitidis* in human brain microvascular endothelial cells. *International Journal of Medical Microbiology* 296, 553–558.

Orihuela, C.J., Mahdavi, J., Thornton, J., Mann, B., Wooldridge, K.G., Abouseada, N., Oldfield, N.J., Self, T., Ala'Aldeen, D.A. and Tuomaneni, E.I. (2009) Laminin receptor initiates bacterial contact with the blood brain barrier in experimental meningitis models. *Journal of Clinical Investigation* 119, 1638–1646.

Oude Weernink, P.A., Han, L., Jakobs, K.H. and Schmidt, M. (2007) Dynamic phospholipid signaling by G protein-coupled receptors. *Biochimica et Biophysica Acta* 1768, 888–900.

Parge, H.E., Forest, K.T., Hickey, M.J., Christensen, D.A., Getzoff, E.D. and Tainer, J.A. (1995) Structure of the fiber-forming protein pilin at 2.6 Ångstrom resolution. *Nature* 378, 32–38.

Pron, B., Taha, M.K., Rambaud, C., Fournet, J.C., Pattey, N., Monnet, J.P., Musilek, M., Beretti, J.L. and Nassif, X. (1997) Interaction of *Neisseria meningitidis* with the components of the blood–brain barrier correlates with an increased expression of PilC. *Journal of Infectious Diseases* 176, 1285–1292.

Pujol, C., Eugene, E., DesaintMartin, L. and Nassif, X. (1997) Interaction of *Neisseria meningitidis* with a polarized monolayer of epithelial cells. *Infection and Immunity* 65, 4836–4842.

Rudel, T., Vanputten, J.P.M., Gibbs, C.P., Haas, R. and Meyer, T.F. (1992) Interaction of two variable proteins (PilE and PilC) required for pilus-mediated adherence of *Neisseria gonorrhoeae* to human epithelial cells. *Molecular Microbiology* 6, 3439–3450.

Rudel, T., Facius, D., Barten, R., Scheuerpflug, I., Nonnenmacher, E. and Meyer, T.F. (1995a) Role of pili and the phase-variable PilC protein in natural competence for transformation of *Neisseria gonorrhoeae*. *Proceedings of the National Academy of Sciences USA* 92, 7986–7990.

Rudel, T., Scheuerpflug, I. and Meyer, T.F. (1995b) *Neisseria* PilC protein identified as Type-4 pilus tip located adhesin. *Nature* 373, 357–359.

Schubert-Unkmeir, A., Konrad, C., Slanina, H., Czapek, F., Hebling, S. and Frosch, M. (2010) *Neisseria meningitidis* induces brain microvascular endothelial cell detachment from the matrix and cleavage of occludin: a role for MMP-8. *PLoS Pathogens* 6, e1000874.

Seib, K., Serruto, D., Oriente, F., Delany, I., Adu-Bobie, J., Veggi, D., Arico, B., Rappuoli, R. and Pizza, M. (2009) Factor H-binding protein is important for meningococcal survival in human whole blood and serum and in the presence of the antimicrobial peptide LL-37. *Infection and Immunity* 77, 292–299.

Skerker, J.M. and Berg, H.C. (2001) Direct observation of extension and retraction of type IV pili. *Proceedings of the National Academy of Sciences USA* 98, 6901–6904.

Stojiljkovic, I., Hwa, V., DesaintMartin, L., Ogaora, P., Nassif, X., Heffron, F. and So, M. (1995) The *Neisseria meningitidis* hemoglobin receptor – its role in iron utilization and virulence. *Molecular Microbiology* 15, 531–541.

Sun, Y.H., Bakshi, S., Chalmers, R. and Tang, C.M. (2000) Functional genomics of *Neisseria meningitidis* pathogenesis. *Nature Medicine* 6, 1269–1273.

Tala, A., Monaco, C., Nagorska, K., Exley, R.M., Corbett, A., Zychlinsky, A., Alifano, P. and Tang, C.M. (2011) Glutamate utilization promotes meningococcal survival *in vivo* through avoidance of the neutrophil oxidative burst. *Molecular Microbiology* 81, 1330–1342.

Uruno, T., Liu, J.L., Zhang, P.J., Fan, Y.X., Egile, C., Li, P., Mueller, S.C. and Zhan, X. (2001) Activation of Arp2/3 complex-mediated actin polymerization by cortactin. *Nature Cell Biology* 3, 259–266.

Virji, M. (1997) Post-translational modifications of meningococcal pili. Identification of common substituents: glycans and α-glycerophosphate – a review. *Gene* 192, 141–147.

Virji, M. (2009) Pathogenic neisseriae: surface modulation, pathogenesis and infection control. *Nature Reviews Microbiology* 7, 274–286.

Virji, M., Makepeace, K., Peak, I., Payne, G., Saunders, J.R., Ferguson, D.J.P. and Moxon, E.R. (1995) Functional implications of the expression of PilC proteins in meningococci. *Molecular Microbiology* 16, 1087–1097.

Winther-Larsen, H.C., Hegge, F.T., Wolfgang, M., Hayes, S.F., van Putten, J.P.M. and Koomey, M. (2001) *Neisseria gonorrhoeae* PilV, a type IV pilus-associated protein essential to human epithelial cell adherence. *Proceedings of the National Academy of Sciences USA* 98, 15276–15281.

Wolfgang, M., Lauer, P., Park, H.S., Brossay, L., Hebert, J. and Koomey, M. (1998) PilT mutations lead to simultaneous defects in competence for natural transformation and twitching motility in piliated *Neisseria gonorrhoeae*. *Molecular Microbiology* 29, 321–330.

Wolfgang, M., van Putten, J.P.M., Hayes, S.F. and Koomey, M. (1999) The *comP* locus of *Neisseria gonorrhoeae* encodes a type IV prepilin that is dispensable for pilus biogenesis but essential for natural transformation. *Molecular Microbiology* 31, 1345–1357.

Wolfgang, M., van Putten, J.P.M., Hayes, S.F., Dorward, D. and Koomey, M. (2000) Components and dynamics of fiber formation define a ubiquitous biogenesis pathway for bacterial pili. *EMBO Journal* 19, 6408–6418.

6 *Streptococcus pneumoniae* Meningitis

Matthias Klein,[1]* Sven Hammerschmidt[2] and Uwe Koedel[1]
[1]*Ludwig-Maximilian-University, Munich, Germany;* [2]*Ernst Moritz Arndt University of Greifswald, Greifswald, Germany*

6.1 Introduction

Up to the beginning of the 20th century, meningitis caused by the Gram-positive organism *Streptococcus pneumoniae* (pneumococcus) was a lethal disease. Antibiotics started to be available during the 1940s and 1950s and improved the prognosis and led to the survival of more than half of patients. Despite early diagnostics and the introduction of new highly effective antibiotics, as well as optimization of supportive intensive care, prognosis has, unfortunately, not changed significantly during recent years. Pneumococcal meningitis is the most common cause of community-acquired bacterial meningitis in Europe and the USA and mortality is still high and reaches 14–30% (Brouwer *et al.*, 2010; Thigpen *et al.*, 2011). Furthermore, up to one-third of survivors suffer from neurological and neuropsychological deficits (Durand *et al.*, 1993; van de Beek *et al.*, 2010). Unfortunate courses of the disease are mainly related to the development of intracranial complications during the acute stage, notably cerebrovascular alterations such as vasculitis, vasospasm and venous thrombosis as well as hydrocephalus and brain oedema (Kastenbauer and Pfister, 2003). These alterations result in hypoperfusion and increased intracranial pressure, frequently leading to stroke and/or cerebral herniation. To study the patho-mechanisms that underlie such intracranial complications, animal models of pneumococcal meningitis have been developed that closely mimic the course of meningitis in humans. The results of these studies have significantly increased our understanding of pneumococcal meningitis and helped to establish a pathophysiological concept of the disease.

6.2 Pathogenesis of Pneumococcal Meningitis

Meningitis is an inflammation of the subarachnoid space (SAS). Bacteria can reach the SAS either by continuous spread, e.g. from a parameningeal focus, by the haematogenous route or, less commonly, by direct inoculation, e.g. after neurosurgical procedures (nosocomial meningitis) and in cases of cerebrospinal fluid (CSF) fistulas or brain trauma. In order to infect the central nervous system (CNS) via the haematogenous route, the causative pathogen has first to colonize and then cross the mucosa of the nasopharynx, survive and proliferate in the bloodstream, pass the blood–brain barrier

*matthias.klein@med.uni-muenchen.de

(BBB) and/or blood–cerebrospinal fluid barrier (BCSFB), and finally replicate in the SAS.

6.2.1 Colonization of the nasopharyngeal mucosa

Pneumococci colonize mucosal surfaces of the nasopharynx using a repertoire of adhesins, secreted polysaccharides and proteins, which interact directly with host cellular receptors or indirectly by exploiting extracellular matrix or serum proteins as a molecular bridge, thereby linking the pathogen with its target cell (Fig. 6.1). Moreover, pneumococci expose a variety of surface proteins for immune evasion and are able to recruit host proteolytic enzymes for their penetration through the extracellular matrix in which mucosal cells are embedded (Gamez and Hammerschmidt, 2012; Voss *et al.*, 2012). Approximately 20% of clinical pneumococcal isolates produce pili, either pilus-1 (PI-1) or pilus-2 (PI-2), each encoded by genes located on different genomic islands (Bagnoli *et al.*, 2008). The major pilin subunit forming the pilus backbone is Rrg (Rlr-regulated gene) B for PI-1 and PitB for PI-2. RrgA and RrgC in PI-1 and PitA in PI-2 are

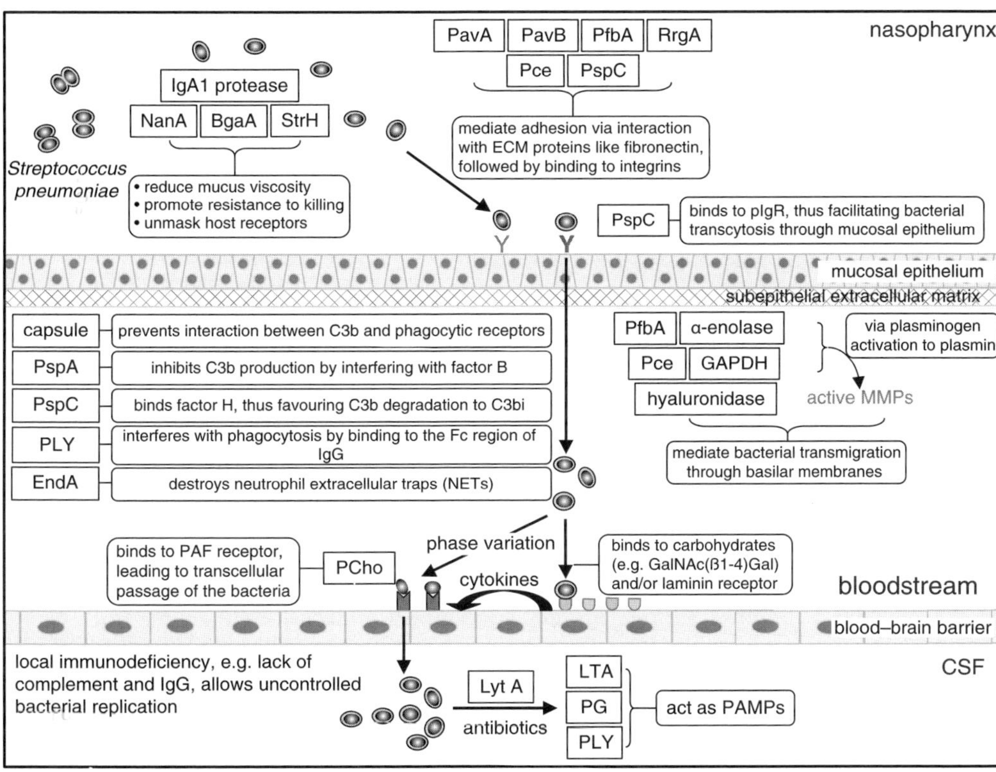

Fig. 6.1. The pathophysiological concept of pneumococcal meningitis. See accompanying text for details. PavA and PavB, pneumococcal adherence and virulence factors A and B; PfbA, plasmin and fibronectin binding protein A; RrgA, Rlr-regulated gene A; Pce, phosphorylcholine esterase; PspA/PspC, pneumococcal surface protein A, C; IgA1 protease; exoglycosidase NanA, neuraminidase A; exoglycosidase BgaA, β-galactosidase A; exoglycosidase StrH, β-*N*-acetylglucosaminidase; pIgR, polymeric immunoglobulin receptor; GADPH, glyceraldehyde-3-phosphate dehydrogenase; MMP, matrix metalloproteinase; PLY, pneumolysin; EndA, endonuclease; PAF, platelet-activating factor; PCho, phosphorylcholine; Lyt A, *N*-acetylmuramoyl-L-alanine amidase; LTA, lipoteichoic acid; PG, peptidoglycan.

ancillary pilus proteins. RrgA is located at the PI-1 pilus tip and the host target proteins for RrgA are fibronectin, laminin, lactoferrin and collagen I (LeMieux *et al.*, 2006). Pili interactions with the mucosal cell surface lead to primary attachment of the bacteria. In addition, uptake of choline from the eukaryotic cell membrane and subsequent binding of choline on teichoic and lipoteichoic acids (LTAs) of the bacterial cell wall allow interaction of pneumococci with platelet activating factor (PAF) receptor and, thus, contribute to adhesion on endothelial cells.

Adhesion on mucosal epithelial cells is also mediated by choline-binding proteins (CBPs), which are attached non-covalently to the cell wall via phosphorylcholine. A highly essential CBP of pneumococci is the multifunctional PspC protein (also known as CbpA or SpsA), which binds directly to the ectodomain of the human polymeric immunoglobulin receptor (pIgR) and also functions as a factor H-binding protein. Strikingly, pneumococci engage unloaded human pIgR for adherence to and transcytosis across mucosal epithelial cells (Hammerschmidt, 2006). Interestingly, PspC directly binds to an integrin receptor for laminin present on the vascular endothelium of the BBB, contributing to the development of pneumococcal meningitis (Orihuela *et al.*, 2009). Recently, PsrP was shown to mediate attachment of *S. pneumoniae* to keratin-10 on human lung epithelium, to be required for pneumococcal persistence in the lungs, and to be relevant to pneumococcal aggregation *in vivo* and biofilm formation (Shivshankar *et al.*, 2009). PavB is another surface protein, anchored in a sortase-dependent manner, which is highly conserved among pneumococci and identified as a pneumococcal adhesin involved in colonization. The core domain of PavB consists of repetitive sequences, the streptococcal surface repeats (SSURE), whose number of repeat units, each of approximately 150 amino acid residues, is variable and strain specific but serotype independent (Jensch *et al.*, 2010). PavB interacts via its SSURE domain with fibronectin and plasminogen. The SSURE domains most likely also interact with a yet unknown cellular receptor. Furthermore, pneumococcal adhesion and colonization of the mucosa can be enhanced by the phosphorylcholine esterase Pce, which functions by increasing the amount of phosphorylcholine on the cell surface.

Other important enzymes involved in colonization are zinc metalloproteases (e.g. IgA1-protease), exoglycosidases (e.g. neuraminidase NanA), the β-galactosidase BgaA and the β-*N*-acetyl glucosaminidase StrH. Together, these enzymes reduce mucus viscosity, promote pneumococcal resistance to opsonophagocytic killing mediated by neutrophils and unmask cryptic host receptors for adherence (Dalia *et al.*, 2010). This can also result in the supply of nutrients that are important for survival of the bacteria. The IgA1-protease is most likely involved in neutralization of the mucosal immune response by deactivating IgA1. After splicing IgA1, the Fab fragment remains bound on the bacterial surface, neutralizes the negative load of the capsule and counteracts the anti-adhesive effect of the capsule.

6.2.2 Invasion of pathogens into the bloodstream

After successful colonization of the mucosal cavity, the pathogen has to reach the bloodstream (Fig. 6.1). Local mucosal plasma cells produce dimeric IgA, which binds to pIgR on the basolateral side of the epithelial cells. The epithelial cells, in turn, mediate the transport of dimeric IgA through the polarized mucosal epithelium and secrete sIgA, consisting of an IgA dimer and the covalently bound ectodomain of pIgR, known as 'secretory component'. The pIgR is transcytosed to the apical cell surface and pneumococi bind via PspC (Hammerschmidt, 2006). The PspC-pIgR-mediated pneumococcal attachment to respiratory epithelial cells triggers cytoskeleton rearrangements, specifically involving protein-tyrosine kinases (PTKs), protein kinase B (Akt) and phosphatidylinositol 3-kinase (PI3K), respectively (Agarwal and Hammerschmidt,

2009). When the unloaded pIgR is recycled, the receptor can be transported on a retrograde pathway from apical to basal membrane. Pneumococci can adopt this retrograde transport machinery of pIgR, and after PspC-mediated binding to pIgR, pneumococci are ingested and transcytosed through mucosal epithelial cells (Elm *et al.*, 2004).

An important enzyme for mediating passage through the subepithelial connective tissue is the pneumococcal hyaluronidase, which dissolves hyaluronic acid in connective tissue. The importance of hyaluronic acid is well demonstrated in a model of nasally induced pneumococcal meningitis: co-administration of hyaluronidase significantly increased the percentage of animals that developed pneumococcal meningitis (Zwijnenburg *et al.*, 2001). Resolution of connective tissue can also be mediated by binding and activation of proteolytic host enzymes. For example, pneumococci recruit plasminogen to surface proteins PavB, Pce, GAPDH (glyceraldehyde-3-phosphate dehydrogenase) or α-enolase, which is subsequently processed by host plasminogen activators to the proteolytically active plasmin. This enhances even further the transmigration of bacteria through basilar membranes as a prerequisite for pneumococcal invasion of the bloodstream and the brain (Bergmann *et al.*, 2003).

6.2.3 Pneumococcal survival in the bloodstream

After pneumococcal adherence to type II pneumocytes of the alveoli, they can spread rapidly into the blood by crossing the vascular endothelium (Tuomanen, 1999), most likely by the intracellular route. However, because the strategies used by pneumococci for translocation are not yet fully elucidated, the paracellular route of entry cannot be excluded as an alternative route. For paracellular invasion, the toxin pneumolysin is a major virulence factor because it inhibits the normal beating of cilia on epithelial and endothelial cells (Steinfort *et al.*, 1989; Zysk *et al.*, 2001). Spread of pneumococci into the bloodstream may also occur from the lymphatic system and lymph nodes as pneumococci are also found in the draining lymphoid tissue (Kirby *et al.*, 2009).

After entering the bloodstream, pneumococcal survival is dependent on resistance to the host immune system (Fig. 6.1). In non-immune hosts, capsule expression hampers phagocytosis of the bacteria by impeding activation of the alternative complement system, thus preventing opsonization of the pathogen by C3b. Pneumococcal surface proteins PspA, PspC and PavA, as well as pneumolysin, protect bacteria from phagocytosis. In experimental mouse models of sepsis and meningitis, PavA, which possesses fibronectin-binding properties, was identified to have key functions for *in vivo* survival of *S. pneumoniae* (Holmes *et al.*, 2001; Pracht *et al.*, 2005; Noske *et al.*, 2009; Kadioglu *et al.*, 2010). PspA inhibits binding of C3a on the pneumococcal cell surface. Furthermore, it inhibits binding of factor B on bound C3b and the production of the C3-convertase, which is necessary for the further production of C3b. PspA also binds lactoferrin, which is important because the iron-depleted form of lactoferrin, apolactoferrin, has bactericidal activity, but this is inhibited due to conformational changes upon binding to PspA. PspC binds the complement regulator factor H, which splices C3b into the biologically inactive form C3bi and, thus, contributes to the inhibition of complement-triggered bacterial lysis. In contrast to other thiol-dependent toxins (such as streptolysin), pneumolysin is located intracellularly but is liberated during bacterial lysis (Tuomanen, 1999). Insertion of pneumolysin into the host cell membrane results in pore formation and subsequent cytolysis. In addition, pneumolysin can activate the classical pathway of the immune system, even without the presence of specific antibodies. This leads to a reduction of opsonization and phagocytosis of pneumococci, which is due to the ability of pneumolysin to bind to the Fc region of IgG. Pneumococci can also subvert the biological functions of 'neutrophil extracellular traps' (NETs) produced by granulocytes (von Kockritz-Blickwede and Nizet, 2009), by producing the surface-bound DNase EndA, which destroys the antibacterial properties of NETs. Furthermore, D-alanylation of LTAs incorporates a positive charge into the cell wall, leading to the release of negative antimicrobial peptides.

6.2.4 Invasion of pneumococci into the SAS

To infect the CNS after bacteraemia, pneumococci have to overcome the BBB/BCSFB (Fig. 6.1). In most cases of blood-borne bacterial meningitis, the exact point of entry into the CSF is unknown, but experimental meningitis models and histopathological studies have provided important information. In animal models, Gram-stained pneumococci were found almost exclusively in close proximity to the leptomeninges in the SAS. This identifies the cerebral endothelium, but not the choroid plexus, as the route for pneumococcal entry into the SAS. But how do pneumococci overcome the endothelial barrier? The following strategies are possible: (i) paracellular passage by destruction of tight junctions or damage of endothelial cells; (ii) transcellular passage by active or passive transcytosis; and (iii) entry into the SAS together with or even within leucocytes ('Trojan horse theory').

For pneumococci, the second strategy appears important. The first step is adhesion of pneumococci to cerebral endothelial cells inside the blood vessel through binding to carbohydrates (e.g. GalNAc(β1-4)Gal) (Krivan *et al.*, 1988) and/or the laminin receptor (via PspC) (Orihuela *et al.*, 2009). Further interaction between pathogen and endothelium requires an activation of the endothelial cell, which is – at least in part – mediated by pneumococcal NanA (Banerjee *et al.*, 2010) and leads to enhancement of PAF receptor expression on the cell surface. Normally, when PAF binds to its receptor, the ligand–receptor complex is internalized by the endothelial cell. The PAF receptor also functions as the binding site for the pneumococcal phosphorylcholine and, by analogy to the uptake of PAF, pneumococci are endocytosed into the cell (Cundell *et al.*, 1995). Pneumococci reside in a membrane-bound vacuole and some of the pneumococci die, while others migrate through the endothelial cell into the SAS (Radin *et al.*, 2005).

6.2.5 Pneumococcal survival in the SAS

The normal CSF is characterized by the presence of low numbers of resident immunocompetent cells such as macrophages and dendritic cells and low concentrations of soluble pathogen recognition receptors (PRRs) such as complement or C-reactive protein (CRP). Initially, this constitutive immunodeficiency allows pathogens to proliferate freely in the SAS until, at higher bacterial concentrations, their presence leads to an activation of local immunocompetent cells with a consecutive upregulation and expression of soluble and cellular PRRs (Bottcher *et al.*, 2003; Rupprecht *et al.*, 2007). Subsequent damage to the BBB/BCSFB through host inflammation allows influx of complement factors and antibodies from the blood into the CSF. However, the resulting increase in complement and antibody is unable to sufficiently opsonize and phagocytose all of the rapidly growing bacteria in the CSF and, thus, the host response in the SAS towards bacterial invasion is inadequate.

6.2.6 Mechanisms of immune activation

The key trigger factor of immune activation is detection of pathogen-associated molecular patterns (PAMPs) through PRRs on and in immunocompetent cells. Early experiments in a rabbit model showed that intracisternal injection of the pneumococcal PAMPs peptidoglycan or LTA can lead to a suppurative inflammatory reaction in the CSF (Tuomanen *et al.*, 1985a,b) (Fig. 6.2). In these experiments, the concentration of PAMPs correlated with the degree of the clinical symptoms. In humans with pneumococcal meningitis, there is also a close relationship between high PAMP levels in the CSF and unfavourable outcome (Schneider *et al.*, 1999). The key PRR molecules in pneumococcal meningitis are the Toll-like

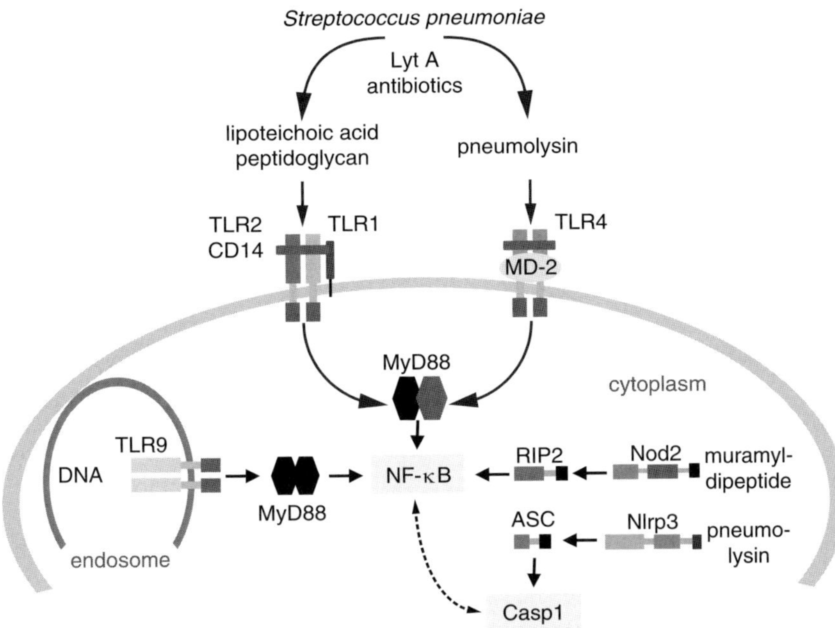

Fig. 6.2. A model for engagement of PRRs by *S. pneumoniae*. See text for details.

receptors (TLRs) and members of the nucleotide-binding oligomerization domain and leucine-rich repeat-containing gene product (NOD)-like receptor (NLR) family.

The involvement of TLRs in the detection of pneumococci by the immune system was shown first by *in vitro* experiments on genetically modified fibroblasts. Fibroblasts that overexpressed TLR2, TLR4 or TLR9 were activated after incubation with pneumococci. TLR2 detects the bacterial cell wall components LTA and peptidoglycan. LTA appears to require an interaction between TLR2, TLR1 and the membrane receptor CD14. TLR9 can be activated by pneumococcal DNA *in vitro*. TLR4 was reported to act as a recognition receptor for pneumolysin *in vitro* and *in vivo* (Malley *et al*., 2003), and the cytokine-inducing activity of pneumolysin on macrophages was described in other experimental studies (Hoegen *et al*., 2011). These findings, however, contrast with data presented by McNeela *et al*. (2010) who demonstrated that pneumolysin by itself exerts no pro-inflammatory effects, but enhances cytokine secretion from dendritic cells and macrophages upon exposure to live bacteria or known TLR ligands in a TLR4-independent manner.

Investigations on isolated macrophages of gene-deficient mice demonstrated that: (i) single deficiency of TLR2, TLR4 or TLR9 did not affect pneumococcal-induced activation of macrophages; (ii) double deficiency of TLR2 and TLR4 was associated with a markedly reduced activation of macrophages; and (iii) macrophages deficient in TLR2, TLR4 and TLR9 were unable to react to pneumococcal stimulation at all. Thus, activation of macrophages by pneumococci requires the concerted action of TLR2, TLR4 and TLR9. However, other PRRs also seem to be involved in the recognition of pneumococci. For example, cells that express NOD2 (but not TLR2, TLR4 and TLR9) can also be stimulated by pneumococci (Klein *et al*., 2008). These *in vitro* results can only partly be transferred to the *in vivo* situation. Experiments using a mouse model of pneumococcal meningitis showed that: (i) genetic deficiency of MyD88, an essential adapter molecule for signalling of all TLRs (except TLR3), was associated with a nearly complete absence of the subarachnoid inflammation; (ii) singular deficiencies of TLR2 or TLR4 did not alter the immune response; and (iii) double deficiency of TLR2 and TLR4 led to a significant reduction of the inflammatory reaction in the SAS. However, a decrease of the immune reaction was not observed in animals with an additional TLR9 deficiency. Thus, NOD2 might be involved in the recognition of pneumococci in the brain. This is supported by the finding that increases of tumour necrosis factor (TNF)-α and the chemokine CCL3 observed in infected wild-type mice were not seen in NOD2-deficient mice after intracerebral infection of animals with pneumococci (Liu *et al.*, 2010). Nevertheless, this observation has to be interpreted carefully as the course of pneumococcal meningitis was not influenced by the genetic lack of RIP2, an essential adapter molecule for NOD1- and NOD2-induced signalling (Hoegen *et al.*, 2011). Thus, TLR9 does not seem to be significant for immune activation during pneumococcal meningitis *in vivo*; the role of NOD2 remains unresolved.

Further *in vivo* experiments revealed the importance of another NOD-like receptor in the recognition of pneumococci in meningitis, namely NLRP3. NLRP3 interacts with the cytoplasmic adapter molecule ASC, which, in turn, is important for the recruitment of pro-caspase 1 into this protein complex. Within the 'NLRP3-inflammasome' multi-protein complex, pro-caspase 1 is transferred into the biologically active cysteine protease caspase-1 that is crucial for the production of active cytokines of the interleukin (IL)-1 family by splicing of their precursor proteins. Activation of NRLP3 can be induced by pneumolysin (McNeela *et al.*, 2010; Witzenrath *et al.*, 2011). Experimental data observed in mice support the relevance of the NRLP3 inflammasome: (i) ASC-, NLRP3- and caspase-1-deficient mice had a markedly diminished immune response in the CSF after intracisternal infection with live pneumococci; (ii) the CSF concentration of IL-1β was lower after challenge of animals with pneumolysin-deficient pneumococci than after challenge with pneumolysin-producing pneumococci; and (iii) pneumolysin was shown to be a highly potent activator of caspase-1 (Hoegen *et al.*, 2011).

Finally, the interaction between pneumococcal PAMPs and TLR molecules leads to a MyD88-dependent activation of the transcription factors NF-κB (Koedel *et al.*, 2000) and AP-1 (Tsuchiya *et al.*, 2007), which regulate the expression of cytokines (e.g. pro-IL-1β), and components of the NLRP3-inflammasome (e.g. NLRP3 and pro-caspase 1) (Koedel *et al.*, 2002a; Nau and Bruck, 2002). As a consequence, invading pneumococci can trigger the activation of caspase-1, which transfers precursor proteins of the IL-1 family into their active form. These cytokines bind to IL-1 family receptors and further activate NF-κB in a MyD88-dependent way, forming a positive feedback loop. This activation of NF-κB seems to be the central engine of the immune response during pneumococcal meningitis: a long-lasting NF-κB activation is observed in the CNS of mice with pneumococcal meningitis and it is found especially in areas of heavy inflammation and along penetrating cortical vessels. Moreover, pharmacological inhibition of NF-κB results in a reduction of the pneumococci-induced cerebral immune activation (Koedel *et al.*, 2000).

6.3 Cytokines in Pneumococcal Meningitis

Immune stimulation through PRRs leads to NF-κB activation and the release of a variety of cytokines and chemokines (Fig. 6.3). LytA (*N*-acetylmuramoyl-L-alanine amidase)-dependent autolysis of the pneumococcus, as well as antibiotic-induced lysis, leads to the release of additional subcapsular bacterial products like LTA, peptidoglycan, muramyl dipeptide and pneumolysin, which further drive and regulate cerebral inflammation.

6.3.1 Inflammatory cytokines

The cytokines IL-1β, IL-18, TNF-α and IL-6 are key mediators for the induction and regulation of acute inflammatory reactions. Notably, they induce the liberation of

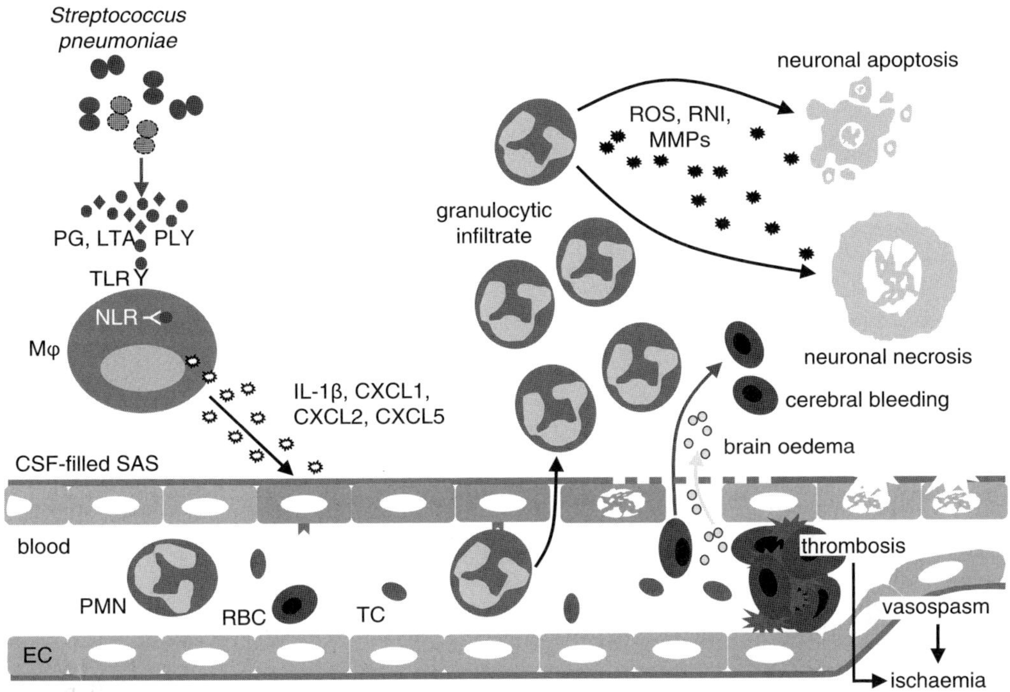

Fig. 6.3. The major pathophysiological steps of pneumococcal meningitis. See text for details. CSF, cerebrospinal fluid-filled SAS, subarachnoid space; PG, peptidoglycan; LTA, lipoteichoic acid; PLY, pneumolysin; Mϕ, macrophages; TLR, Toll-like receptor; NLR, nucleotide-binding domain and leucine-rich repeat containing gene product family receptor; PMN, polymorphonuclear neutrophil; ROS, reactive oxygen species; RNI, reactive nitrogen intermediates; MMP, matrix metalloproteinase; RBC, red blood cell; TC, thrombocyte.

chemokines, reactive oxygen species (ROS) and reactive nitrogen species (RNS), which are all relevant in the immune response during pneumococcal meningitis. These cytokines are produced by cells of the immune system and cells of the CNS, such as cerebrovascular endothelial cells, astrocytes and microglial cells. In CSF samples from patients with acute bacterial meningitis, increased concentrations of IL-1β, IL-6 and TNF-α have been observed (Kastenbauer *et al.*, 2005). The CSF concentrations of IL-1β (but not of IL-6 and TNF-α) correlate with an unfavourable course of the disease (Zwijnenburg *et al.*, 2006). In animal models of pneumococcal meningitis, increases of IL-1β, IL-6 and TNF-α mRNA and protein expression were noted during the acute stage of the disease. To further analyse the function of these cytokines, experiments on genetically deficient mice were undertaken. By genetic depletion of TNF-α or its receptors TNFR1 and TNFR2, the pneumococcal-induced cerebral immune response was only mildly reduced, which did not alter bacterial killing or meningitis-associated brain damage (Wellmer *et al.*, 2001). In infected IL-6-deficient animals, significantly higher levels of IL-1β, TNF-α and the CXC chemokine CXCL-2 were found in the brain as compared with infected wild-type mice. This higher expression of pro-inflammatory proteins was associated with an increase in CSF pleocytosis in IL-6-deficient mice (Paul *et al.*, 2003). However, experiments on the lack of IL-1β in pneumococcal meningitis are missing, but studies on mice with caspase-1 and IL-1 receptor (IL-1R) deficiencies have been published. During experimental pneumococcal meningitis, a significant upregulation of caspase-1 mRNA and protein expression has been observed. This was associated with an increase in IL-1β concentrations in the brain. By genetic depletion of caspase-1, the meningitis-induced increase of IL-1β levels was significantly reduced (Koedel *et al.*, 2002b), which in turn was associated with a decreased inflammatory reaction. Genetic depletion of murine IL-1R1 also decreased cerebral expression of TNF-α and the CXC chemokines CXCL-1 and CXCL-2. Microscopic assessment of the brains of infected animals also showed a reduced inflammatory infiltrate in the SAS of IL-1R1-deficient mice as compared with wild-type mice.

These results show that: (i) TNF-α plays a minor pro-inflammatory role; (ii) IL-6 exerts an anti-inflammatory effect, and (iii) the caspase-1–IL-1β–IL-1R1 signalling pathway is of central importance for the introduction and maintenance of the cerebral immune response during pneumococcal meningitis.

6.3.2 Chemokines

Pro-inflammatory cytokines like IL-1β stimulate the expression of chemokines and adhesion molecules that steer the migration of leucocytes from the bloodstream to the SAS during pneumococcal meningitis. In CSF samples from patients with bacterial meningitis, increased concentrations of CXCL-1, CXCL-5, CXCL-8, CCL-2, CCL-3, CCL-4 and CCL-20 have been observed (Kastenbauer *et al.*, 2005). In the mouse model of pneumococcal meningitis, upregulation of CXC chemokines CXCL-1, CXCL-2 and CXCL-5 was found in the brain during the acute stage of the disease. Furthermore, increased concentrations of other CXCL chemokines (such as CXCL-12 and CXCL-16) and CCL chemokines (such as CCL-2, CCL-9 and CCL-12) were observed as the disease progressed. By intracisternal injection of recombinant CXCL-1 and/or CXCL2, suppurative meningitis could be evoked in rats (Wells *et al.*, 2003). Moreover, pharmacological blockage and genetic depletion of CXCR2, a receptor for CXCL-1 and CXCL-2, as well as neutralization of CXCL-1 and CXCL-2, were associated with a significant reduction of leucocyte influx into the SAS in pneumococcal meningitis (Echchannaoui *et al.*, 2005; Woehrl *et al.*, 2011). These results demonstrate a central role for ELR (glutamic acid-leucine-arginene) CXC chemokines in the recruitment of leucocytes into the SAS during pneumococcal meningitis.

Experiments in mice show that intracisternal inoculation of IL-1β and TNF-α leads to a significant extravasation of polymorphonuclear leucocytes (PMNLs) into the SAS. In mice that lack P-selectin, the cytokine-induced pleocytosis was diminished, as compared with wild-type mice. Mice lacking P-selectin and E-selectin did not develop inflammation in the SAS. Furthermore, in rabbits and rats with pneumococcal meningitis, treatment with the selectin blocker fucoidin and antibodies against MAC-1 or ICAM-1 significantly reduced inflammation in the CSF (Granert *et al.*, 1998, 1999). Inhibition of the leucocyte–endothelium interaction was associated with a reduction of intracranial complications and tissue damage. Other studies have shown that depletion of PMNLs could reduce meningitis-associated brain damage (Hoffmann *et al.*, 2007; Koedel *et al.*, 2009). Thus, PMNLs that migrate to the SAS seem to be crucial in the development of brain damage during pneumococcal meningitis.

6.4 Mediators of Brain Damage During Pneumococcal Meningitis

Activated leucocytes produce and secrete a large arsenal of potentially cytotoxic agents (Fig. 6.3). During the last two decades, numerous studies have been published on the importance of ROS, RNS and matrix metalloproteinases (MMPs) as potential effector molecules during the development of meningitis-associated tissue damage.

6.4.1 MMPs

MMPs are zinc-dependent endopeptidases that degrade extracellular matrix proteins during tissue reconstruction under physiological conditions. Extracellular matrix proteins such as collagen IV and fibronectin are essential components of the subendothelial basal lamina of cerebral blood vessels and contribute significantly to the integrity of the BBB/BCSFB. Thus, the observation that intracerebral injection of MMPs leads to damage of the BBB is not surprising. Furthermore, PMNLs are known to use their MMPs to cross the subendothelial basal lamina.

In CSF samples of patients with bacterial meningitis, increased concentrations of MMP-8 and MMP-9 were detected. An association was found between a high MMP-9 concentration in the CSF and disruption of the BBB/BCSFB and the development of neurological sequelae (Leppert *et al.*, 2001). Similarly, in animal models of pneumococcal meningitis, upregulation of MMP-3, -7, -8 and -9 has been reported. Treatment of animals with MMP inhibitors significantly decreased meningitis-associated intracranial complications, such as BBB/BCSFB damage, and improved the clinical course of the disease: mortality and the frequency of neurological sequelae, such as cognitive deficits, were reduced (Leib *et al.*, 2001). Overall, the studies support the concept of a central role of MMPs (especially MMP-9) during meningitis-associated brain damage.

6.4.2 ROS and RNS

ROS and RNS play a central role in the pathophysiology and neuropathology of pneumococcal meningitis (Klein *et al.*, 2006a). *In vitro*, PMNLs, microglial cells and cerebral endothelial cells (but not astrocytes and neurons) produce superoxide radicals after exposure to pneumococci. Immunohistochemical analysis of rat brains with pneumococcal meningitis showed signs of ROS production, mainly within the inflammatory infiltrate and along penetrating cortical vessels. Nitric oxide (NO) is derived from the conversion of L-arginine to L-citrulline by NO synthase (NOS). At present, three different forms of NOS have been identified: the neuronal NOS (nNOS) and the endothelial NOS (eNOS), which are both expressed constitutively, and the inducible NOS (iNOS). In CSF samples from patients with bacterial meningitis, increased levels of nitrite and nitrate (stable metabolites of NO) have been measured. In addition, cell culture experiments have shown that microglial cells, astrocytes and endothelial cells produce increased amounts of NO after stimulation with pneumococcal cell-wall components. Furthermore, animal experiments using various NOS inhibitors, given in the early and late stages of infection, have underscored the importance of NO during pneumococcal meningitis. When given during the early stage of infection, inhibition of NOS leads to a reduction of meningeal inflammation and pathophysiological alterations. However, when given during later stages of the disease, the results vary from an anti-inflammatory and neuroprotective effect to an increase of cerebral hypoperfusion and neuronal damage. These contrary results might be due to problems with specificity, side effects and bioavailability of inhibitors of the different NOS isoforms. The varying roles can be studied by using animals that lack single NOS isoforms. In experimental pneumococcal meningitis, the lack of iNOS led to a significant reduction of the expression of pro-inflammatory mediators (Winkler *et al.*, 2001). This anti-inflammatory effect was associated with a significant reduction of meningitis-associated BBB damage. In contrast, eNOS-deficient mice with pneumococcal meningitis developed an increase in cerebral inflammation and intracranial complications (Koedel *et al.*, 2001). Thus, the functional role of NO in bacterial meningitis seems dependent on the site of production. While NO that is produced by iNOS seems to mediate pro-inflammatory and cytotoxic effects, NO production by eNOS has anti-inflammatory and neuroprotective effects.

The reaction of ROS and NO generates the strong oxidant peroxynitrite ($ONOO^-$). High concentrations of nitrotyrosine, a footprint and marker of peroxynitrite, are associated with an unfavourable clinical outcome. Increased concentrations of nitrotyrosine were found in the CSF of patients with pneumococcal meningitis, localized to the inflammatory infiltrate in the SAS and along penetrating cortical vessels (Kastenbauer *et al.*, 2002). Experimental studies showed an identical staining pattern for nitrotyrosine. Functionally, treatment with peroxynitrite scavengers (e.g. MnTBAP and uric acid) not only decreased the production of nitrotyrosine but also reduced meningitis-associated intracranial and cochlear complications and tissue damage (Kastenbauer *et al.*, 2001; Klein *et al.*, 2003).

ROS and RNS such as peroxynitrite can be cytotoxic through multiple independent mechanisms (Pacher *et al.*, 2007). Cytotoxic effects include inactivation of several enzymes (especially of the mitochondrial respiratory chain), damage to ion transporters and the induction of lipid peroxidation. ROS can attack unsaturated lipid acids by initiating lipid peroxidation, which leads to the loss of membrane function and integrity and finally cell death. In CSF samples of patients with bacterial meningitis (but not in the CSF of control patients), an increased concentration of malondialdehyde (MDA) and 4-hydroxynonenal (4-HNE) – the reaction products of lipid peroxidation – was detected. In concordance, an increase of these markers was also noted in the brain of animals with experimental bacterial meningitis. Using immunohistochemistry, MDA and 4-HNE were found in the inflammatory infiltrate of the brain and along penetrating cortical vessels of patients and mice suffering from pneumococcal meningitis (Schaper *et al.*, 2002). This staining pattern corresponds to the nitrotyrosine staining pattern. Furthermore, treatment with the inhibitor of lipid peroxidation U74389F leads to a significant reduction of meningitis-associated intracranial complications in rats (Lorenzl *et al.*, 1995). Thus, peroxynitrite-induced lipid peroxidation appears to be important in the development of meningitis-associated tissue damage.

Another mechanism of oxidant cytotoxicity is the induction of DNA single-strand breaks with a consecutive activation of the nuclear enzyme poly-(ADP-ribose)-polymerase (PARP). Experimental studies have shown that: (i) intense PARP activation and consecutive cellular energy depletion plays an essential role during endothelial cell death evoked by pneumococci *in vitro*; (ii) PARP is activated in the brains of mice with pneumococcal meningitis; and (iii) genetic PARP deficiency and pharmacological inhibition of PARP reduces the cerebral immune reaction and intracranial complications in pneumococcal meningitis (Koedel *et al.*, 2002c).

6.5 Neuropathology of Pneumococcal Meningitis

The usual findings in brains of patients who have died from pneumococcal meningitis are the typical suppurative infiltrate in the (leptomeningeal) SAS and a variety of cerebrovascular and intraparenchymatose alterations (Dodge and Swartz, 1965; Nau *et al.*, 1999, 2004). During the acute stage, swollen endothelial cells and subintimal infiltrates of PMNLs can be seen in the region of small and mid-sized arteries and veins. Later during the disease, a diffuse inflammation of the whole vessel wall with focal necrosis and small thrombi can present. Finally, arteriitis with perivascular bleeding and occlusion of the vessel volumes are frequently present. In the brain parenchyma, especially in superficial layers of the cortex, an infiltrate of PMNLs, reactive astrocytosis and activation of microglia are observed. Furthermore, neuronal death is described in affected regions of the cortex that is attributed mainly to ischaemia. Similarly, in infected adult rats, areas of necrosis with a vascular pattern can be found in the cortex, and vasculitis of small cerebral vessels, cerebral haemorrhages and abscess formation are common. Similar results were obtained in adult mice with experimental meningitis (Gerber *et al.*, 2001; Klein *et al.*, 2006b). The development of such complications is dependent on the causative pneumococcal strain that is being used for the induction of experimental meningitis (Ostergaard *et al.*, 2004). Furthermore, in a rabbit model of pneumococcal meningitis, neuronal apoptosis was regularly observed in the dentate gyrus as early as 24 h after infection (Braun *et al.*, 1999). Neuronal apoptosis in the dentate gyrus is also found in infant rats with pneumococcal meningitis (Leib and Tauber, 1999). However, the degree of apoptotic brain injury is less severe in infant rats than in rabbits. The infant rat model also shows focal necrosis of cortical neurons on the basis of vasculitis. In an infant mouse model of pneumococcal meningitis, the incidence of hippocampal apoptosis and cortical necrosis was considerably lower than in infant rats and also differed between mouse strains (Grandgirard *et al.*, 2007). In adult rat and mouse models, apoptotic neurons in the dentate gyrus are found only occasionally and in low numbers (Klein *et al.*, 2006b). The heterogeneity in brain pathology may be related to differences in: (i) the vulnerability to brain injury among different species, strains and age groups; as well as (ii) the neuropathogenicity of different bacterial strains/serotypes.

Another important hallmark of brains from patients with meningitis and in animal models is ventricle enlargement and brain swelling (Klein *et al.*, 2006b). These pathological findings correlate with the most common acute intracranial complications found during pneumococcal meningitis, namely ischaemic stroke, venous thrombosis, hydrocephalus and brain oedema (Klein *et al.*, 2009).

6.6 Novel Treatment Strategies for Pneumococcal Meningitis

Studying the underlying mechanisms that lead to intracranial complications during pneumococcal meningitis allows the development of new adjunctive therapies. The main tenet for these treatment strategies is to reduce CNS inflammation by interfering at different steps of the inflammation cascade with the following.

6.6.1 Non-bacteriolytic antibiotics

During conventional treatment of pneumococcal meningitis with β-lactam antibiotics, large amounts of pneumococcal cell wall components and pneumolysin are liberated into the CSF. Consequently, the immune response is boosted (inflammatory burst) leading to an initial worsening of the disease. Use of the non-bacteriolytic antibiotics rifampicin and daptomycin has been shown to reduce CSF inflammation and improve clinical outcome in animal models of pneumococcal meningitis (Grandgirard *et al.*, 2010). Neither daptomycin nor rifampicin can be recommended as monotherapy in pneumococcal meningitis (daptomycin lacking efficacy against pneumococcal meningitis and rifampicin leading to rapid resistance). However, a combination therapy of ceftriaxone and daptomycin or rifampicin might be of interest, but clinical studies on both treatment strategies are still lacking.

6.6.2 Inhibition of pro-inflammatory cytokine release

Genetic depletion of caspase-1 and pharmacological inhibition of the IL-1 receptor significantly decreased brain inflammation and improved outcome in a mouse model of pneumococcal meningitis (Hoegen *et al.*, 2011). However, data on the long-term effects in a clinically relevant mouse model are still missing, as are human data.

6.6.3 Reducing the burden of ROS, RNS and MMPs

Detoxification of ROS and RNS by administration of the strong antioxidant and radical scavenger acetylcysteine reduced meningitis-associated CNS complications (e.g. cerebral hypoperfusion and brain oedema) and neuronal damage in rats and improved pneumococcal meningitis-associated hearing loss (Auer *et al.*, 2000; Christen *et al.*, 2001; Klein *et al.*, 2003). This is important because hearing loss is the most common long-term sequelae of pneumococcal meningitis. The advantage of this treatment strategy is direct activity against the effector molecules that mediate collateral damage. However, the experimental benefit of an adjunctive antioxidant therapy that actually translates into a clinical benefit in humans has yet to be determined. Inhibition of MMPs during meningitis also seems an interesting, albeit not yet wholly evaluated, approach to improve the prognosis of pneumococcal meningitis. However, administration of the MMP inhibitor and antibiotic doxycycline has led to both beneficial and harmful effects in pneumococcal meningitis (Meli *et al.*, 2006). In contrast, data on several MMP inhibitors that inhibit a variety of convertases protected the hippocampus from apoptotic damage and improved long-term outcome in infant rats with pneumococcal meningitis (Leib *et al.*, 2001; Meli *et al.*, 2004).

6.6.4 Accelerating the resolution of inflammation

Many intracranial complications of pneumococcal meningitis occur after therapy has already been initiated, and the long lifespan of PMNLs in the CSF during infection contributes to this phenomenon. In a mouse model of pneumococcal meningitis, reduction of this PMNL lifespan by adjunctive therapy with roscovitine significantly reduced CSF pleocytosis, mortality and brain damage (Koedel *et al.*, 2009). Roscovitine inhibits cyclin-dependent kinases and, thus, enhances resolution of inflammation by promoting PMNL apoptosis. However, clinical data on the effects of roscovitine in pneumococcal meningitis do not exist.

6.7 Conclusions

During the past two decades, most data on the pathophysiological mechanisms of meningitis have been obtained in models of pneumococcal meningitis. As outlined in this chapter, these data have been summarized in a pathophysiological concept. Using this concept, several novel treatment strategies have been developed and the first results from experimental studies are promising. However, we must accept that humans with pneumococcal meningitis are severely ill and patient numbers are limited. Thus, a thorough examination and comparison of single agents in clinically relevant animal models needs to be done before such drugs can be taken into clinical trials and eventually recommended for treatment of humans with pneumococcal meningitis.

References

Agarwal, V. and Hammerschmidt, S. (2009) Cdc42 and the phosphatidylinositol 3-kinase-Akt pathway are essential for PspC-mediated internalization of pneumococci by respiratory epithelial cells. *Journal of Biological Chemistry* 284, 19427–19436.

Auer, M., Pfister, L.A., Leppert, D., Tauber, M.G. and Leib, S.L. (2000) Effects of clinically used antioxidants in experimental pneumococcal meningitis. *Journal of Infectious Diseases* 182, 347–350.

Bagnoli, F., *et al.* (2008) A second pilus type in *Streptococcus pneumoniae* is prevalent in emerging serotypes and mediates adhesion to host cells. *Journal of Bacteriology* 190, 5480–5492.

Banerjee, A., van Sorge, N.M., Sheen, T.R., Uchiyama, S., Mitchell, T.J. and Doran, K.S. (2010) Activation of brain endothelium by pneumococcal neuraminidase NanA promotes bacterial internalization. *Cellular Microbiology* 12, 1576–1588.

Bergmann, S., Wild, D., Diekmann, O., Frank, R., Bracht, D., Chhatwal, G.S. and Hammerschmidt, S. (2003) Identification of a novel plasmin(ogen)-binding motif in surface displayed α-enolase of *Streptococcus pneumoniae*. *Molecular Microbiology* 49, 411–423.

Bottcher, T., von Mering, M., Ebert, S., Meyding-Lamade, U., Kuhnt, U., Gerber, J. and Nau, R. (2003) Differential regulation of Toll-like receptor mRNAs in experimental murine central nervous system infections. *Neuroscience Letters* 344, 17–20.

Braun, J.S., Novak, R., Herzog, K.H., Bodner, S.M., Cleveland, J.L. and Tuomanen, E.I. (1999) Neuroprotection by a caspase inhibitor in acute bacterial meningitis. *Nature Medicine* 5, 298–302.

Brouwer, M.C., Tunkel, A.R. and van de Beek, D. (2010) Epidemiology, diagnosis, and antimicrobial treatment of acute bacterial meningitis. *Clinical Microbiology Reviews* 23, 467–492.

Christen, S., Schaper, M., Lykkesfeldt, J., Siegenthaler, C., Bifrare, Y.D., Banic, S., Leib, S.L. and Tauber, M.G. (2001) Oxidative stress in brain during experimental bacterial meningitis: Differential effects of α-phenyl-tert-butyl nitrone and *N*-acetylcysteine treatment. *Free Radical Biology and Medicine* 31, 754–762.

Cundell, D.R., Gerard, N.P., Gerard, C., Idanpaan-Heikkila, I. and Tuomanen, E.I. (1995) *Streptococcus pneumoniae* anchor to activated human cells by the receptor for platelet-activating factor. *Nature* 377, 435–438.

Dalia, A.B., Standish, A.J. and Weiser, J.N. (2010) Three surface exoglycosidases from *Streptococcus pneumoniae*, NanA, BgaA, and StrH, promote resistance to opsonophagocytic killing by human neutrophils. *Infection and Immunity* 78, 2108–2116.

Dodge, P.R. and Swartz, M.N. (1965) Bacterial meningitis: a review of selected aspects. II. Special neurologic problems, postmeningitic complications and clinicopathologlcal correlations (concluded). *New England Journal of Medicine* 272, 1003–1010.

Durand, M.L., Calderwood, S.B., Weber, D.J., Miller, S.I., Southwick, F.S., Caviness, V.S. and Swartz, M.N. (1993) Acute bacterial meningitis in adults – a review of 493 episodes. *New England Journal of Medicine* 328, 21–28.

Echchannaoui, H., Frei, K., Letiembre, M., Strieter, R.M., Adachi, Y. and Landmann, R. (2005) CD14 deficiency leads to increased MIP-2 production, CXCR2 expression, neutrophil transmigration, and early death in pneumococcal infection. *Journal of Leukocyte Biology* 78, 705–715.

Elm, C., Braathen, R., Bergmann, S., Frank, R., Vaerman, J.P., Kaetzel, C.S., Chhatwal, G.S., Johansen, F.E. and Hammerschmidt, S. (2004) Ectodomains 3 and 4 of human polymeric immunoglobulin receptor (hpIgR) mediate invasion of *Streptococcus pneumoniae* into the epithelium. *Journal of Biological Chemistry* 279, 6296–6304.

Gamez, G. and Hammerschmidt, S. (2012) Combat pneumococcal infections: adhesins as candidates for protein-based vaccine development. *Current Drug Targets* 13, 323–337.

Gerber, J., Raivich, G., Wellmer, A., Noeske, C., Kunst, T., Werner, A., Bruck, W. and Nau, R. (2001) A mouse model of *Streptococcus pneumoniae* meningitis mimicking several features of human disease. *Acta Neuropathologica* 101, 499–508.

Grandgirard, D., Steiner, O., Taeuber, M.G. and Leib, S.L. (2007) An infant mouse model of brain damage in pneumococcal meningitis. *Acta Neuropathologica* 114, 609–617.

Grandgirard, D., Burri, M. and Oberson, K., Buhlmann, A., Simon, F. and Leib, S.L. (2010) In infant rat pneumococcal meningitis, ceftriaxone plus daptomycin versus ceftriaxone attenuates brain damage and hearing loss while ceftriaxone plus rifampicin does not. In: *19th European Congress of Clinical Mircrobiology and Infectious Diseases*, 16–19 May 2009, Helsinki, Finland. Abstract O381.

Granert, C., Raud, J. and Lindquist, L. (1998) The polysaccharide fucoidin inhibits the antibiotic-induced inflammatory cascade in experimental pneumococcal meningitis. *Clinical and Diagnostic Laboratory Immunology* 5, 322–324.

Granert, C., Raud, J., Waage, A. and Lindquist, L. (1999) Effects of polysaccharide fucoidin on cerebrospinal fluid interleukin-1 and tumor necrosis factor alpha in pneumococcal meningitis in the rabbit. *Infection and Immunity* 67, 2071–2074.

Hammerschmidt, S. (2006) Adherence molecules of pathogenic pneumococci. *Current Opinion in Microbiology* 9, 12–20.

Hoegen, T., Tremel, N., Klein, M., Angele, B., Wagner, H., Kirschning, C., Pfister, H.W., Fontana, A., Hammerschmidt, S. and Koedel, U. (2011) The NLRP3 inflammasome contributes to brain injury in pneumococcal meningitis and is activated through ATP-dependent lysosomal cathepsin B release. *Journal of Immunology* 187, 5440–5451.

Hoffmann, O., Priller, J., Prozorovski, T., Schulze-Topphoff, U., Baeva, N., Lunemann, J.D., Aktas, O., Mahrhofer, C., Stricker, S., Zipp, F. and Weber, J.R. (2007) TRAIL limits excessive host immune responses in bacterial meningitis. *Journal of Clinical Investigation* 117, 2004–2013.

Holmes, A.R., McNab, R., Millsap, K.W., Rohde, M., Hammerschmidt, S., Mawdsley, J.L. and Jenkinson, H.F. (2001) The *pavA* gene of *Streptococcus pneumoniae* encodes a fibronectin-binding protein that is essential for virulence. *Molecular Microbiology* 41, 1395–1408.

Jensch, I., Gamez, G., Rothe, M., Ebert, S., Fulde, M., Somplatzki, D., Bergmann, S., Petruschka, L., Rohde, M., Nau, R. and Hammerschmidt, S. (2010) PavB is a surface-exposed adhesin of *Streptococcus pneumoniae* contributing to nasopharyngeal colonization and airways infections. *Molecular Microbiology* 77, 22–43.

Kadioglu, A., Brewin, H., Haertel, T., Brittan, J., Klein, M., Hammerschmidt, S. and Jenkinson, H. (2010) Pneumococcal protein PavA is important for nasopharyngeal carriage and development of sepsis. *Molecular Oral Microbiology* 25, 50–60.

Kastenbauer, S. and Pfister, H.W. (2003) Pneumococcal meningitis in adults – spectrum of complications and prognostic factors in a series of 87 cases. *Brain* 126, 1015–1025.

Kastenbauer, S., Koedel, U., Becker, B.F. and Pfister, H.W. (2001) Experimental meningitis in the rat: protection by uric acid at human physiological blood concentrations. *European Journal of Pharmacology* 425, 149–152.

Kastenbauer, S., Koedel, U., Becker, B.F. and Pfister, H.W. (2002) Oxidative stress in bacterial meningitis in humans. *Neurology* 58, 186–191.

Kastenbauer, S., Angele, B., Sporer, B., Pfister, H.W. and Koedel, U. (2005) Patterns of protein expression in infectious meningitis: a cerebrospinal fluid protein array analysis. *Journal of Neuroimmunology* 164, 134–139.

Kirby, A.C., Coles, M.C. and Kaye, P.M. (2009) Alveolar macrophages transport pathogens to lung draining lymph nodes. *Journal of Immunology* 183, 1983–1989.

Klein, M., Koedel, U., Pfister, H.W. and Kastenbauer, S. (2003) Meningitis-associated hearing loss: protection by adjunctive antioxidant therapy. *Annals of Neurology* 54, 451–458.

Klein, M., Koedel, U. and Pfister, H.W. (2006a) Oxidative stress in pneumococcal meningitis: a future target for adjunctive therapy? *Progress in Neurobiology* 80, 269–280.

Klein, M., Paul, R., Angele, B., Popp, B., Pfister, H.W. and Koedel, U. (2006b) Protein expression pattern in experimental pneumococcal meningitis. *Microbes and Infection* 8, 974–983.

Klein, M., Obermaier, B., Angele, B., Pfister, H.W., Wagner, H., Koedel, U. and Kirschning, C.J. (2008) Innate immunity to pneumococcal infection of the central nervous system depends on Toll-like receptor (TLR) 2 and TLR4. *Journal of Infectious Diseases* 198, 1028–1036.

Klein, M., Pfister, H., Leib, S. and Koedel, U. (2009) Therapy of community-acquired acute bacterial meningitis: the clock is running. *Expert Opinion on Pharmacotherapy* 10, 2609–2623.

Koedel, U., Bayerlein, I., Paul, R., Sporer, B. and Pfister, H.W. (2000) Pharmacologic interference with NF-κB activation attenuates central nervous system complications in experimental pneumococcal meningitis. *Journal of Infectious Diseases* 182, 1437–1445.

Koedel, U., Paul, R., Winkler, F., Kastenbauer, S., Huang, P.L. and Pfister, H.W. (2001) Lack of endothelial nitric oxide synthase aggravates murine pneumococcal meningitis. *Journal of Neuropathology and Experimental Neurology* 60, 1041–1050.

Koedel, U., Scheld, W.M. and Pfister, H.W. (2002a) Pathogenesis and pathophysiology of pneumococcal meningitis. *Lancet Infectious Diseases* 2, 721–736.

Koedel, U., Winkler, F., Angele, B., Fontana, A., Flavell, R.A. and Pfister, H.W. (2002b) Role of caspase-1 in experimental pneumococcal meningitis: evidence from pharmacologic caspase inhibition and caspase-1-deficient mice. *Annals of Neurology* 51, 319–329.

Koedel, U., Winkler, F., Angele, B., Fontana, T. and Pfister, H.W. (2002c) Meningitis-associated central nervous system complications are mediated by the activation of poly(ADP-ribose) polymerase. *Journal of Cerebral Blood Flow and Metabolism* 22, 39–49.

Koedel, U., Frankenberg, T., Kirschnek, S., Obermaier, B., Hacker, H., Paul, R. and Hacker, G. (2009) Apoptosis is essential for neutrophil functional shutdown and determines tissue damage in experimental pneumococcal meningitis. *PLoS Pathogens* 5, e1000461.

Krivan, H.C., Roberts, D.D. and Ginsburg, V. (1988) Many pulmonary pathogenic bacteria bind specifically to the carbohydrate sequence Galnac-β-1-4Gal found in some glycolipids. *Proceedings of the National Academy of Sciences USA* 85, 6157–6161.

Leib, S.L. and Tauber, M.G. (1999) Pathogenesis of bacterial meningitis. *Infectious Disease Clinics of North America* 13, 527–548.

Leib, S.L., Clements, J.M., Lindberg, R.L.P., Heimgartner, C., Loeffler, J.M., Pfister, L.A., Tauber, M.G. and Leppert, D. (2001) Inhibition of matrix metalloproteinases and tumour necrosis factor α converting enzyme as adjuvant therapy in pneumococcal meningitis. *Brain* 124, 1734–1742.

LeMieux, J., Hava, D.L., Basset, A. and Camilli, A. (2006) RrgA and RrgB are components of a multisubunit pilus encoded by the *Streptococcus pneumoniae* rlrA pathogenicity islet. *Infection and Immunity* 74, 2453–2456.

Leppert, D., Lindberg, R.L.P., Kappos, L. and Leib, S.L. (2001) Matrix metalloproteinases: multifunctional effectors of inflammation in multiple sclerosis and bacterial meningitis. *Brain Research Reviews* 36, 249–257.

Liu, X., Chauhan, V.S., Young, A.B. and Marriott, I. (2010) NOD2 mediates inflammatory responses of primary murine glia to *Streptococcus pneumoniae*. *Glia* 58, 839–847.

Lorenzl, S., Koedel, U., Frei, K., Bernatowicz, A., Fontana, A. and Pfister, H.W. (1995) Protective effect of a 21-aminosteroid during experimental pneumococcal meningitis. *Journal of Infectious Diseases* 172, 113–118.

Malley, R., Henneke, P., Morse, S.C., Cieslewicz, M.J., Lipsitch, M., Thompson, C.M., Kurt-Jones, E., Paton, J.C., Wessels, M.R. and Golenbock, D.T. (2003) Recognition of pneumolysin by Toll-like receptor 4 confers resistance to pneumococcal infection. *Proceedings of the National Academy of Sciences USA* 100, 1966–1971.

McNeela, E.A., *et al.* (2010) Pneumolysin activates the NLRP3 inflammasome and promotes proinflammatory cytokines independently of TLR4. *PLoS Pathogens* 6, e1001191.

Meli, D.N., Loeffler, J.M., Baumann, P., Neumann, U., Buhl, T., Leppert, D. and Leib, S.L. (2004) In pneumococcal meningitis a novel water-soluble inhibitor of matrix metalloproteinases and TNF-α converting enzyme attenuates seizures and injury of the cerebral cortex. *Journal of Neuroimmunology* 151, 6–11.

Meli, D.N., Coimbra, R.S., Erhart, D.G., Loquet, G., Bellac, C.L., Tauber, M.G., Neumann, U. and Leib, S.L. (2006) Doxycycline reduces mortality and injury to the brain and cochlea in experimental pneumococcal meningitis. *Infection and Immunity* 74, 3890–3896.

Nau, R. and Bruck, W. (2002) Neuronal injury in bacterial meningitis: mechanisms and implications for therapy. *Trends in Neurosciences* 25, 38–45.

Nau, R., Soto, A. and Bruck, W. (1999) Apoptosis of neurons in the dentate gyrus in humans suffering from bacterial meningitis. *Journal of Neuropathology and Experimental Neurology* 58, 265–274.

Nau, R., Gerber, J., Bunkowski, S. and Bruck, W. (2004) Axonal injury, a neglected cause of CNS damage in bacterial meningitis. *Neurology* 62, 509–511.

Noske, N., Kaemmerer, U., Rohde, M. and Hammerschmidt, S. (2009) Pneumococcal interaction with human dendritic cells: phagocytosis, survival, and induced adaptive immune response are manipulated by PavA. *Journal of Immunology* 183, 1952–1963.

Orihuela, C.J., Mahdavi, J., Thornton, J., Mann, B., Wooldridge, K.G., Abouseada, N., Oldfield, N.J., Self, T., Ala'Aldeen, D.A. and Tuomaneni, E.I. (2009) Laminin receptor initiates bacterial contact with the blood brain barrier in experimental meningitis models. *Journal of Clinical Investigation* 119, 1638–1646.

Ostergaard, C., Brandt, C., Konradsen, H.B. and Samuelsson, S. (2004) Differences in survival, brain damage, and cerebrospinal fluid cytokine kinetics due to meningitis caused by 3 different *Streptococcus pneumoniae* serotypes: evaluation in humans and in 2 experimental models. *Journal of Infectious Diseases* 190, 1212–1220.

Pacher, P., Beckman, J.S. and Liaudet, L. (2007) Nitric oxide and peroxynitrite in health and disease. *Physiological Reviews* 87, 315–424.

Paul, R., Koedel, U., Winkler, F., Kieseier, B.C., Fontana, A., Kopf, M., Hartung, H.P. and Pfister, H.W. (2003) Lack of IL-6 augments inflammatory response but decreases vascular permeability in bacterial meningitis. *Brain* 126, 1873–1882.

Pracht, D., Elm, C., Gerber, J., Bergmann, S., Rohde, M., Seiler, M., Kim, K.S., Jenkinson, H.F., Nau, R. and Hammerschmidt, S. (2005) PavA of *Streptococcus pneumoniae* modulates adherence, invasion, and meningeal inflammation. *Infection and Immunity* 73, 2680–2689.

Radin, J.N., Orihuela, C.J., Murti, G., Guglielmo, C., Murray, P.J. and Tuomanen, E.I. (2005) β-arrestin 1 participates in platelet-activating factor receptor-mediated endocytosis of *Streptococcus pneumoniae*. *Infection and Immunity* 73, 7827–7835.

Rupprecht, T.A., Angele, B., Klein, M., Heesemann, J., Pfister, H.W., Botto, M. and Koedel, U. (2007) Complement C1q and C3 are critical for the innate immune response to *Streptococcus pneumoniae* in the central nervous system. *Journal of Immunology* 178, 1861–1869.

Schaper, M., Gergely, S., Lykkesfeldt, J., Zbaren, J., Leib, S.L., Tauber, M.G. and Christen, S. (2002) Cerebral vasculature is the major target of oxidative protein alterations in bacterial meningitis. *Journal of Neuropathology and Experimental Neurology* 61, 605–613.

Schneider, O., Michel, U., Zysk, G., Dubuis, O. and Nau, R. (1999) Clinical outcome in pneumococcal meningitis correlates with CSF lipoteichoic acid concentrations. *Neurology* 53, 1584–1587.

Shivshankar, P., Sanchez, C., Rose, L.F. and Orihuela, C.J. (2009) The *Streptococcus pneumoniae* adhesin PsrP binds to Keratin 10 on lung cells. *Molecular Microbiology* 73, 663–679.

Steinfort, C., Wilson, R., Mitchell, T., Feldman, C., Rutman, A., Todd, H., Sykes, D., Walker, J., Saunders, K., Andrew, P.W., Boulnois, G.J. and Cole, P.J. (1989) Effect of *Streptococcus pneumoniae* on human respiratory epithelium in vitro. *Infection and Immunity* 57, 2006–2013.

Thigpen, M.C., *et al.* (2011) Bacterial meningitis in the United States, 1998–2007. *New England Journal of Medicine* 364, 2016–2025.

Tsuchiya, K., Toyama, K., Tsuprun, V., Hamajima, Y., Kim, Y., Ondrey, F.G. and Lin, J. (2007) Pneumococcal peptidoglycan-polysaccharides induce the expression of interleukin-8 in airway epithelial cells by way of nuclear factor-κB, nuclear factor interleukin-6, or activation protein-1 dependent mechanisms. *Laryngoscope* 117, 86–91.

Tuomanen, E. (1999) Molecular and cellular biology of pneumococcal infection. *Current Opinion in Microbiology* 2, 35–39.

Tuomanen, E., Liu, H., Hengstler, B., Zak, O. and Tomasz, A. (1985a) The induction of meningeal inflammation by components of the pneumococcal cell wall. *Journal of Infectious Diseases* 151, 859–868.

Tuomanen, E., Tomasz, A., Hengstler, B. and Zak, O. (1985b) The relative role of bacterial cell wall and capsule in the induction of inflammation in pneumococcal meningitis. *Journal of Infectious Diseases* 151, 535–540.

van de Beek, D., *et al.* (2010) Adjunctive dexamethasone in bacterial meningitis: a meta-analysis of individual patient data. *Lancet Neurology* 9, 254–263.

von Kockritz-Blickwede, M. and Nizet, V. (2009) Innate immunity turned inside-out: antimicrobial defense by phagocyte extracellular traps. *Journal of Molecular Medicine* 87, 775–783.

Voss, S., Gamez, G. and Hammerschmidt, S. (2012) Impact of pneumococcal microbial surface components recognizing adhesive matrix molecules on colonization. *Molecular Oral Microbiology* 27, 246–256.

Wellmer, A., Gerber, J., Ragheb, J., Zysk, G., Kunst, T., Smirnov, A., Bruck, W. and Nau, R. (2001) Effect of deficiency of tumor necrosis factor alpha or both of its receptors on *Streptococcus pneumoniae* central nervous system infection and peritonitis. *Infection and Immunity* 69, 6881–6886.

Wells, C.A., Ravasi, T., Faulkner, G.J., Carninci, P., Okazaki, Y., Hayashizaki, Y., Sweet, M., Wainwright, B.J. and Hume, D.A. (2003) Genetic control of the innate immune response. *BMC Immunology* 4, 5.

Winkler, F., Koedel, U., Kastenbauer, S. and Pfister, H.W. (2001) Differential expression of nitric oxide synthases in bacterial meningitis: role of the inducible isoform for blood–brain barrier breakdown. *Journal of Infectious Diseases* 183, 1749–1759.

Witzenrath, M., *et al.* (2011) The NLRP3 inflammasome is differentially activated by pneumolysin variants and contributes to host defense in pneumococcal pneumonia. *Journal of Immunology* 187, 434–440.

Woehrl, B., Brouwer, M.C., Murr, C., Heckenberg, S.G., Baas, F., Pfister, H.W., Zwinderman, A.H., Morgan, B., Barnum, S.R., van der Ende, A., Koedel, U. and van de Beek, D. (2011) Complement component 5 contributes to poor disease outcome in humans and mice with pneumococcal meningitis. *Journal of Clinical Investigation* 121, 3943–3953.

Zwijnenburg, P.J., van der Poll, T., Florquin, S., van Deventer, S.J., Roord, J.J. and Van Furth, A.M. (2001) Experimental pneumococcal meningitis in mice: a model of intranasal infection. *Journal of Infectious Diseases* 183, 1143–1146.

Zwijnenburg, P.J.G., van der Poll, T., Roord, J.J. and van Furth, A.M. (2006) Chemotactic factors in cerebrospinal fluid during bacterial meningitis. *Infection and Immunity* 74, 1445–1451.

Zysk, G., Schneider-Wald, B.K., Hwang, J.H., Bejo, L., Kim, K.S., Mitchell, T.J., Hakenbeck, R. and Heinz, H.P. (2001) Pneumolysin is the main inducer of cytotoxicity to brain microvascular endothelial cells caused by *Streptococcus pneumoniae*. *Infection and Immunity* 69, 845–852.

7 *Haemophilus influenzae* Meningitis

Darryl J. Hill[1] and Myron Christodoulides[2]*
[1]*School of Cellular and Molecular Medicine, University of Bristol, Bristol, UK;*
[2]*University of Southampton Faculty of Medicine, Southampton General Hospital, Southampton, UK*

7.1 Introduction

Historically, isolates of *Haemophilus influenzae* (Hi) are divided into capsule expressing (typeable, THi) and non-capsule expressing (non-typeable, NTHi) serotypes based on agglutination with type-specific sera. Both THi and NTHi isolates of Hi are capable of causing a range of pathologies. The most common infections caused by NTHi strains are those of the middle ear (otitis media) and sinus (sinusitis). In addition, Hi exacerbates chronic obstructive pulmonary disease (COPD) leading to increased morbidity and mortality. Other localized infections include conjunctivitis, pneumonia, chronic cough, epiglottitis, cellulitis and infections in patients with cystic fibrosis (Agrawal and Murphy, 2011). From initial colonization of the nasopharynx, Hi can disseminate to cause a range of invasive pathologies such as septicaemia, meningitis and septic arthritis. Strains expressing type b capsule (Hib) are the most common cause of invasive Hi disease globally.

The epidemiology of invasive disease due to Hi has altered dramatically following the introduction of the Hib vaccine in the 1990s. While overall case numbers of invasive disease have significantly decreased in countries where the vaccine is now used, invasive disease due to serotypes other than b, as well as due to NTHi strains, is still reported. For example, a study in Canada noted strain replacement of Hib, which prior to introduction of the vaccine accounted for approximately 65% of total invasive disease. However, in the post-vaccination era, Hib accounted for less than 10% of the total disease, with increased disease observed due to Hif (~14%) and NTHi (~70%) strains (Adam *et al.*, 2010). Over a 2-year period (2008–2009) in British Columbia, 66% of cases of invasive Hi disease were attributed to NTHi bacteria, while Hia and Hif accounted for 20% of cases (Shuel *et al.*, 2011). The majority of studies of Hi invasive disease have focused on Hib rather than NTHi strains. In this chapter, the pathophysiology of Hib meningitis at the cellular and molecular levels will be discussed. Surprisingly, many aspects of the molecular mechanisms that allow Hib to enter the cerebrospinal fluid (CSF) to cause meningitis remain unclear.

7.2 A Model of *Haemophilus influenzae* Meningitis

The pathogenesis of Hib meningitis is a multi-step process that begins with: (i) colonization of the nasopharynx; (ii) subsequent invasion

*mc4@soton.ac.uk

into the blood, which leads to haematogenous dissemination; (iii) bacterial penetration of the blood–cerebrospinal fluid barrier (BCSFB)/blood–brain barrier (BBB) and entry into the subarachnoid space (SAS); which leads to (iv) a compartmentalized host inflammatory response, meningitis. Normally, Hi is a transient commensal of the upper respiratory tract: why only certain individuals succumb to invasive Hi disease remains unclear, but this may involve a combination of bacterial virulence factor expression, host genetic susceptibility and co-infection. Here we propose a model for Hib meningitis, which is based on our current knowledge of bacterial virulence factors and host cell receptor recognition of these ligands. Importantly, animal models have provided valuable information on the pathology of Hib meningitis, in particular the infant rat. The cardinal events of bacterial colonization of the nasopharynx, haematogenous dissemination of bacteria and the subsequent development of purulent leptomeningitis are common to meningitis occurring in rats and humans.

7.2.1 Colonization of the nasopharynx

Hi colonize mucosal epithelial cells of the nasopharynx and a variety of surface structures are involved.

Role of the capsule

THi can express one of six capsule types, designated a to f. Capsulated Hi isolates do adhere to human epithelial cells, but the absence or reduction of capsule expression allows increased bacterial adherence and invasion of human cells via surface molecules that may not be accessible in fully encapsulated phenotypes (St Geme and Falkow, 1991). Growth phase and environment also influence the levels of capsulation observed and the subsequent ability of Hi to adhere to epithelial cells (St Geme and Cutter, 1996). True acapsulate (NT) isolates of Hi lack the genetic information to produce a capsule, while some type b strains can become acapsulate through deletion within the *cap* locus (St Geme *et al.*, 1994).

Role of lipopolysaccharide

Lipopolysaccharide (LPS, strictly a lipo-oligosaccharide), of Hi can be decorated with molecules that promote bacterial adhesion to epithelial cells. For example, the addition of phosphorylcholine (ChoP) to LPS enables the bacteria to adhere to and invade human epithelial cells via the platelet-activating factor (PAF) receptor. Interaction via PAF also triggers host signalling events that may have broader implications than simply facilitating bacterial invasion (Swords *et al.*, 2001). Addition of ChoP to LPS has also been shown to aid bacterial survival through promoting resistance to antimicrobial peptides at the epithelium (Lysenko *et al.*, 2000).

Role of type IV and haemagglutinating (HA) pili

Common to other pathogens that are capable of colonizing exposed mucosal surfaces, the haemagglutinating (HA) pili of Hib (Stull *et al.*, 1984) are also important adhesins. HA pili of THi differ from the type IV pili expressed by NTHi strains for which the structure of the PilA subunit has recently been solved (Kolappan *et al.*, 2012). HA pili are encoded by the *hif* gene cluster comprising five genes in a *hifA–E* cluster. The main pilin subunit, HifA (M_r ~23 kDa), is encoded by the *hifA* gene and the product is assembled into a polymeric rod with HifD and HifE located at the pilus tip (McCrea *et al.*, 1997). The adhesive function of HA pili has been ascribed to HifE (Gilsdorf *et al.*, 1997). HifB functions as a molecular chaperone facilitating pilus subunit stability in the periplasmic space, while HifC facilitates translocation across the outer membrane (Watson *et al.*, 1994). HA pili of THi are subject to phase variation, enabling expression to change in different physiological locations.

It is important to note that, during nasopharyngeal colonization, both pilus-expressing and non-expressing strains can be isolated. One study identified that the vast majority of NTHi isolates from respiratory tract infection possess the *hifA* gene (Nakamura *et al.*, 2006), suggesting a role in non-typeable pathogenesis. The type IV pilus of NTHi strains mediate bacterial attachment to normal human bronchial epithelial cells and enable colonization of the respiratory tract in a chinchilla model of infection (Jurcisek *et al.*, 2007). HA pili have been shown to interact with several human molecules including the Anton (AnWj) antigen expressed on the surface of erythrocytes (van Alphen *et al.*, 1987). Sialic acid-containing lactosyl ceramides, as well as gangliosides GM1, GM2, GM3 and GD1a, have been demonstrated to inhibit Hib adhesion to epithelial cells and erythrocytes (van Alphen *et al.*, 1991).

Role of outer-membrane proteins (OMPs)

Differential solubility studies of the Hi OMPs identified six major proteins designated P1–P6, present in multiple invasive isolates. A number of studies have identified roles for OMPs in mediating Hi interactions with human cells. P2 (M_r ~37 kDa) is the most prominent of these OMPs and is expressed by both THi and NTHi strains. P2 is a trimeric porin, each monomer of which is a 16-stranded β-barrel presenting eight surface-exposed loops (Klingman *et al.*, 1988). The protein is highly immunogenic during carriage and infection and has long been considered a potential non-capsular vaccine antigen for Hi. P2 demonstrates variation in both sequence and size among different NTHi strains (Forbes *et al.*, 1992). In isolates from patients with otitis media or COPD, loops 2, 4, 5 and 8 of P2 were identified as hypervariable (Duim *et al.*, 1993). Additionally, sequential isolation of Hi from a patient with chronic bronchitis revealed antigenic variation of P2 predominating in loop 6 (Duim *et al.*, 1994). An animal model using subcutaneous tissue cages in rabbits to study persistent infection of Hi also identified longitudinal antigenic variation of P2. Selection occurred more quickly through immunization with the carriage strain than with a heterologous strain (Duim *et al.*, 1996). In this study, again the majority of changes were within loop 6 of P2. Loop 5 has also been identified as immunodominant, yet produces strain-specific antibodies due to sequence variation, an important consideration in the potential use of P2 as a vaccine antigen. The P2 OMP mediates adherence of Hi to mucin purified from the human respiratory tract (Reddy *et al.*, 1996). By contrast, in a separate study, no interaction of purified P2 to chinchilla mucosal epithelium was observed (Miyamoto and Bakaletz, 1996). These conflicting observations may suggest a role in species specificity for P2.

P5 has also been identified as one of the surface proteins capable of binding to sialic acid of mucins from human nasopharynx and middle ear (Reddy *et al.*, 1996). Thus, like P2, P5 may have a role in early colonization of Hi in the respiratory tract. THi and NTHi strains target members of the carcinoembryonic antigen-related cell adhesion molecule (CEACAM) family (Virji *et al.*, 2000). Of the CEACAM family, CEACAM1 has the widest expression profile, being produced by epithelial and endothelial cells as well as cells of the immune system. THi and NTHi strains bind soluble recombinant as well as cell-expressed CEACAM1 via P5. In addition, complementation of a non-binding NTHi strain with P5 from a THi strain conferred the ability to bind to CEACAM1 (Hill *et al.*, 2001). The Hi P5 targets a region on the non-glycosylated face of human CEACAM1 centred on isoleucine 91 (Villullas *et al.*, 2007). Besides P5, a second ligand on some Hi strains has the capacity to bind to cell-expressed CEACAMs, although the nature of this ligand remains to be determined (Hill *et al.*, 2001). CEACAM expression increases in inflammatory situations in response to cytokines such as gamma interferon (IFN-γ). Cytokine (INF-γ) challenge of epithelial cells has been shown to increase cellular invasion of Opa-expressing capsulate *Neisseria meningitidis* via *de novo* expression of CEACAM1 (Griffiths *et al.*, 2007). Although unproven, it is also possible that cytokine production in the nasopharynx induced by P5 expressing Hi that leads to CEACAM1 upregulation, aiding bacterial dissemination from the mucosal epithelium.

Like P2, OMP P5 is expressed by both THi and NTHi strains, and variation is observed within the surface-exposed loops of P5 between strains of Hi. Loops 1–3 appear to be hypervariable within sequences from different strains of Hi, while loop 4 is largely conserved (Webb and Cripps, 1998). During the course of persistent bronchitis caused by NTHi strains, variation was observed between the P5 surface-exposed loops. Notably, in sequential isolates of the same strain, mutation resulted in a premature stop codon due to the loss of a single A nucleotide in a poly(A) tract within the *p5* gene (Duim *et al.*, 1997). Thus, P5 appears to be both antigenically variable and phase variable.

The OMP P5 also binds to intracellular adhesion molecule (ICAM)-1. Purified LPS from Hi can induce the expression of ICAM-1 by primary human bronchial epithelial cells (Khair *et al.*, 1994). Subsequently, Frick *et al.* (2000) described upregulation of ICAM-1 following binding of both THi and NTHi strains to human respiratory epithelial cells (A549). However, in contrast to the previous studies, LPS alone was insufficient to induce ICAM-1 expression. In the same study, Hi caused human umbilical vein endothelial cells (HUVECs) to upregulate ICAM-1, and in this instance LPS alone was sufficient to induce ICAM-1 expression. Mutational analyses did not attribute ICAM-1 upregulation in A549 cells to the presence of high-molecular-weight, Hap or Hia proteins. In keeping with previous studies, Hi adhesion to A549 cells resulted in an upregulation of ICAM-1: hence, Hi in this instance upregulates its own receptor (Avadhanula *et al.*, 2006).

Other surface proteins involved in interactions with human cells

Non-pilus *Haemophilus* surface fibrils (Hsf, M_r ~245 kDa) are encoded by a single gene, belong to the autotransporter adhesin family and remain attached to the cell surface (St Geme *et al.*, 1996). Hsf has been shown to mediate attachment to human Chang conjunctival epithelial cells (St Geme and Cutter, 1995) via two distinct binding domains (HsfBD1 and HsfBD2), which share homology with regions of Hia, a smaller autotransporter expressed by around a quarter of NTHi strains (Barenkamp and St Geme, 1996; Cotter *et al.*, 2005). The two binding domains (BDs) differ in affinity, with HsfBD1 having a higher affinity than HsfBD2. By using a HeLa cell-binding model, this difference in affinity has been attributed to an Asp (BD1)–Glu (BD2) residue change within the acidic binding clefts of Hsf (Radin *et al.*, 2009). Despite the detailed molecular knowledge of Hsf binding, the human receptor(s) targeted by this adhesin remain(s) unknown. However, Hsf can bind to the serum protein vitronectin (Hallstrom *et al.*, 2006). Hia (~115 kDa) also possesses two binding domains, HiaBD1 and HiaBD2, which target the same human cell moiety with differing affinities (Yeo *et al.*, 2004), but this recognition receptor has not yet been identified.

The *Haemophilus* adhesion and penetration protein (Hap) of NTHi is an autotransporter that shares significant homology with the IgA proteases of both *Neisseria* and *Haemophilus* spp. Hap, unlike other Hi autotransporters, appears to retain autocatalytic cleavage activity, allowing a M_r ~110 kDa soluble protein (Hap_S) to be released from the bacterial surface. The adhesive properties of Hap reside within this Hap_S region. However, the full-length (M_r ~150 kDa) Hap can be retained at the bacterial surface, and host factors, such as secretory leucocyte protease inhibitor, have been shown to inhibit the release of Hap_S, thus potentiating host interaction (Hendrixson and St Geme, 1998). The C-terminal 311 amino acid region of Hap_S mediates the interaction of Hi with Chang and A549 cells. In addition, the Hap_S terminal 511 amino acid region mediates the interaction with the extracellular matrix (ECM) proteins fibronectin, laminin and collagen IV. The terminal 311 amino acid region of Hap_S may also be important for bacterial intercellular interactions during micro-colony and biofilm formation (Hendrixson and St Geme, 1998; Fink *et al.*, 2003). The structure of Hap_S has been solved to 2.2 Å and elegantly revealed how structural features of the β-helix domain permit Hap–Hap multimeric interactions that overcome repulsive effects between bacterial cells (Meng *et al.*, 2011).

The majority (~80%) of NTHi strains lack Hia but express high-molecular-weight proteins, HMW1 and HMW2. Both proteins bind to NCI-H292 and HaCaT cells. In contrast to HMW2, HMW1 also bound to Chang and HEp-2 cells (Buscher *et al.*, 2004). HMW1 appears to target sialic acid, α2,3-linked to as yet undetermined glycoprotein(s) on the cell surface, while the specific binding partner for HMW2 remains to be identified. Both HMW1 and HMW2 have been implicated in carriage (Cholon *et al.*, 2008) and localized disease such as otitis media; however, no specific role for these proteins has been defined for invasive disease, with invasive isolates of Hi displaying variable expression of these proteins.

The phase variable cell envelope opacity associated protein A (OapA) conveys an opaque phenotype to Hi colonies on agar and has been identified as an adhesin. OapA is highly conserved among THi and NTHi strains and mutants lacking OapA bound to Chang epithelial cells in lower numbers than the corresponding parent isolates (Prasadarao *et al.*, 1999). In the same study, recombinant OapA was able to diminish binding of diverse Hi strains to Chang cells by up to 50%. OapA has been purported to function in mucosal colonization rather than invasion in infant rat infection models (Weiser *et al.*, 1995).

Intra- and inter-epithelial cell barrier penetration

The use of oropharyngeal organ culture models has revealed that Hib can penetrate between epithelial cells at sites of injury and separation of tight junctions (Farley *et al.*, 1990). In this study, increased invasion of a non-piliated phenotype was observed. Subsequent studies also revealed NTHi penetration between epithelial cells in a model using a cultured human lung epithelial cell line, H292, in a process referred to as paracytosis (van Schilfgaarde *et al.*, 1995). In support of this mode of barrier penetration, downregulation of epithelial genes associated with tight junction formation, including claudin 7 and 10, was observed in a murine model of NTHi infection (Clarke *et al.*, 2011). The same study showed this response to be mediated via Toll-like receptor (TLR)-triggered signalling. Hi invasion into primary human and chinchilla epithelial cells was associated with a rearrangement of the actin cytoskeleton (Holmes and Bakaletz, 1997). Cytoskeletal rearrangement results in macropinocytic uptake of Hi into primary human epithelial cells and the presence of intracellular bacteria within vesicles (Ketterer *et al.*, 1999). Other studies have indicated that intracellular Hi appear to be in a state of degradation. The significance of intracellular and intercellular barrier penetration in pathogenesis versus survival in the host remain to be fully appreciated (Clementi and Murphy, 2011). However, the increased invasion of acapsulate versus capsule-expressing Hi (St Geme and Falkow, 1991) is likely to involve many of the subcapsular antigens described above, e.g. ChoP-modified LPS and P5.

7.2.2 Invasion into the blood, and haematogenous spread

Studies with the infant rat model have provided considerable information on the early events of colonization and entry into the blood by Hib. Both the intraperitoneal route and, more appropriate to human infection, the intranasal route have been used to induce bacteraemia and meningitis in infant rats (Smith *et al.*, 1973; Moxon *et al.*, 1974; Moxon and Ostrow, 1977). Intranasal inoculation leads to nasopharyngeal colonization by Hib, after which the bacteria are visualized on oral, nasopharyngeal and nasal epithelial surfaces. Invasion of the nasal mucosa occurs within 5 min of intranasal instillation and this is accompanied by an acute inflammatory response consisting of polymorphonuclear leucocytes (PMNLs) presenting in the mucosa and sometimes in the perineural spaces of the olfactory nerves. By 3 h after instillation, inflammation is more extensive and PMNLs are found in large numbers in the olfactory perineural spaces beneath the cribriform plate and in the SAS immediately superior to the plate (Ostrow *et al.*, 1979). However, the CSF at this stage is sterile, and any inflammation in the SAS is probably an extension of the acute nasopharyngeal response. Although Hib were observed in the perineural space of olfactory neurons, direct spread to the SAS is unlikely to occur via this route as bacterial migration was limited and too few bacteria survived natural clearance. More likely, Hib reach the submucosal lymphatics and from here enter the systemic circulation at the interface. Bacteraemia is established within 3–12 h of instillation in the infant rat and, as in humans, intense bacteraemia is a prerequisite for the development of meningitis. Significantly, age-related susceptibility to bacteraemia and bacterial invasion of the CSF are features of both natural human and experimental rat infection. Thus, Hib reach the meninges by haematogenous spread and not directly from the nasopharynx, although nasopharyngitis leading to non-specific inflammation above the cribriform plate probably facilitates invasion at this site (Ostrow *et al.*, 1979).

The presence of type b capsule is essential for the intravascular survival of Hi strains in the infant rat and humans. Capsule expression decreases the deposition of complement C3 on the bacterial surface: indeed, increased copy number of the type b *cap* locus decreased complement deposition and opsonophagocytosis of Hi even further (Noel *et al.*, 1996). While capsulate phenotypes of Hi are generally more resistant to complement-mediated killing than acapsulate phenotypes, strains of NTHi have been isolated that show decreased deposition/activity of C3 on their surface, which may aid their survival during dissemination in the blood (Williams *et al.*, 2001).

Besides the capsule, several other structural features of Hi have roles in evasion of the immune response. For example, LPS can aid bacterial evasion of the host immune system through molecular mimicry. The LPS of Hi contains moieties that mimic human structures, including variations of globotetraose and sialyl-lactose. Through molecular mimicry, the bacterial surface can be protected from complement deposition and antibody binding, which may aid bacterial survival in the blood during dissemination. In addition, variation complexities arise through phase variation of the various enzymes involved in the addition of moieties to the core LPS backbone (Weiser *et al.*, 1989). Furthermore, the presence of ChoP on LPS alters antibody binding to the bacterial surface, thereby aiding resistance to bactericidal killing (Clark *et al.*, 2012). LPS can also be modified by the addition of sialic acid or disialic acid (Fox *et al.*, 2006). A lack of LPS sialylation leads to attenuation of virulence of Hi, whereas the presence of sialic acid promotes survival of bacteria *in vitro* and *in vivo* (Bouchet *et al.*, 2003). The lipid A moiety of LPS anchors the molecule to the bacterial outer membrane and is responsible for the majority of invasive disease symptoms following bacterial cell lysis.

Both capsule and LPS also play a role in Hi survival in macrophages (Williams *et al.*, 1991). Capsulated Hi can survive and replicate within macrophages, whereas acapsulate mutants are killed after ingestion. Differences in LPS structure, introduced by mutation, also affect the ability of capsulated Hi to survive in macrophages. The P2 OMP has been reported to induce tumour necrosis factor-α and interleukin (IL)-6 production from murine macrophages and human monocytes, which was dependent on a functional TLR2/MyD88 pathway (Galdiero *et al.*, 2004). Thus, Hi interactions with macrophages not only enhance the persistence of bacteraemia and contribute to intravascular inflammation but may also be important for bacterial entry into the CSF by a 'Trojan horse mechanism', although this remains to be confirmed.

Vitronectin inhibits the terminal process of the complement cascade, and by binding vitronectin via Hsf, Hi are able to increase resistance to serum-mediated killing (Hallstrom *et al.*, 2006). This possibly enhances bacteraemia, but no studies have identified if the Hsf–vitronectin binding event supports the adhesion of Hib to endothelial cells and subsequent bacterial invasion. Unlike Hsf or THi, no direct interaction of Hia with vitronectin has been demonstrated, although early studies reported that both THi and NTHi strains bind to vitronectin equally. NTHi protein E, a surface lipoprotein of M_r 16 kDa, has also been shown to bind to vitronectin (Hallstrom *et al.*, 2009). Strains lacking protein E, through mutation, are still able to bind to vitronectin, albeit to a lesser extent. This suggests that other surface proteins, which may include Hia, are capable of mediating NTHi binding to vitronectin. Whilst Hsf and protein E of Hi promote bacterial survival in the blood, one study indicates that this attribute is also present in strains isolated from the nasopharynx (Hallstrom *et al.*, 2010).

In rat models of infection, intravenous injection of OMP P2 loop 7 can disrupt normal physiological coagulation and fibrinolytic functions, measured by increased levels of plasminogen activator inhibitor 1 (Vitiello *et al.*, 2008). Of note, levels of E-cadherin, a marker of endothelial damage, were also increased in this model of infection. Thus, P2 may contribute to pathology during haematogenous dissemination of Hi.

7.2.3 Penetration into the central nervous system (CNS)

Bacteraemia is a prerequisite for the development of classical meningeal inflammation. Undoubtedly, the route of meningeal invasion in the infant rat model, by either the intraperitoneal or intranasal route of infection, is from the bloodstream, and several hypotheses can be proposed. Several observations support entry through the dorsal longitudinal and lateral sinuses: Hib are found first in these sinuses, dural inflammation is greatest around these draining sites and pachymeningitis occurs before leptomeningitis and is more severe. Alternatively, Hib could arrive in the SAS via thin-walled meningeal veins and venules: in support of this route is the fact that CSF flows naturally from the SAS to the dorsal longitudinal sinus. Thus, invading Hib would seed the dura, initiate inflammation and then spread to the leptomeninges.

Invasion of the CSF from the blood is dependent on Hib penetration of the BCSFB/BBB, which is provided by the endothelium of blood vessels. In support of the pathological findings from human and infant rat post-mortem, *in vitro* culture models have provided some insight into the mechanisms by which Hib interact with endothelial cells. Whilst pili clearly have a role in epithelial adhesion, human brain microvascular endothelial cells (HBMECs) contain lactosyl ceramide and GM3 as well as low levels of GM1, GM2 and GD1a. Furthermore, lipid raft endocytosis involving GM1 has been implicated in *Cryptococcus neoformans* internalization into HBMECs. Hib expressing HA pili could enable entry into the CSF. However, piliated strains of Hib possess no apparent advantage over non-piliated strains for colonization or invasion of infant rats (Kaplan *et al.*, 1983). In rats infected with piliated, adherent Hib strains, isolates recovered from the blood and CSF were found to be non-adherent and non-piliated, and these findings correspond to observations of children with Hib meningitis. Thus, downregulation of HA pili may be an important prerequisite for CSF invasion by Hib strains.

Type IV pili of NTHi strains could enable endothelial cell invasion in a manner similar to type IV pili expressed by *Streptococcus agalactiae*. This organism expresses PilA, which interacts with collagen and engages integrin α2-β1 expressed on BMECs, using collagen as a molecular bridge. In murine models, integrin binding by *S. agalactiae* stimulates the upregulation of inflammatory mediator release, such as IL-8, which results in neutrophil influx and increases the permeability of the brain endothelium (Banerjee *et al.*, 2011).

The precise role of Hap during invasive disease remains unclear. However, the *hap* gene was ubiquitous in isolates obtained from disseminated infection, including meningitis (Rodriguez *et al.*, 2003). Furthermore, the ECM protein interactions of Hap suggest a role for adhesion to endothelial cells via pertinent integrin and non-integrin matrix protein receptors, e.g. laminin, expressed on microvascular endothelial cells. In addition to promoting survival during haematogenous dissemination, protein E has been shown to mediate adhesion to the ECM via interactions with vitronectin and also laminin (Hallstrom *et al.*, 2011). A role for the vitronectin-binding proteins Hsf/Hia and protein E in invasive disease remains to be elucidated, but it may be possible that, through interaction with matrix proteins, strains of Hi are able to invade endothelial cells via integrins and the laminin receptor.

OMP P2 may also have a role during invasive disease and penetration of the BCSFB/BBB. Hi interactions with the non-integrin 67 kDa laminin receptor have been demonstrated *in vitro* (Orihuela *et al.*, 2009). In the same study, using recombinant laminin receptor and knock-out mutants of Hi, P2 was shown to mediate this interaction. Following situations mimicking inflammatory conditions such as septicaemia, laminin receptor was upregulated on human cerebral endothelial cells, which in turn could increase Hi targeting of the BCSFB during disseminated infection. Notably, laminin receptor is also targeted by other pathogens capable of causing CNS infection, including equine encephalitic virus, *Streptococcus pneumoniae* and *N. meningitidis* as well as prion proteins. While the region of P2 responsible for laminin receptor interaction remains to be determined, in a study using synthetic peptides, the surface-exposed loops 5–7 of P2 were shown to mediate signalling via the mitogen-activated protein kinase (MAPK) pathway in the monocytic lymphoma cell line U937 (Galdiero *et al.*, 2003). Within the context of CNS infection, the MAPK signalling cascade is activated in the glioblastoma astrocytoma cell line U87-MG in response to challenge with P2 or synthetic loop 7 (Vitiello *et al.*, 2011). Given that endothelial cells express CEACAM1, inflammation of BMECs may also lead to increased CEACAM1 expression and subsequent cellular invasion by Hi via P5 expressed in both THi and NTHi strains.

Using HUVECs, acapsulate Hi are better able to adhere and invade than capsule-expressing bacteria (Virji *et al.*, 1991). In this study, internalized bacteria were quantified by a gentamicin exclusion assay, indicating that viability was maintained. In addition, bacteria within vesicles were observed by electron microscopy. Such adhesion to and invasion of endothelium may facilitate not only direct traversal of the endothelial barrier, but also indirect barrier penetration through pro-inflammatory damage.

7.2.4 Lessons from the infant rat model of Hib meningitis correlate with human pathology

Infant rats injected intranasally or intraperitoneally with Hib share essentially the same histopathology and remarkable similarities to human post-mortem observations. There is widespread purulent and fibrinous pachymeningitis and leptomeningitis, and bacteria are present in all inflammatory foci. Sampling of CSF from the *cisterna magna* of the rat demonstrates that, once present in the CSF, bacterial numbers increase rapidly, and this is accompanied by an increase in the number of inflammatory cells. Accumulation of PMNLs in the dura, SAS and leptomeninges is the dominant inflammatory feature, with the cellular infiltrate ranging from 10^5 to 10^7 PMNLs per gram of brain (Moxon *et al.*, 1974). The exudate ranges in thickness from small periarterial accumulations of inflammatory cells to filling the SAS. Apart from predominant PMNLs in the early stages, macrophages, lymphocytes and rare plasma cells are also increasingly present with time, and fibrin deposition is observed between inflammatory cells. Cellular infiltration occurs first in the dorsal portion of the dura mater around the rostral dorsal longitudinal sinus, and pachymeningitis occurs before leptomeningitis and is more severe. Leptomeningitis is present mostly in the dorsal longitudinal fissure, basilar frontal regions and around the lateral aspects of the pons. The inflammatory exudate is largely contained in the SAS, with PMNLs found in the superficial cortex only occasionally. Nuclear fragmentation of neurons is also an infrequent event. In both models, other brain structures including the choroid plexi, ventricles, ependyma, cerebellum, midbrain, thalamus, medulla, cerebral white and grey matters and meningeal vessels do not show histological lesions.

The infant rat model has also shed light on the pathogenesis of Hib-induced labyrinthitis, where PMNL inflammation reaches the inner ear by spreading from the SAS (Wiedermann *et al.*, 1986). PMNLs accumulate in the perilymphatic space of the vestibule and in the scalae tympani and vestibule, but the cochlea and organ of Corti, utricle, saccule and semicircular canals remain intact. These observations support human autopsy studies (Prosnitz, 1964), which have suggested that deafness associated with pyogenic bacterial meningitis occurs when inflammation spreads from the meninges/SAS to the cochlea via the cochlea aqueduct.

Although the histopathology of meningitis observed in infant rats is similar to that reported in humans (Adams *et al.*, 1948), only humans show leptomeningeal vasculitis, vascular necrosis, cortical necrosis, microgliosis, astrocytosis in the *glia limitans superficialis*, neuronal necrosis related to ischaemia and subependymal perivascular inflammation.

7.3 Conclusions

A plethora of studies have contributed to our understanding of the interactions of Hi with eukaryotic cells and tissues and have identified individual host components to which bacterial surface proteins bind. We recognize a dynamic interplay between multiple bacterial and human components as bacteria colonize, disseminate, penetrate into the CNS and induce an inflammatory response. Nevertheless, we still have more to learn regarding how Hi overcome the numerous challenges and niche variations encountered during invasive disease.

References

Adam, H.J., Richardson, S.E., Jamieson, F.B., Rawte, P., Low, D.E. and Fisman, D.N. (2010) Changing epidemiology of invasive *Haemophilus influenzae* in Ontario, Canada: evidence for herd effects and strain replacement due to Hib vaccination. *Vaccine* 28, 4073–4078.

Adams, R.D., Kubik, C.S. and Bonner, F.J. (1948) The clinical and pathological aspects of influenzal meningitis. *Archives of Pediatrics* 65, 408–441.

Agrawal, A. and Murphy, T.F. (2011) *Haemophilus influenzae* infections in the *H. influenzae* type b conjugate vaccine era. *Journal of Clinical Microbiology* 49, 3728–3732.

Avadhanula, V., Rodriguez, C.A., Ulett, G.C., Bakaletz, L.O. and Adderson, E.E. (2006) Nontypeable *Haemophilus influenzae* adheres to intercellular adhesion molecule 1 (ICAM-1) on respiratory epithelial cells and upregulates ICAM-1 expression. *Infection and Immunity* 74, 830–838.

Banerjee, A., Kim, B.J., Carmona, E.M., Cutting, A.S., Gurney, M.A., Carlos, C., Feuer, R., Prasadarao, N.V. and Doran, K.S. (2011) Bacterial pili exploit integrin machinery to promote immune activation and efficient blood–brain barrier penetration. *Nature Communications* 2, 462.

Barenkamp, S.J. and St Geme, J.W. (1996) Identification of a second family of high-molecular-weight adhesion proteins expressed by non-typable *Haemophilus influenzae*. *Molecular Microbiology* 19, 1215–1223.

Bouchet, V., Hood, D.W., Li, J., Brisson, J.R., Randle, G.A., Martin, A., Li, Z., Goldstein, R., Schweda, E.K., Pelton, S.I., Richards, J.C. and Moxon, E.R. (2003) Host-derived sialic acid is incorporated into *Haemophilus influenzae* lipopolysaccharide and is a major virulence factor in experimental otitis media. *Proceedings of the National Academy of Sciences USA* 100, 8898–8903.

Buscher, A.Z., Burmeister, K., Barenkamp, S.J. and St Geme, J.W. (2004) Evolutionary and functional relationships among the nontypeable *Haemophilus influenzae* HMW family of adhesins. *Journal of Bacteriology* 186, 4209–4217.

Cholon, D.M., Cutter, D., Richardson, S.K., Sethi, S., Murphy, T.F., Look, D.C. and St Geme, J.W. (2008) Serial isolates of persistent *Haemophilus influenzae* in patients with chronic obstructive pulmonary disease express diminishing quantities of the HMW1 and HMW2 adhesins. *Infection and Immunity* 76, 4463–4468.

Clark, S.E., Snow, J., Li, J., Zola, T.A. and Weiser, J.N. (2012) Phosphorylcholine allows for evasion of bactericidal antibody by *Haemophilus influenzae*. *PLoS Pathogens* 8, e1002521.

Clarke, T.B., Francella, N., Huegel, A. and Weiser, J.N. (2011) Invasive bacterial pathogens exploit TLR-mediated downregulation of tight junction components to facilitate translocation across the epithelium. *Cell Host Microbe* 9, 404–414.

Clementi, C.F. and Murphy, T.F. (2011) Non-typeable *Haemophilus influenzae* invasion and persistence in the human respiratory tract. *Frontiers in Cellular and Infection Microbiology* 1, 1.

Cotter, S.E., Yeo, H.J., Juehne, T. and St Geme, J.W. (2005) Architecture and adhesive activity of the *Haemophilus influenzae* Hsf adhesin. *Journal of Bacteriology* 187, 4656–4664.

Duim, B., Dankert, J., Jansen, H.M. and van Alphen, L. (1993) Genetic analysis of the diversity in outer membrane protein P2 of non-encapsulated *Haemophilus influenzae*. *Microbial Pathogenesis* 14, 451–462.

Duim, B., van Alphen, L., Eijk, P., Jansen, H.M. and Dankert, J. (1994) Antigenic drift of non-encapsulated *Haemophilus influenzae* major outer membrane protein P2 in patients with chronic bronchitis is caused by point mutations. *Molecular Microbiology* 11, 1181–1189.

Duim, B., Vogel, L., Puijk, W., Jansen, H.M., Meloen, R.H., Dankert, J. and van Alphen, L. (1996) Fine mapping of outer membrane protein P2 antigenic sites which vary during persistent infection by *Haemophilus influenzae*. *Infection and Immunity* 64, 4673–4679.

Duim, B., Bowler, L.D., Eijk, P.P., Jansen, H.M., Dankert, J. and van Alphen, L. (1997) Molecular variation in the major outer membrane protein P5 gene of nonencapsulated *Haemophilus influenzae* during chronic infections. *Infection and Immunity* 65, 1351–1356.

Farley, M.M., Stephens, D.S., Kaplan, S.L. and Mason, E.O. Jr (1990) Pilus- and non-pilus-mediated interactions of *Haemophilus influenzae* type b with human erythrocytes and human nasopharyngeal mucosa. *Journal of Infectious Diseases* 161, 274–280.

Fink, D.L., Buscher, A.Z., Green, B., Fernsten, P. and St Geme, J.W. (2003) The *Haemophilus influenzae* Hap autotransporter mediates microcolony formation and adherence to epithelial cells and extracellular matrix via binding regions in the C-terminal end of the passenger domain. *Cellular Microbiology* 5, 175–186.

Forbes, K.J., Bruce, K.D., Ball, A. and Pennington, T.H. (1992) Variation in length and sequence of porin (*ompP2*) alleles of non-capsulate *Haemophilus influenzae*. *Molecular Microbiology* 6, 2107–2112.

Fox, K.L., Cox, A.D., Gilbert, M., Wakarchuk, W.W., Li, J., Makepeace, K., Richards, J.C., Moxon, E.R. and Hood, D.W. (2006) Identification of a bifunctional lipopolysaccharide sialyltransferase in *Haemophilus influenzae*: incorporation of disialic acid. *Journal of Biological Chemistry* 281, 40024–40032.

Frick, A.G., Joseph, T.D., Pang, L., Rabe, A.M., St Geme, J.W. and Look, D.C. (2000) *Haemophilus influenzae* stimulates ICAM-1 expression on respiratory epithelial cells. *Journal of Immunology* 164, 4185–4196.

Galdiero, S., Capasso, D., Vitiello, M., D'Isanto, M., Pedone, C. and Galdiero, M. (2003) Role of surface-exposed loops of *Haemophilus influenzae* protein P2 in the mitogen-activated protein kinase cascade. *Infection and Immunity* 71, 2798–2809.

Galdiero, M., Galdiero, M., Finamore, E., Rossano, F., Gambuzza, M., Catania, M.R., Teti, G., Midiri, A. and Mancuso, G. (2004) *Haemophilus influenzae* porin induces Toll-like receptor 2-mediated cytokine production in human monocytes and mouse macrophages. *Infection and Immunity* 72, 1204–1209.

Gilsdorf, J.R., McCrea, K.W. and Marrs, C.F. (1997) Role of pili in *Haemophilus influenzae* adherence and colonization. *Infection and Immunity* 65, 2997–3002.

Griffiths, N.J., Bradley, C.J., Heyderman, R.S. and Virji, M. (2007) IFN-γ amplifies NFκB-dependent *Neisseria meningitidis* invasion of epithelial cells via specific upregulation of CEA-related cell adhesion molecule 1. *Cellular Microbiology* 9, 2968–2983.

Hallstrom, T., Trajkovska, E., Forsgren, A. and Riesbeck, K. (2006) *Haemophilus influenzae* surface fibrils contribute to serum resistance by interacting with vitronectin. *Journal of Immunology* 177, 430–436.

Hallstrom, T., Blom, A.M., Zipfel, P.F. and Riesbeck, K. (2009) Nontypeable *Haemophilus influenzae* protein E binds vitronectin and is important for serum resistance. *Journal of Immunology* 183, 2593–2601.

Hallstrom, T., Resman, F., Ristovski, M. and Riesbeck, K. (2010) Binding of complement regulators to invasive nontypeable *Haemophilus influenzae* isolates is not increased compared to nasopharyngeal isolates, but serum resistance is linked to disease severity. *Journal of Clinical Microbiology* 48, 921–927.

Hallstrom, T., Singh, B., Resman, F., Blom, A.M., Morgelin, M. and Riesbeck, K. (2011) *Haemophilus influenzae* protein E binds to the extracellular matrix by concurrently interacting with laminin and vitronectin. *Journal of Infectious Diseases* 204, 1065–1074.

Hendrixson, D.R. and St Geme, J.W. (1998) The *Haemophilus influenzae* Hap serine protease promotes adherence and microcolony formation, potentiated by a soluble host protein. *Molecular Cell* 2, 841–850.

Hill, D.J., Toleman, M.A., Evans, D.J., Villullas, S., van Alphen, L. and Virji, M. (2001) The variable P5 proteins of typeable and non-typeable

Haemophilus influenzae target human CEACAM1. *Molecular Microbiology* 39, 850–862.

Holmes, K.A. and Bakaletz, L.O. (1997) Adherence of non-typeable *Haemophilus influenzae* promotes reorganization of the actin cytoskeleton in human or chinchilla epithelial cells *in vitro*. *Microbial Pathogenesis* 23, 157–166.

Jurcisek, J.A., Bookwalter, J.E., Baker, B.D., Fernandez, S., Novotny, L.A., Munson, R.S. Jr and Bakaletz, L.O. (2007) The PilA protein of non-typeable *Haemophilus influenzae* plays a role in biofilm formation, adherence to epithelial cells and colonization of the mammalian upper respiratory tract. *Molecular Microbiology* 65, 1288–1299.

Kaplan, S.L., Mason, E.O. Jr and Wiedermann, B.L. (1983) Role of adherence in the pathogenesis of *Haemophilus influenzae* type b infection in infant rats. *Infection and Immunity* 42, 612–617.

Ketterer, M.R., Shao, J.Q., Hornick, D.B., Buscher, B., Bandi, V.K. and Apicella, M.A. (1999) Infection of primary human bronchial epithelial cells by *Haemophilus influenzae*: macropinocytosis as a mechanism of airway epithelial cell entry. *Infection and Immunity* 67, 4161–4170.

Khair, O.A., Devalia, J.L., Abdelaziz, M.M., Sapsford, R.J., Tarraf, H. and Davies, R.J. (1994) Effect of *Haemophilus influenzae* endotoxin on the synthesis of IL-6, IL-8, TNF-α and expression of ICAM-1 in cultured human bronchial epithelial cells. *European Respiratory Journal* 7, 2109–2116.

Klingman, K.L., Jansen, E.M. and Murphy, T.F. (1988) Nearest neighbor analysis of outer membrane proteins of nontypeable *Haemophilus influenzae*. *Infection and Immunity* 56, 3058–3063.

Kolappan, S., Tracy, E.N., Bakaletz, L.O., Munson, R.S. Jr and Craig, L. (2012) Expression, purification, crystallization and preliminary crystallographic analysis of PilA from the nontypeable *Haemophilus influenzae* type IV pilus. *Acta Crystallographica Section F Structural Biology and Crystallization Communications* 68, 284–287.

Lysenko, E.S., Gould, J., Bals, R., Wilson, J.M. and Weiser, J.N. (2000) Bacterial phosphorylcholine decreases susceptibility to the antimicrobial peptide LL-37/hCAP18 expressed in the upper respiratory tract. *Infection and Immunity* 68, 1664–1671.

McCrea, K.W., Watson, W.J., Gilsdorf, J.R. and Marrs, C.F. (1997) Identification of two minor subunits in the pilus of *Haemophilus influenzae*. *Journal of Bacteriology* 179, 4227–4231.

Meng, G., Spahich, N., Kenjale, R., Waksman, G. and St Geme, J.W. (2011) Crystal structure of the *Haemophilus influenzae* Hap adhesin reveals an intercellular oligomerization mechanism for bacterial aggregation. *EMBO Journal* 30, 3864–3874.

Miyamoto, N. and Bakaletz, L.O. (1996) Selective adherence of non-typeable *Haemophilus influenzae* (NTHi) to mucus or epithelial cells in the chinchilla eustachian tube and middle ear. *Microbial Pathogenesis* 21, 343–356.

Moxon, E.R. and Ostrow, P.T. (1977) *Haemophilus influenzae* meningitis in infant rats: role of bacteremia in pathogenesis of age-dependent inflammatory responses in cerebrospinal fluid. *Journal of Infectious Diseases* 135, 303–307.

Moxon, E.R., Smith, A.L., Averill, D.R. and Smith, D.H. (1974) *Haemophilus influenzae* meningitis in infant rats after intranasal inoculation. *Journal of Infectious Diseases* 129, 154–162.

Nakamura, M., Asaka, T., Kirita, A., Miyazaki, H., Senda, Y., Fujita, S., Fukushima, R., Watanabe, K., Karasawa, T., Kawahara, E., Shimura, S. and Yamagishi, T. (2006) Occurrence of the fimbria gene *hifA* in clinical isolates of nonencapsulated *Haemophilus influenzae*. *Microbiology and Immunology* 50, 327–329.

Noel, G.J., Brittingham, A., Granato, A.A. and Mosser, D.M. (1996) Effect of amplification of the Cap b locus on complement-mediated bacteriolysis and opsonization of type b *Haemophilus influenzae*. *Infection and Immunity* 64, 4769–4775.

Orihuela, C.J., Mahdavi, J., Thornton, J., Mann, B., Wooldridge, K.G., Abouseada, N., Oldfield, N.J., Self, T., Ala'Aldeen, D.A. and Tuomanen, E.I. (2009) Laminin receptor initiates bacterial contact with the blood brain barrier in experimental meningitis models. *Journal of Clinical Investigation* 119, 1638–1646.

Ostrow, P.T., Moxon, E.R., Vernon, N. and Kapko, R. (1979) Pathogenesis of bacterial meningitis. Studies on the route of meningeal invasion following *Hemophilus influenzae* inoculation of infant rats. *Laboratory Investigation* 40, 678–685.

Prasadarao, N.V., Lysenko, E., Wass, C.A., Kim, K.S. and Weiser, J.N. (1999) Opacity-associated protein A contributes to the binding of *Haemophilus influenzae* to chang epithelial cells. *Infection and Immunity* 67, 4153–4160.

Prosnitz, L.R. (1964) Deafness following *Hemophilus influenzae* meningitis. *Archives of Internal Medicine* 113, 415–417.

Radin, J.N., Grass, S.A., Meng, G., Cotter, S.E., Waksman, G. and St Geme, J.W. (2009) Structural basis for the differential binding affinities of the HsfBD1 and HsfBD2 domains in the *Haemophilus influenzae* Hsf adhesin. *Journal of Bacteriology* 191, 5068–5075.

Reddy, M.S., Bernstein, J.M., Murphy, T.F. and Faden, H.S. (1996) Binding between outer membrane proteins of nontypeable *Haemophilus influenzae* and human nasopharyngeal mucin. *Infection and Immunity* 64, 1477–1479.

Rodriguez, C.A., Avadhanula, V., Buscher, A., Smith, A.L., St Geme, J.W. and Adderson, E.E. (2003) Prevalence and distribution of adhesins in invasive non-type b encapsulated *Haemophilus influenzae. Infection and Immunity* 71, 1635–1642.

Shuel, M., Hoang, L., Law, D.K. and Tsang, R. (2011) Invasive *Haemophilus influenzae* in British Columbia: non-Hib and non-typeable strains causing disease in children and adults. *International Journal of Infectious Diseases* 15, e167–173.

Smith, A.L., Smith, D.H., Averill, D.R. Jr, Marino, J. and Moxon, E.R. (1973) Production of *Haemophilus influenzae* b meningitis in infant rats by intraperitoneal inoculation. *Infection and Immunity* 8, 278–290.

St Geme, J.W. and Cutter, D. (1995) Evidence that surface fibrils expressed by *Haemophilus influenzae* type b promote attachment to human epithelial cells. *Molecular Microbiology* 15, 77–85.

St Geme, J.W. and Cutter, D. (1996) Influence of pili, fibrils, and capsule on *in vitro* adherence by *Haemophilus influenzae* type b. *Molecular Microbiology* 21, 21–31.

St Geme, J.W. and Falkow, S. (1991) Loss of capsule expression by *Haemophilus influenzae* type b results in enhanced adherence to and invasion of human cells. *Infection and Immunity* 59, 1325–1333.

St Geme, J.W., Takala, A., Esko, E. and Falkow, S. (1994) Evidence for capsule gene sequences among pharyngeal isolates of nontypeable *Haemophilus influenzae. Journal of Infectious Diseases* 169, 337–342.

St Geme, J.W., Cutter, D. and Barenkamp, S.J. (1996) Characterization of the genetic locus encoding *Haemophilus influenzae* type b surface fibrils. *Journal of Bacteriology* 178, 6281–6287.

Stull, T.L., Mendelman, P.M., Haas, J.E., Schoenborn, M.A., Mack, K.D. and Smith, A.L. (1984) Characterization of *Haemophilus influenzae* type b fimbriae. *Infection and Immunity* 46, 787–796.

Swords, W.E., Ketterer, M.R., Shao, J., Campbell, C.A., Weiser, J.N. and Apicella, M.A. (2001) Binding of the non-typeable *Haemophilus influenzae* lipooligosaccharide to the PAF receptor initiates host cell signalling. *Cellular Microbiology* 3, 525–536.

van Alphen, L., Poole, J., Geelen, L. and Zanen, H.C. (1987) The erythrocyte and epithelial cell receptors for *Haemophilus influenzae* are expressed independently. *Infection and Immunity* 55, 2355–2358.

van Alphen, L., Geelen-van den Broek, L., Blaas, L., van Ham, M. and Dankert, J. (1991) Blocking of fimbria-mediated adherence of *Haemophilus influenzae* by sialyl gangliosides. *Infection and Immunity* 59, 4473–4477.

van Schilfgaarde, M., van Alphen, L., Eijk, P., Everts, V. and Dankert, J. (1995) Paracytosis of *Haemophilus influenzae* through cell layers of NCI-H292 lung epithelial cells. *Infection and Immunity* 63, 4729–4737.

Villullas, S., Hill, D.J., Sessions, R.B., Rea, J. and Virji, M. (2007) Mutational analysis of human CEACAM1: the potential of receptor polymorphism in increasing host susceptibility to bacterial infection. *Cellular Microbiology* 9, 329–346.

Virji, M., Kayhty, H., Ferguson, D.J., Alexandrescu, C. and Moxon, E.R. (1991) Interactions of *Haemophilus influenzae* with cultured human endothelial cells. *Microbial Pathogenesis* 10, 231–245.

Virji, M., Evans, D., Griffith, J., Hill, D., Serino, L., Hadfield, A. and Watt, S.M. (2000) Carcinoembryonic antigens are targeted by diverse strains of typable and non-typable *Haemophilus influenzae. Molecular Microbiology* 36, 784–795.

Vitiello, M., Galdiero, S., D'Isanto, M., D'Amico, M., Di Filippo, C., Cantisani, M., Galdiero, M. and Pedone, C. (2008) Pathophysiological changes of Gram-negative bacterial infection can be reproduced by a synthetic peptide mimicking loop L7 sequence of *Haemophilus influenzae* porin. *Microbes and Infection* 10, 657–663.

Vitiello, M., Finamore, E., Cantisani, M., Bevilacqua, P., Incoronato, N., Falanga, A., Galdiero, E. and Galdiero, M. (2011) P2 porin and loop L7 from *Haemophilus influenzae* modulate expression of IL-6 and adhesion molecules in astrocytes. *Microbiology and Immunology* 55, 347–356.

Watson, W.J., Gilsdorf, J.R., Tucci, M.A., McCrea, K.W., Forney, L.J. and Marrs, C.F. (1994) Identification of a gene essential for piliation in *Haemophilus influenzae* type b with homology to the pilus assembly platform genes of Gram-negative bacteria. *Infection and Immunity* 62, 468–475.

Webb, D.C. and Cripps, A.W. (1998) Secondary structure and molecular analysis of interstrain variability in the P5 outer-membrane protein of non-typable *Haemophilus influenzae* isolated from diverse anatomical sites. *Journal of Medical Microbiology* 47, 1059–1067.

Weiser, J.N., Love, J.M. and Moxon, E.R. (1989) The molecular mechanism of phase variation of *H. influenzae* lipopolysaccharide. *Cell* 59, 657–665.

Weiser, J.N., Chong, S.T., Greenberg, D. and Fong, W. (1995) Identification and characterization of a cell envelope protein of *Haemophilus influenzae* contributing to phase variation in colony opacity and nasopharyngeal colonization. *Molecular Microbiology* 17, 555–564.

Wiedermann, B.L., Hawkins, E.P., Johnson, G.S., Lamberth, L.B., Mason, E.O. and Kaplan, S.L. (1986) Pathogenesis of labyrinthitis associated with *Haemophilus influenzae* type b meningitis in infant rats. *Journal of Infectious Diseases* 153, 27–32.

Williams, A.E., Maskell, D.J. and Moxon, E.R. (1991) Relationship between intracellular survival in macrophages and virulence of *Haemophilus influenzae* type b. *Journal of Infectious Diseases* 163, 1366–1369.

Williams, B.J., Morlin, G., Valentine, N. and Smith, A.L. (2001) Serum resistance in an invasive, nontypeable *Haemophilus influenzae* strain. *Infection and Immunity* 69, 695–705.

Yeo, H.J., Cotter, S.E., Laarmann, S., Juehne, T., St Geme, J.W. and Waksman, G. (2004) Structural basis for host recognition by the *Haemophilus influenzae* Hia autotransporter. *EMBO Journal* 23, 1245–1256.

8 *Escherichia coli* Meningitis

Kwang Sik Kim*
Johns Hopkins University School of Medicine, Baltimore, USA

8.1 Introduction

Gram-negative bacillary meningitis (GNBM) continues to be an important cause of mortality and morbidity throughout the world. Case fatality rates have ranged between 15% and 40%, and approximately 50% of the survivors sustain neurological sequelae. A major contributing factor to such mortality and morbidity is our incomplete understanding of the pathogenesis of this disease (Kim, 2001, 2002, 2003, 2008, 2010, 2012). Both clinical and experimental data indicate limited efficacy with antimicrobial therapy alone for the treatment of GNBM (Kim, 2010). *Escherichia coli* is a common cause of GNBM, particularly during the neonatal period. Post-mortem studies of infants with the acute stages of *E. coli* meningitis revealed the presence of bacteria in the subarachnoid space (SAS) with predominant infiltration of polymorphonuclear leucocytes (PMNLs) and vasculitis in meningeal vessels, but the detailed histopathological findings are surprisingly lacking (Berman and Banker, 1966).

Given the plethora of *E. coli* serotypes, it is striking that *E. coli* strains possessing the K1 capsular polysaccharide are predominant (approximately 80%) among isolates from neonatal *E. coli* meningitis. Most of these K1 isolates are associated with a limited number of O serotypes (e.g. O1, O7, O16, O18, O45) belonging to phylogenetic group B2 and to a lesser extent to group D (Sarff *et al.*, 1975; Bonacorsi *et al.*, 2003). The basis of this association of phylogenetic groups B2 and D with *E. coli* meningitis has not been elucidated.

An emergence of antibiotic resistance is an additional contributing factor to mortality and morbidity associated with *E. coli* meningitis. Recent reports of neonatal meningitis caused by *E. coli* producing CTX-M-type or TEM-type extended-spectrum β-lactamases are a particular concern (Moissenet *et al.*, 2010; Blanco *et al.*, 2011). Drug-resistant clonal group ST131 is prevalent among *E. coli* strains causing extra-intestinal infection and some carried CTX-M-type extended-spectrum β-lactamases (Blanco *et al.*, 2011). These findings indicate that a novel strategy is needed to identify new targets for prevention and therapy of *E. coli* meningitis.

8.2 The Role of the Blood–Brain Barrier (BBB) in *Escherichia coli* Meningitis

Several lines of evidence from human cases of *E. coli* meningitis and animal models of experimental haematogenous meningitis

*kwangkim@jhmi.edu

indicate that *E. coli* invasion into the brain follows a high level of bacteraemia, and that cerebral capillaries are the portal of entry into the brain (Kim *et al.*, 1992). However, the mechanisms remain incompletely understood.

The BBB is a structural and functional barrier that is formed by brain microvascular endothelial cells (BMECs), astrocytes and pericytes (Kim, 2008). It regulates the passage of molecules into and out of the brain to maintain the neural microenvironment, and astrocytes and pericytes help maintain the barrier property of BMECs. The BBB protects the brain from microbes circulating in the blood, but meningitis-causing pathogens have been shown to traverse the BBB transcellularly, paracellularly and/or by means of infected phagocytic cells ('Trojan horse mechanism') (Kim, 2008). However, the contributions of astrocytes and pericytes to *E. coli* translocation of the BBB are minimal, whereas interactions with the endothelial barrier are critical steps for the development of *E. coli* meningitis.

The *in vitro* BBB model has been developed with human brain microvascular endothelial cells (HBMECs) (Stins *et al.*, 1997). Upon cultivation on collagen-coated Transwell inserts, these HBMECs exhibit morphological and functional properties of tight junction formation as well as a polarized monolayer. These are shown by the demonstrations of tight junction proteins (claudin 5 and ZO-1) and adherens junction proteins (VE-cadherin and β-catenin) and their spatial separation, as well as high transendothelial electrical resistance.

The *in vivo* BBB model has been developed by inducing haematogenous meningitis in infant rats and mice. In this animal model, *E. coli* is administered orally, subcutaneously, intracardially or intravenously, resulting in bacteraemia and subsequent entry into the central nervous system (CNS) (Kim *et al.*, 1992; Huang *et al.*, 1995, 1999; Wang *et al.*, 1999; Hoffman *et al.*, 2000; Khan *et al.*, 2002; Wang and Kim, 2002; Zhu *et al.*, 2010a,b). Studies in experimental haematogenous meningitis models indicate that the primary site of entry into the CNS for circulating *E. coli* is the cerebral vasculature, not the choroid plexus (Kim *et al.*, 1992).

8.3 *E. coli* Penetration of the BBB

The development of both *in vitro* and *in vivo* models of the BBB has facilitated our investigations on the mechanisms of microbial translocation of the BBB. Several studies have demonstrated that meningitis-causing *E. coli* K1 strains exhibit the ability to traverse the BBB by transcellular penetration without altering barrier permeability and to then induce meningitis in the SAS (Kim, 2008). Our electron microscopy studies have shown that meningitis-causing *E. coli* K1 strains internalize into HBMECs and transmigrate the monolayer within an enclosed membrane-bound vacuole without intracellular multiplication and without any change in the integrity of the HBMEC monolayer. No free bacteria are found in the cytoplasm of HBMECs or between adjacent HBMECs (Stins *et al.*, 1999; Kim, 2003).

E. coli entry into the CNS of infant rats with experimental haematogenous meningitis has been documented without any change in BBB permeability and without concomitant infiltration of host inflammatory cells (e.g. PMNLs, macrophages) (Kim *et al.*, 1992, 1997). This excludes the possibility that *E. coli* penetrates into the brain using the paracellular mechanism or the Trojan horse mechanism via transmigration of *E. coli*-infected phagocytic cells. It is also important to point out that *E. coli* is an enteric organism, and there are no data supporting the hypotheses that *E. coli* meningitis occurs following inhalation or intranasal spread (Mittal *et al.*, 2010) or that exposure to nicotine via passive smoking increases the development of disease (Chi *et al.*, 2011).

Studies with the *in vitro* and *in vivo* models of the BBB have revealed that successful traversal of the BBB by circulating *E. coli* requires: (i) a threshold level of bacteraemia; (ii) *E. coli* binding to and invasion of HBMECs; and (iii) traversal of the BBB as live bacteria. Notably, specific microbial–host factor interactions are involved in this sequence of events, as described below.

8.3.1 A threshold level of bacteraemia

Several studies in humans and experimental animals point to a relationship between the magnitude of bacteraemia and the development of *E. coli* meningitis (Dietzman *et al.*, 1974; Kim *et al.*, 1992). For example, a significantly higher incidence of *E. coli* meningitis was noted in neonates who had bacterial counts in blood > 10^3 colony forming units (CFU)/ml (six out of 11 neonates), compared with those with blood bacterial counts < 10^3 CFU/ml (one out of 19 neonates). A high degree of bacteraemia is a primary determinant for meningeal invasion by circulating *E. coli* K1 in neonatal and adult animals with experimental haematogenous *E. coli* meningitis (Kim *et al.*, 1992). However, an approximately 10^6-fold greater inoculum of *E. coli* K1 is required to induce a similar high-level bacteraemia in adult animals compared with neonatal animals. These findings suggest that the age dependency of *E. coli* meningitis is most likely due to the relative resistance of adults to high-level bacteraemia and less likely due to greater invasion of meningitis-causing *E. coli* in HBMECs derived from neonates, compared with those from adults. This concept is shown by our demonstration that the abilities of meningitis-causing *E. coli* K1 to bind and invade BMECs are similar between BMECs derived from young and old rats as well as HBMECs derived from different ages (Stins *et al.*, 1999). Thus, one of the reasons for the close association of meningitis-causing *E. coli* strains with neonatal meningitis is their ability to escape from host defences and then to achieve a threshold level of bacteraemia necessary for invasion of the meninges. These findings indicate that the prevention of bacterial multiplication in the blood, which is required for penetration into the brain, would be one potential approach for prevention of *E. coli* meningitis.

E. coli K1 capsular polysaccharide provides serum resistance and anti-phagocytic properties (Kim, 2001). Expression of the K1 capsule and O-lipopolysaccharide (LPS) are critical for induction of a high degree of bacteraemia (Kim *et al.*, 1992), but the feasibility of using the K1 capsule and O-LPS for the prevention of *E. coli* bacteraemia has been shown to be limited (Kim, 2008). However, recent studies using functional *E. coli* genome approaches have identified several other *E. coli* factors that contribute to bactaeremia (Xie *et al.*, 2006b; Moriel *et al.*, 2010). Studies are in progress to determine the nature of the protective and broadly conserved antigens that can be used in multi-epitope subunit vaccines against *E. coli* infections (Moriel *et al.*, 2010).

8.3.2 *E. coli* binding to and invasion of HBMEC

A high degree of bacteraemia is necessary but not sufficient for *E. coli* penetration of the BBB *in vivo*, and *E. coli* binding to and invasion of HBMECs is a prerequisite for penetration into the SAS (Kim, 2008) and the development of meningitis. This was shown by the demonstration in infant rats with experimental haematogenous meningitis that several isogenic mutants of meningitis-causing *E. coli* K1 strain RS218, deleted of factors contributing to HBMEC binding, e.g. outer membrane protein (OMP) A, and invasion, e.g. Ibe (named after Invasion of brain endothelial cell) proteins and cytotoxic necrotizing factor (CNF1), were significantly less able to induce meningitis than the parent strain, despite similar levels of bacteraemia (Table 8.1). These findings indicate that those *E. coli* factors contributing to HBMEC binding and invasion are necessary for penetration into the SAS *in vivo*. However, these *E. coli* K1 factors do not influence the release of chemokines such as interleukin (IL-)8 from HBMECs and a neurotropism is exhibited, because the meningitis-causing *E. coli* K1 strain RS218 does not induce IL-8 release from non-brain endothelial cells, e.g. from umbilical veins (Galanakis *et al.*, 2006).

E. coli *factors contributing to HBMEC binding*

Infections caused by pathogenic *E. coli* are often initiated by binding of the bacteria to the host cell surface, and this concept is likely to be important for circulating *E. coli* to

Table 8.1. Development of bacteraemia (mean ± SD) and meningitis (defined as positive cerebrospinal fluid (CSF) cultures) in infant rats receiving meningitis-causing *E. coli* K1 strain RS218 or its deletion mutants. (Modified from Kim, 2001.)

E. coli strain	No. of animals	Bacteraemia (log_{10} CFU/ml blood)	% of animals with positive CSF
RS218	19	7.18±0.63	12 (63)
Δ*ompA*	22	7.05±0.49	6 (27)[a]
RS218	24	7.51±1.25	16 (67)
Δ*ibeA*	25	6.97±1.21	4 (16)[a]
RS218	27	7.01±1.17	15 (56)
Δ*ibeB*	25	7.06±1.29	4 (16)[a]
RS218	24	7.53±0.40	18 (75)
Δ*ibeC*	24	7.80±0.67	10 (42)[a]
RS218	17	7.50±0.32	14 (82)
Δ*aslA*	22	7.60±0.49	7 (32)[a]
RS218	26	7.64±1.00	20 (77)
Δ*cnf1*	27	7.24±1.60	12 (44)[a]

[a]Significantly reduced compared with RS218.

withstand blood flow and shear stress *in vivo* and cross the BBB. Several *E. coli* factors are identified to be involved in binding to HBMECs that subsequently affects cellular invasion, including type 1 fimbriae (FimH), flagella (FliC), OmpA and lipoprotein NlpI. The roles of these *E. coli* factors in HBMEC binding were confirmed by deletion and complementation experiments. Thus, isogenic deletion mutants showed reduced binding to HBMECs and their binding capacity was restored to the level of the parent strain by complementation with respective wild-type genes.

Type 1 fimbriae: Our experiments with an *E. coli* DNA microarray, comparing the gene expression patterns of HBMEC-associated against non-associated *E. coli* K1, revealed that type 1 fimbriae play an important role in *E. coli* K1 binding to HBMECs (Teng *et al.*, 2005). The HBMEC-associated *E. coli* K1 showed significantly higher expression levels of the *fim* cluster genes compared with non-associated bacteria. Expression of type 1 fimbriae in wild-type *E. coli* is regulated by phase variation in which each bacterium can alternate between fimbriated and non-fimbriated states, so-called phase-ON and phase-OFF, respectively. We have shown that *E. coli* K1 associated with HBMECs are predominantly type 1 fimbriae phase-ON bacteria. From our *E. coli* DNA microarray experiments, we also identified a novel site-specific recombinase, HbiF, which inverted the molecular switch *fimS* independently of the two known recombinases, FimB and FimE, that invert *fimS* and control the expression of the downstream *fim* operon (Xie *et al.*, 2006a). Discovery of HbiF-mediated *fimS* switching provides a new opportunity for regulating type 1 fimbriae expression, which will help in developing a novel strategy for the prevention and therapy of *E. coli* bacteraemia and meningitis.

We also identified that FimH interacts with a glycosylphosphatidylinositol-anchored receptor, CD48, on the surface of HBMECs. The FimH–CD48 interaction contributes to *E. coli* binding to HBMECs and increases intracellular calcium $[Ca^{2+}]i$ (Khan *et al.*, 2007), which was confirmed by the demonstration that CD48 antibody blocks

FimH-mediated binding and FimH-induced $[Ca^{2+}]i$ changes in HBMECs.

S fimbriae, which bind to terminal NeuAc α2,3-galactose sequences present on glycoproteins, have been implicated in *E. coli* binding to HBMECs. Purified S fimbriae or a recombinant *E. coli* strain HB101 expressing S fimbriae were shown to bind to the luminal surfaces of the brain vascular endothelium in neonatal rat brain tissues (Parkkinen *et al.*, 1988). We have previously shown using S fimbriated transformants of *E. coli* strain HB101 that S fimbriae allowed this *E. coli* laboratory strain to bind to HBMECs. However, in-frame deletion of the S fimbriae operon in meningitis-causing *E. coli* K1 did not affect *E. coli* binding to and invasion of HBMECs, and also did not affect *E. coli* K1 penetration into the CNS in the experimental haematogenous meningitis animal model. Thus, S fimbriae are not critical for either HBMEC binding *in vitro* or traversal of the BBB *in vivo* by meningitis-causing *E. coli* K1.

Flagella: The external whip-like structures involved in bacterial motility have been shown to contribute to the virulence of many enteric bacteria, including meningitis-causing *E. coli*. The *E. coli* DNA microarray experiments demonstrated that flagella play an important role in *E. coli* K1 binding to HBMECs (Parthasarathy *et al.*, 2007). The flagellum is synthesized from three classes of genes. The class I region consists of the master operon *flhDC*, the class II region comprises the genes involved in the synthesis of the flagella basal body and hook, and the class III region consists of genes involved in flagella synthesis and motility. Using defined deletion mutants constructed for each class of genes, the mutants deleted of the flagella structure exhibited significant defects in HBMEC binding and invasion, while deletion of genes affecting only motility did not influence binding to and invasion of HBMECs (Parthasarathy *et al.*, 2007). In addition, recombinant flagellin (FliC) has been shown to bind directly to the surface of HBMECs and addition of exogenous recombinant flagellin decreased *E. coli* K1 binding to HBMECs.

OmpA: this major outer membrane protein and its N-terminal domain cross the outer membrane eight times in anti-parallel β-strands with four hydrophilic surface-exposed loops and short periplasmic turns. The N-terminal portion of OmpA and its surface-exposed loops contribute to binding to HBMECs (Prasadarao *et al.*, 1996b; Maruvada and Kim, 2011) and OmpA interacts with HBMECs through *N*-acetylglucosamine (GlcNAc) residues of gp96 (Khan *et al.*, 2003). Administration of chitooligomers (GlcNAc β1, 4-GlcNAc oligomers) and chitohexose can block traversal of the BBB by meningitis-causing *E. coli* K1 (Prasadarao *et al.*, 1996a; Maruvada and Kim, 2011). Of interest, gp96 is also a cellular receptor for another CNS-infecting bacterium, *Listeria monocytogenes* Vip (Cabanes *et al.*, 2005) (Table 8.2).

However, our study with the *E. coli* DNA microarray, which compared the *ompA* deletion mutant with its parent *E. coli* K1 strain RS218, revealed that the mutant exhibited significantly lower expression of both the *fim* cluster genes and type 1 fimbriae on the bacterial surface (Teng *et al.*, 2006). Thus, decreased binding of the *ompA* deletion mutant may be related to its lower expression of type 1 fimbriae. Importantly, the *ompA* deletion mutant was less efficient in its penetration into the brain *in vivo* compared with the parent *E. coli* K1 strain (Wang and Kim, 2002). Additional studies are needed to determine whether these *in vitro* and *in vivo* defects of the *ompA* deletion mutant are in part

Table 8.2. BBB receptors used by *E. coli* and other CNS-infecting microorganisms. (Modified from Kim, 2008, 2010.)

Receptor	Organism and ligand
gp96	*E. coli* OmpA
	L. monocytogenes Vip
37LRP	*E. coli* CNF1
	N. meningitidis PilQ/PorA
	S. pneumoniae CbpA
	H. influenzae type b Omp2
	Prion protein
	Viruses (sindbis, dengue, tick-borne encephalitis, Venezuelan equine encephalitis, adeno-associated)

related to its decreased expression of type 1 fimbriae and also to understand how *ompA* deletion affects type 1 fimbriae expression.

NlpI: This is an outer membrane-anchored lipoprotein that enables evasion of serum-mediated killing through regulation of the complement regulator C4bp deposition on the bacterial surface (Tseng *et al.*, 2012). NlpI is an important factor used by Crohn's disease-associated *E. coli* strain LF82 (O83:H1) bacteria to interact with intestinal epithelial cells (Barnich *et al.*, 2004). Deletion of *nlpI* in *E. coli* strain LF82 decreased expression of type 1 fimbriae and flagella. NlpI also contributes to meningitis-causing *E. coli* K1 binding to and invasion of HBMECs (Teng *et al.*, 2010). However, unlike strain LF82, deletion of *nlpI* in meningitis-causing *E. coli* did not affect the expression of type 1 fimbriae, flagella and OmpA, indicating that the contribution of NlpI to HBMEC binding and invasion is independent of those bacterial factors in meningitis-causing *E. coli*. This was shown by the demonstration that mutants deleted of type 1 fimbriae, OmpA and NlpI exhibited significantly decreased HBMEC binding and invasion, compared with mutants deleted of individual factors or a combination of the two factors (Teng *et al.*, 2010). Type 1 fimbriae, OmpA and NlpI are likely, therefore, to contribute independently to HBMEC binding and invasion. However, it still remains unclear how and why several factors of meningitis-causing *E. coli* are involved in HBMEC binding.

E. coli *structures contributing to invasion of HBMECs*

Previous studies using Tn*phoA* mutagenesis, signature-tagged mutagenesis and differential fluorescence induction with screening of a green fluorescent protein fusion library identified several *E. coli* determinants contributing to invasion of HBMECs, such as Ibe proteins and CNF1. Isogenic deletion mutants of these proteins were less invasive in HBMECs and less able to penetrate into the SAS/brain *in vivo* (Table 8.1) and their invasive defects were restored to the levels of the parent strain by complementation with respective wild-type genes.

Ibe proteins: Ibe A, B and C proteins were identified via Tn*phoA* mutagenesis of meningitis-causing *E. coli* K1 strain RS218 and screening of the mutants for loss of invasion, using both *in vitro* and *in vivo* BBB models (Kim, 2001). Exogenous recombinant Ibe proteins were shown to inhibit meningitis-causing *E. coli* K1 invasion of HBMECs (Huang *et al.*, 1995, 1999), suggesting that Ibe proteins contribute to HBMEC invasion by bacterial ligand–host cell receptor interactions. This concept was supported by the demonstration of a HBMEC 45 kDa albumin-like surface protein interactive with IbeA, and a polyclonal antibody raised against this receptor protein inhibited *E. coli* K1 invasion of HBMECs (Kim, 2001). The gene, *ibeA*, was shown to be prevalent in meningitis-causing *E. coli* K1 of phylogenetic B2 group, while *ibeB* and *ibeC* were found to have homologues in non-meningitis isolates of *E. coli*. It remains unclear whether the *ibeB* and *ibeC* homologues from non-meningitis isolates will exhibit the HBMEC invasion phenotype of meningitis-causing *E. coli* K1 strains. However, the mechanisms involved with IbeA, IbeB and IbeC proteins in *E. coli* K1 invasion of HBMECs appear to be similar and their contributions to HBMEC invasion are likely to be redundant. This is shown by the fact that HBMEC invasion frequencies did not differ among mutants deleted of *ibeA*, *ibeB* and *ibeC* versus mutants deleted of single or double genes (Kim, 2002). Additional studies are needed to elucidate the mechanisms involved with IbeA, IbeB and IbeC for their contribution to *E. coli* meningitis.

Cytotoxic necrotizing factor 1 (CNF1): This is a bacterial virulence factor associated with extra-intestinal pathogenic *E. coli* strains causing urinary tract infection and meningitis. CNF1 is an AB-type toxin, composed of an N-terminal cell-binding domain and a C-terminal domain that catalyses the site-specific deamination of a glutamine residue to a glutamate. CNF1 has been shown to activate RhoGTPases such as RhoA and to induce the uptake, by macropinocytosis, of latex beads, bacteria and apoptotic bodies into non-professional phagocytes such as epithelial and endothelial cells.

CNF1 contributes to *E. coli* K1 invasion of HBMECs *in vitro* and traversal of the BBB *in vivo*, and both of these events are dependent upon RhoA activation (Khan *et al.*, 2002). This was shown by: (i) the decreased invasion and RhoA activation with the CNF1 deletion mutant compared to the parent strain in HBMECs; and (ii) restoration of the CNF1 mutant's invasion frequency to the level of the parent strain in HBMECs expressing constitutively active RhoA.

Internalization of CNF1 has been suggested to occur via receptor-mediated endocytosis upon binding to a cell surface receptor. Yeast two-hybrid screening of a HBMEC cDNA library with the N-terminal cell-binding domain of CNF1 as 'bait' has identified the HBMEC receptor for CNF1 as the 37 kDa laminin receptor precursor (37LRP) (Chung *et al.*, 2003). This receptor interacted with N-terminal CNF1 and full-length CNF1, but not with C-terminal CNF1 CNF1-mediated RhoA activation and bacterial uptake were inhibited by 37LRP antisense oligodeoxynucleotides, whereas they were increased in 37LRP-overexpressing cells, demonstrating a correlation between the effects of CNF1 and levels of 37LRP expression in HBMECs (Chung *et al.*, 2003). These findings indicate that the CNF1–37LRP interaction is the initial step required for CNF1-mediated RhoA activation and bacterial uptake in eukaryotic cells.

37LRP is a ribosome-associated cytoplasmic protein and a precursor of the 67 kDa laminin receptor (67LR). It is unclear how 67LR is matured and synthesized from the 37LRP, but mature 67LR was shown to be present on the cell surface and functions as a membrane receptor for the adhesive basement membrane protein laminin. Incubation of HBMECs with CNF1-expressing *E. coli* K1 upregulates 67LR expression and recruits 67LR to the site of invading *E. coli* K1 in a CNF1-dependent manner (Kim, 2003), supporting the participation of 67LR in CNF1-expressing *E. coli* K1 invasion of HBMECs. 37LRP is also a cellular target for other ligands found on CNS-infecting microorganisms (Table 8.2). However, the exact mechanisms by which ligand interactions with the same receptor lead to CNS penetration by different organisms remain to be established.

E. coli *invasion of HBMECs involves host cell actin cytoskeleton rearrangements*

Pathogenic microbes can exploit various strategies to penetrate host cells (Kim, 2008). Microbial internalization into non-professional phagocytes such as endothelial and epithelial cells occurs mainly via two different mechanisms involving host cell actin cytoskeleton rearrangements: a 'zipper' mechanism, involving the formation of cell protrusions in contact with the pathogens, and a 'trigger' mechanism, involving the formation of membrane ruffling around the pathogens. Scanning and transmission electron microscopy studies have shown that internalization of meningitis-causing *E. coli* K1 into HBMECs is associated with microvilli-like protrusions at the entry site on the surface of HBMECs (Prasadarao *et al.*, 1999; Kim, 2003), suggesting the involvement of HBMEC actin cytoskeleton rearrangement in bacterial invasion. This is supported by the observation that F-actin condensation occurs with invading bacteria, and blockade of actin condensation with microfilament-disrupting agents such as cytochalasin D inhibits *E. coli* K1 invasion.

Meningitis-causing E. coli *K1 strains exploit host signalling molecules for invasion of HBMECs*

Several host signal transduction pathways have been shown to be involved in *E. coli* K1 invasion of HBMECs. These include focal adhesion kinase (FAK), paxillin, phosphatidylinositol 3-kinase (PI3K), Src kinase, signal transducers and activators of transcription 3 (STAT3), Rho GTPases (RhoA and Rac1), cytosolic phospholipase A2 (cPLA2), 5-lipoxygenase and cysteinyl leukotrienes, vascular endothelial growth factor (VEGF) receptor-1, ezrin, radixin and moesin (ERM), calmodulin-dependent myosin light-chain kinase and protein kinase C (PKC) (Kim, 2008; Zhao *et al.*, 2010; Zhu *et al.*, 2010a,b; Maruvada and Kim, 2011, 2012). However, the underlying host cell–microbial interactions are not completely understood.

It is important to note that activation of these host cell signalling molecules is influenced by the provenance of the host cell and the nature of the microbial pathogen. For example, FimH of meningitis-causing *E. coli* has been shown to induce RhoA activation, but not FAK activation in HBMECs (Khan *et al.*, 2007). In contrast, FimH of uropathogenic *E. coli* induces FAK activation in bladder epithelial cells (Martinez *et al.*, 2000). A similar concept is shown with host receptors, e.g. gp96 functions as the receptor for *E. coli* OmpA and *L. monocytogenes* Vip. The OmpA–gp96 interaction resulted in FAK activation in HBMECs (Reddy *et al.*, 2000), but no FAK activation occurred with the Vip–gp96 interaction in mouse fibroblasts (Cabanes *et al.*, 2005).

Our current knowledge on the underlying mechanisms involved with these host cell signalling molecules for their contribution to HBMEC invasion has been derived from the following two approaches: (i) identification of the *E. coli* factors participating in specific host cell signalling molecules; and (ii) examination of the interrelationship of the host cell signalling molecules involved in *E. coli* invasion of HBMECs. For example, OmpA and Ibe proteins of meningitis-causing *E. coli* K1 are involved in FAK and PI3K activation, OmpA and IbeA in STAT3 and Rac1 activation, FimH and CNF1 in RhoA activation, OmpA and NlpI in cPLA2 and PKC activations, and CNF1 in ERM activation (Fig. 8.1). This information has been useful for elucidating why and how several bacterial factors contribute to *E. coli* binding to and invasion

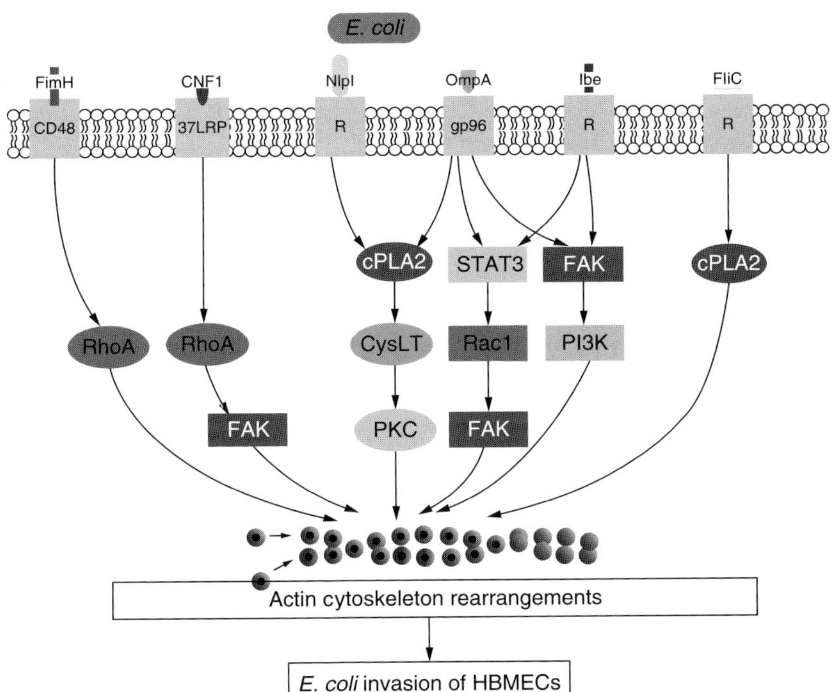

Fig. 8.1. Host signalling molecules involved in HBMEC actin cytoskeleton rearrangements and *E. coli* K1 invasion of the BBB. *E. coli* K1 invasion of the BBB requires specific bacterial factors (FimH, CNF1, NlpI, OmpA, Ibe proteins and FliC) and their interactions with host factors (CD48, 37LRP, R, gp96) on HBMECs, involving Rho GTPases (RhoA and Rac1), focal adhesion kinase (FAK), cytosolic phospholipase A2α (cPLA2α), cysteinyl leukotrienes (CysLT), protein kinase C (PKC), signal transducers and activators of transcription 3 (STAT3), and phosphatidylinositol 3-kinase (PI3K). CNF1, cytotoxic necrotizing factor 1; 37LRP, 37κDa laminin receptor precursor; R, receptor; gp96, glycoprotein 96.

of HBMECs, and also whether or not their contributions are redundant. For example, Rac1 activation occurs in response to OmpA or IbeA, and RhoA activation occurs in response to CNF1 or FimH, while cPLA2 activation occurs in response to OmpA or NlpI (Khan *et al.*, 2007; Teng *et al.*, 2010; Maruvada and Kim, 2011, 2012). Mutants deficient in OmpA and CNF1, OmpA and FimH, or FimH and NlpI exhibit greater defects in invasion of HBMECs compared with individual deletion mutants, whereas mutants deleted of OmpA and Ibe alone do not. Thus, the reasons for the additive (non-redundant) versus indifferent (redundant) effects of different bacterial factors in *E. coli* binding to and invasion of HBMECs can be in part explained by their underlying host cell signalling mechanisms (e.g. involving different or the same host signalling molecules and pathways, respectively).

Meningitis-causing *E. coli* K1 also exploits FAK and PI3K for cell invasion, as shown by decreased invasion in HBMECs expressing dominant-negative FAK and PI3K as well as pharmacological inhibition of both molecules. In addition, FAK is upstream of PI3K in *E. coli* invasion of HBMECs, which is shown by the fact that PI3K activation is abolished in HBMECs expressing dominant-negative FAK (Reddy *et al.*, 2000). Similarly, both STAT3 and Rac1 are involved in meningitis-causing *E. coli* invasion of HBMECs, but STAT3 is upstream of Rac1, as shown by blockade of Rac1 activation in HBMEC expressing dominant-negative STAT3 (Maruvada and Kim, 2012). Also, cPLA2 and PKC are involved in meningitis-causing *E. coli* invasion of HBMECs, but cPLA2 is upstream of PKC, as shown by the demonstration that inhibition of cPLA2 prevents PKC activation in response to meningitis-causing *E. coli* K1 in HBMECs (Zhu *et al.*, 2010b).

It should also be noted that host cell actin cytoskeleton rearrangements are required for HBMEC invasion by meningitis-causing bacteria such as *E. coli*, Group B *Streptococcus* and *L. monocytogenes* (Kim, 2001), but the host cell signalling mechanisms involved in actin cytoskeleton rearrangements and HBMEC invasion are different among these organisms. For example, *E. coli* K1 invasion of HBMECs depends on activation of FAK, Src and cPLA2. In contrast, Group B *Streptococcus* and *L. monocytogenes* invasion of HBMECs was independent of Src, and FAK and cPLA2 activation, respectively.

Arachidonic acid metabolism pathways also contribute to the invasion of HBMECs and subsequent penetration specifically into the SAS/brain by meningitis-causing *E. coli* K1 strains of phlyogenetic groups B2 and D (Zhu *et al.*, 2010a). Gene deletion and pharmacological inhibition of arachidonic acid metabolism pathways prevents *E. coli* penetration specifically into the CNS, without affecting the level of bacteraemia and penetration into other organs such as the kidney, spleen and lung. These findings suggest that determination of the microbial/host factors contributing to arachidonic acid metabolism pathways-mediated penetration of the BBB is likely to inform the neurotropism of *E. coli* and the development of novel targets for prevention and therapy of *E. coli* meningitis.

8.3.3 *E. coli* traversal of the BBB as live bacteria

E. coli K1 has been shown to traverse the BBB as live bacteria without altering the integrity of the HBMEC monolayer and without affecting barrier permeability (Kim, 2001). These are critical factors for the development of meningitis. As indicated above, internalized *E. coli* bacteria are located within membrane-bound vacuoles of HBMECs that transmigrate the HBMEC monolayer. HBMECs have the complete intracellular trafficking machinery required to deliver the microbe-containing vacuoles to cathepsin D-containing lysosomes (Kim *et al.*, 2003). For example, vacuoles containing *E. coli* K1 capsule deletion mutant interact sequentially with early endosomal marker proteins, such as early endosomal auto-antigen 1 and transferrin receptor, and then with late endosome and late endosome/lysosomal markers, such as Rab7 and lysosome-associated membrane proteins. These interactions enable lysosomal fusion with subsequent degradation inside vacuoles. In contrast, the K1 capsule modulates the maturation process of vacuoles containing encapsulated bacteria in early and late endosomes and prevents their fusion with lysosomes. This process allows *E. coli* K1 to cross the BBB as live bacteria (Kim *et al.*, 2003), but additional studies are needed to understand the molecular basis by which the K1 capsule modulates this intracellular trafficking and whether similar events occur with other capsulated bacteria causing meningitis.

8.4 Functional Genomics of *E. coli*

Genome sequencing of meningitis-causing microorganisms provides new tools for elucidating the pathogenesis of meningitis. For example, comparative genome analysis of the prototypic meningitis-causing *E. coli* K1 strain RS218 (O18:K1) versus laboratory K-12 strain MG1655 identified 22 RS218-derived islands (RDIs) that are larger than 10 kb but are absent in strain MG1655 (Xie *et al.*, 2006b). The total length of these RDIs is approximately 793 kb, which replaced approximately 80 kb of MG1655-specific sequences, resulting in an approximately 713 kb larger chromosome size in RS218. These 22 RDIs have been shown to be located at different regions of the *E. coli* K1 RS218 chromosome (Xie *et al.*, 2006b).

Using RDI deletion mutants constructed from strain RS218, eight RDIs have been shown to be involved in the induction of high-grade bacteraemia and binding to HBMECs and subsequent invasion. Two RDIs include a P4-family integrase and are directly adjacent to tRNAs (RDI 4-*serX* and RDI 21-*leuX*) and four RDIs have markedly lower GC percentages compared with the whole RS218 genome (Xie *et al.*, 2006b), suggesting that these RDIs are acquired through a horizontal gene transfer. Further identification and characterization of microbial determinants from those RDIs that are involved in the pathogenesis of *E. coli* meningitis should help in elucidating microbial factors involved in the development of *E. coli* meningitis.

At present, the microbial factors identified from prototypic meningitis-causing O18:K1 *E. coli* strains such as RS218 and C5 have been used to study the pathogenesis of meningitis (Xie *et al.*, 2006b; Kim, 2008). However, it is unclear whether the information derived from these *E. coli* K1 strains is relevant to other *E. coli* K1 strains isolated from CSF. A comparative genomic hybridization (CGH) with an *E. coli* DNA microarray was used to examine the basis of meningitis caused by representative *E. coli* K1 strains isolated from CSF and belonging to phlyogenetic groups B2 and D (Yao *et al.*, 2006). These strains included RS218 (O18:K1, B2 group), C5 (18:K1, B2 group), IHE3034 (O18:K1, B2 group), EC10 (O7:K1, D group), A90 (O1:K1, B2 group), RS168 (O1:K1, D group), RS167 (O16:K1, B2 group), S88 (O45:K1, B2 group) and S95 (O45:K1, B2 group). Hierarchical clustering revealed that these strains can be categorized into two groups. Group 1 includes strains RS218, C5, IHE3034, A90, RS167, S88 and S95, while strains EC10 and RS168 belong to group 2. All group 1 strains belong to the phylogenetic group B2, which is predominant in CSF isolates, and group 2 strains belong to less common phylogenetic groups A and D (Yao *et al.*, 2006). Of interest, a type III secretion system was found in group 2 strains of *E. coli*, but not in group 1 strains isolated from neonatal meningitis, and was shown to contribute to *E. coli* invasion of HBMECs and to intracellular bacterial survival (Yao *et al.*, 2009). The existence of a type III secretion system as well as its effectors and homologues was verified by genome sequencing of strain EC10. This is the first demonstration of a type III secretion system in meningitis-causing *E. coli*, but its contribution to *E. coli* meningitis remains to be established.

CGH was also used to examine the distribution of the eight RDIs that are known to be involved in the pathogenesis of *E. coli* meningitis among representative *E. coli* K1 strains (Xie *et al.*, 2006b). RDI 16 harbours the K1 capsule biosynthesis gene cluster and, as expected, is present in all of the *E. coli* K1 strains. The other pathogenic RDIs exist in strains belonging to our group 1 and phylogenetic group B2. For example, RDI 1, 7, 13, 20 and 22 are widely distributed among this group of *E. coli* K1 strains. Previous studies using PCR, dot blot and Southern blot suggest that PAI III_{536}-like, PAI II_{J96}-like and GimA-like ectochromosomal DNA domains (ECDNAs) are prevalent among O18:K1 strains, the most common serogroup in meningitis-causing *E. coli* (Bonacorsi *et al.*, 2003). Based on their virulence signatures, those ECDNAs correspond to RDI 4, 21 and 22, respectively (Xie *et al.*, 2006b). The distribution of these three islands among O18:K1 strains based on CGH is consistent with previous findings (Bonacorsi *et al.*, 2003; Xie *et al.*, 2006b).

CGH analysis also revealed that type VI secretion system (T6SS)-like gene clusters, including the *icmF*-like component, *clpV*, *dotU* and *hcp2*, are present in RDI 1. The T6SS clusters have two *hcp*-like genes located next to each other in the chromosome of strain RS218, and the two Hcp family proteins have different roles in meningitis-causing *E. coli* K1 infection. They coordinately contribute to *E. coli* binding to and invasion of HBMECs as well as release of IL-6 and IL-8 cytokines (Zhou *et al.*, 2012).

In addition, microbial DNA microarrays offer new opportunities for exploring microbial gene expression profiles during microbial–host cell interactions. For example, using *E. coli* DNA microarray analysis with microarray-grade bacterial RNA isolated from *E. coli* K1 interacting with HBMECs, it was reported that the expression of the type 1 fimbriae and flagella genes is significantly greater for *E. coli* associated with HBMECs compared with *E. coli* not associated with HBMECs.

8.5 Strategies for Preventing *E. coli* Penetration into the Brain

Penetration into the SAS/brain by meningitis-causing *E. coli* K1 requires bacterial binding to and invasion of HBMECS, which involves specific microbial ligand–host cell interactions leading to host cell signalling molecule involvement (Kim, 2008, 2010, 2012). Pharmacological inhibition of these pathways might be a novel strategy for preventing *E. coli* meningitis. For example, CNF1-mediated *E. coli* uptake and RhoA activation in HBMECs were inhibited by 37LRP antisense oligodeoxynucleotides, whereas they were increased in 37LRP-overexpressing cells (Chung *et al.*, 2003). In addition, pharmacological inhibition and gene deletion of host cell signalling molecules, e.g. cPLA2, 37LRP and cysteinyl leukotrienes, was efficient in preventing *E. coli* penetration into the SAS/brain (Zhu *et al.*, 2010b). Another strategy is to modulate the expression and/or secretion of the microbial factors contributing to *E. coli* binding to HBMECs and subsequent invasion. For example, CNF1 is a key *E. coli* invasin, but the protein is cytoplasmic and must be secreted to exert its biological function. However, no signal peptide is present in the CNF1 sequence and it is unclear how CNF1 secretion occurs across the bacterial inner and outer membranes as well as into OM vesicles. Recently, the involvement of ferredoxin in CNF1 secretion across the bacterial inner membrane and of YgfZ in CNF1 secretion into outer-membrane vesicles has been reported (Yu and Kim, 2010, 2012). Elucidating the mechanisms involved in CNF1 secretion, or of type III and type VI secretion systems, will increase our knowledge of the pathogenesis of *E. coli* meningitis and lead to the development of novel targeted therapies.

8.6 Conclusion

Knowledge of the pathogenesis and pathophysiology of *E. coli* meningitis is still incomplete, despite the significant advances that *in vitro* and *in vivo* BBB models have made in illuminating the mechanisms of microbial entry into the CSF-filled SAS. A complete understanding of the microbial-host factors that are involved in *E. coli* pathogenesis will help develop new strategies for prevention and therapy of meningitis and associated neuronal injury.

Acknowledgements

This work was supported by NIH grants R01 NS 26310 and AI 84984.

References

Barnich, N., Bringer, M.A., Claret, L. and Darfeuille-Michaud, A. (2004) Involvement of lipoprotein NlpI in the virulence of adherent invasive *Escherichia coli* strain LF82 isolated from a patient with Crohn's disease. *Infection and Immunity* 72, 2484–2493.

Berman, P.H. and Banker, B.Q. (1966) Neonatal meningitis: a clinical and pathological study of 29 cases. *Pediatrics* 38, 6–24.

Blanco, J., *et al.* (2011) National survey of *Escherichia coli* causing extraintestinal infections reveals the spread of drug-resistant clonal groups O25b:H4-B2-ST131, O15:H1-D-ST393 and CGA-D-ST69 with high virulence gene content in Spain. *Journal of Antimicrobial Chemotherapy* 66, 2011–2021.

Bonacorsi, S., Clermont, O., Houdouin, W., Cordevant, C., Brahimi, N., Marecat, A., Tinsley, C., Nassif, X., Lange, M. and Bingen, E. (2003) Molecular analysis and experimental virulence of French and North American *Escherichia coli* neonatal meningitis isolates: identification of a new virulent clone. *Journal of Infectious Diseases* 187, 1895–1906.

Cabanes, D., Sousa, S., Cebria, A., Lecuit, M., Garcia-del Portillo, F. and Cossart, P. (2005) Gp96 is a receptor for a novel *Listeria monocytogenes* virulence factor, Vip, a surface protein. *EMBO Journal* 24, 2827–2838.

Chi, F., Wang, L., Zheng, X., Wu, C.H., Jong, A., Sheard, M.A., Shi, W. and Huang, S.H. (2011) Meningitic *Escherichia coli* K1 penetration and neutrophil transmigration across the blood–brain barrier are modulated by α7 nicotinic receptor. *PLoS One* 6, e25016.

Chung, J.W., Hong, S.J., Kim, K.J., Goti, D., Stins, M.F., Shin, S., Dawson, V.L., Dawson, T.M. and Kim, K.S. (2003) 37-kDa laminin receptor precursor modulates cytotoxic necrotizing factor 1-mediated RhoA activation and bacterial uptake. *Journal of Biological Chemistry* 278, 16857–16862.

Dietzman, D.E., Fischer, G.W. and Schoenkn, F.D. (1974) Neonatal *Escherichia coli* septicemia bacterial counts in blood. *Journal of Pediatrics* 85, 128–130.

Galanakis, E., Di Cello, F., Paul-Satyaseela, M. and Kim, K.S. (2006) *Escherichia coli* K1 induces IL-8 expression in human brain microvascular endothelial cells. *European Cytokine Network* 17, 260–265.

Hoffman, J.A., Badger, J.L., Zhang, Y., Huang, S.H. and Kim, K.S. (2000) *Escherichia coli* K1 *aslA* contributes to invasion of brain microvascular endothelial cells in vitro and in vivo. *Infection and Immunity* 68, 5062–5067.

Huang, S.H., Wass, C., Fu, Q., Prasadarao, N.V., Stins, M. and Kim, K.S. (1995) *Escherichia coli* invasion of brain microvascular endothelial cells in vitro and in vivo – molecular cloning and characterization of invasion gene *ibe10*. *Infection and Immunity* 63, 4470–4475.

Huang, S.H., Chen, Y.H., Fu, Q., Stins, M., Wang, Y., Wass, C. and Kim, K.S. (1999) Identification and characterization of an *Escherichia coli* invasion gene locus, *ibeB*, required for penetration of brain microvascular endothelial cells. *Infection and Immunity* 67, 2103–2109.

Khan, N.A., Wang, Y., Kim, K.J., Chung, J.W., Wass, C.A. and Kim, K.S. (2002) Cytotoxic necrotizing factor-1 contributes to *Escherichia coli* K1 invasion of the central nervous system. *Journal of Biological Chemistry* 277, 15607–15612.

Khan, N.A., Shin, S., Chung, J.W., Kim, K.J., Elliott, S., Wang, Y. and Kim, K.S. (2003) Outer membrane protein A and cytotoxic necrotizing factor-1 use diverse signaling mechanisms for *Escherichia coli* K1 invasion of human brain microvascular endothelial cells. *Microbial Pathogenesis* 35, 35–42.

Khan, N.A., Kim, Y., Shin, S. and Kim, K.S. (2007) FimH-mediated *Escherichia coli* K1 invasion of human brain microvascular endothelial cells. *Cellular Microbiology* 9, 169–178.

Kim, K.J., Elliott, S.J., Di Cello, F., Stins, M.F. and Kim, K.S. (2003) The K1 capsule modulates trafficking of *E. coli*-containing vacuoles and enhances intracellular bacterial survival in human brain microvascular endothelial cells. *Cellular Microbiology* 5, 245–252.

Kim, K.S. (2001) *Escherichia coli* translocation at the blood–brain barrier. *Infection and Immunity* 69, 5217–5222.

Kim, K.S. (2002) Strategy of *Escherichia coli* for crossing the blood–brain barrier. *Journal of Infectious Diseases* 186, S220–S224.

Kim, K.S. (2003) Pathogenesis of bacterial meningitis: from bacteraemia to neuronal injury. *Nature Reviews Neuroscience* 4, 376–385.

Kim, K.S. (2008) Mechanisms of microbial traversal of the blood–brain barrier. *Nature Reviews Microbiology* 6, 625–634.

Kim, K.S. (2010) Acute bacterial meningitis in infants and children. *Lancet Infectious Diseases* 10, 32–42.

Kim, K.S. (2012) Current concepts on the pathogenesis of *Escherichia coli* meningitis: implications for therapy and prevention. *Current Opinion in Infectious Diseases* 25, 273–278.

Kim, K.S., Itabashi, H., Gemski, P., Sadoff, J., Warren, R.L. and Cross, A.S. (1992) The K1 capsule is the critical determinant in the development of *Escherichia coli* meningitis in the rat. *Journal of Clinical Investigation* 90, 897–905.

Kim, K.S., Wass, C.A. and Cross, A.S. (1997) Blood–brain barrier permeability during the development of experimental bacterial meningitis in the rat. *Experimental Neurology* 145, 253–257.

Martinez, J.J., Mulvey, M.A., Schilling, J.D., Pinkner, J.S. and Hultgren, S.J. (2000) Type 1 pilus-mediated bacterial invasion of bladder epithelial cells. *EMBO Journal* 19, 2803–2812.

Maruvada, R. and Kim, K.S. (2011) Extracellular loops of the *Eschericia coli* outer membrane protein A contribute to the pathogenesis of meningitis. *Journal of Infectious Diseases* 203, 131–140.

Maruvada, R. and Kim, K.S. (2012) IbeA and OmpA of *Escherichia coli* K1 exploit Rac1 activation for invasion of human brain microvascular endothelial cells. *Infection and Immunity* 80, 2035–2041.

Mittal, R., Gonzalez-Gomez, I., Panigrahy, A., Goth, K., Bonnet, R. and Prasadarao, N.V. (2010) IL-10 administration reduces PGE-2 levels and promotes CR3-mediated clearance of *Escherichia coli* K1 by phagocytes in meningitis. *Journal of Experimental Medicine* 207, 1307–1319.

Moissenet, D., Salauze, B., Clermont, O., Bingen, E., Arlet, G., Denamur, E., Merens, A., Mitanchez, D. and Vu-Thien, H. (2010) Meningitis caused by *Escherichia coli* producing TEM-52 extended-spectrum β-lactamase within an extensive outbreak in a neonatal ward: epidemiological investigation and characterization of the strain. *Journal of Clinical Microbiology* 48, 2459–2463.

Moriel, D.G., *et al.* (2010) Identification of protective and broadly conserved vaccine antigens from the genome of extraintestinal pathogenic *Escherichia coli. Proceedings of the National Academy of Sciences USA* 107, 9072–9077.

Parkkinen, J., Korhonen, T.K., Pere, A., Hacker, J. and Soinila, S. (1988) Binding sites in the rat brain for *Escherichia coli* S fimbriae associated with neonatal meningitis. *Journal of Clinical Investigation* 81, 860–865.

Parthasarathy, G., Yao, Y. and Kim, K. (2007) Flagella promote *Escherichia coli* K1 association with and invasion of human brain microvascular endothelial cells. *Infection and Immunity* 75, 2937–2945.

Prasadarao, N.V., Wass, C.A. and Kim, K.S. (1996a) Endothelial cell GlcNAc β1-4GlcNAc epitopes for outer membrane protein A enhance traversal of *Escherichia coli* across the blood–brain barrier. *Infection and Immunity* 64, 154–160.

Prasadarao, N.V., Wass, C.A., Weiser, J.N., Stins, M.F., Huang, S.H. and Kim, K.S. (1996b) Outer membrane protein A of *Escherichia coli* contributes to invasion of brain microvascular endothelial cells. *Infection and Immunity* 64, 146–153.

Prasadarao, N.V., Wass, C.A., Stins, M.F., Shimada, H. and Kim, K.S. (1999) Outer membrane protein A-promoted actin condensation of brain microvascular endothelial cells is required for *Escherichia coli* invasion. *Infection and Immunity* 67, 5775–5783.

Reddy, M.A., Prasadarao, N.V., Wass, C.A. and Kim, K.S. (2000) Phosphatidylinositol 3-kinase activation and interaction with focal adhesion kinase in *Escherichia coli* K1 invasion of human brain microvascular endothelial cells. *Journal of Biological Chemistry* 275, 36769–36774.

Sarff, L.D., McCracken, G.H., Schiffer, M.S., Glode, M.P., Robbins, J.B., Orskov, I. and Orskov, F. (1975) Epidemiology of *Escherichia coli* K1 in healthy and diseased newborns. *Lancet* 1, 1099–1104.

Stins, M.F., Gilles, F. and Kim, K.S. (1997) Selective expression of adhesion molecules on human brain microvascular endothelial cells. *Journal of Neuroimmunology* 76, 81–90.

Stins, M.F., Nemani, P.V., Wass, C. and Kim, K.S. (1999) *Escherichia coli* binding to and invasion of brain microvascular endothelial cells derived from humans and rats of different ages. *Infection and Immunity* 67, 5522–5525.

Teng, C.H., Cai, M., Shin, S., Xie, Y., Kim, K.J., Khan, N.A., Di Cello, F. and Kim, K.S. (2005) *Escherichia coli* K1 RS218 interacts with human brain microvascular endothelial cells via type 1 fimbria bacteria in the fimbriated state. *Infection and Immunity* 73, 2923–2931.

Teng, C.H., Xie, Y., Shin, S., Di Cello, F., Paul-Satyaseela, M., Cai, M. and Kim, K.S. (2006) Effects of *ompA* deletion on expression of type 1 fimbriae in *Escherichia coli* K1 strain RS218 and on the association of *E. coli* with human brain microvascular endothelial cells. *Infection and Immunity* 74, 5609–5616.

Teng, C.H., Tseng, Y.T., Maruvada, R., Pearce, D., Xie, Y., Paul-Satyaseela, M. and Kim, K.S. (2010) NlpI contributes to *Escherichia coli* K1 strain RS218 interaction with human brain microvascular endothelial cells. *Infection and Immunity* 78, 3090–3096.

Tseng, Y.T., Wang, S.W., Kim, K.S., Wang, Y.H., Yao, Y., Chen, C.C., Chiang, C.W., Hsieh, P.C. and Teng, C.H. (2012) NlpI facilitates deposition of C4bp on *Escherichia coli* by blocking classical complement-mediated killing, resulting in high level bacteremia. *Infection and Immunity* 80, 3669–3678.

Wang, Y. and Kim, K.S. (2002) Role of OmpA and IbeB in *Escherichia coli* K1 invasion of brain microvascular endothelial cells in vitro and in vivo. *Pediatric Research* 51, 559–563.

Wang, Y., Huang, S.H., Wass, C.A., Stins, M.F. and Kim, K.S. (1999) The gene locus *yijP* contributes to *Escherichia coli* K1 invasion of brain microvascular endothelial cells. *Infection and Immunity* 67, 4751–4756.

Xie, Y., Yao, Y.F., Kolisnychenko, V., Teng, C.H. and Kim, K.S. (2006a) HbiF regulates type 1 fimbriation independently of FimB and FimE. *Infection and Immunity* 74, 4039–4047.

Xie, Y., Kolisnychenko, V., Paul-Satyaseela, M., Elliott, S., Parthasarathy, G., Yao, Y., Plunkett, G., III, Blattner, F.R. and Kim, K.S. (2006b) Identification and characterization of *Escherichia coli* RS218-derived islands in the pathogenesis of *E. coli* meningitis. *Journal of Infectious Diseases* 194, 358–364.

Yao, Y., Xie, Y. and Kim, K.S. (2006) Genomic comparison of *Escherichia coli* K1 strains isolated from the cerebrospinal fluid of patients with meningitis. *Infection and Immunity* 74, 2196–2206.

Yao, Y., Xie, Y., Perace, D., Zhong, Y., Lu, J., Tao, J., Guo, X. and Kim, K.S. (2009) The type III secretion system is involved in the invasion and intracellular survival of *Escherichia coli* K1 in human brain microvascular endothelial cells. *FEMS Microbiology Letters* 300, 18–24.

Yu, H. and Kim, K.S. (2010) Ferredoxin is involved in secretion of cytotoxic necrotizing factor 1 across the cytoplasmic membrane in *Escherichia coli* K1. *Infection and Immunity* 78, 838–844.

Yu, H. and Kim, K.S. (2012) YgfZ contributes to secretion of cytotoxic necrotizing factor 1 into outer-membrane vesicles in *Escherichia coli*. *Microbiology* 158, 612–621.

Zhao, W.D., Liu, W., Fang, W. G., Kim, K.S. and Chen, Y.H. (2010) Vascular endothelial growth factor receptor 1 contributes to *Escherichia coli* K1 invasion of human brain microvascular endothelial cells through the phosphatidylinositol 3-kinase/Akt signaling pathway. *Infection and Immunity* 78, 4809–4816.

Zhou, Y., Tao, J., Yu, H., Ni, J., Zeng, L., Teng, Q., Kim, K.S., Zhao, G.P., Guo, X. and Yao, Y. (2012) Hcp family proteins secreted via the Type VI secretion system coordinately regulate *Escherichia coli* K1 interaction with human brain microvascular endothelial cells. *Infection and Immunity* 80, 1243–1251.

Zhu, L., Maruvada, R., Sapirstein, A., Malik, K.U., Peters-Golden, M. and Kim, K.S. (2010a) Arachidonic acid metabolism regulates *Escherichia coli* penetration of the blood–brain barrier. *Infection and Immunity* 78, 4302–4310.

Zhu, L., Pearce, D. and Kim, K.S. (2010b) Prevention of *Escherichia coli* K1 penetration of the blood–brain barrier by counteracting the host cell receptor and signaling molecule involved in *E. coli* invasion of human brain microvascular endothelial cells. *Infection and Immunity* 78, 3554–3559.

9 Group B *Streptococcus* Meningitis

Victor Nizet[1] and Kelly S. Doran[1,2*]
[1]*University of California at San Diego, California, USA;* [2]*San Diego State University, San Diego, USA*

9.1 Introduction

Streptococcus agalactiae (Group B *Streptococcus*, GBS) is a Gram-positive encapsulated bacterium possessing an array of virulence factors that render it capable of producing serious disease in susceptible hosts, in particular the human newborn (Maisey *et al.*, 2008a). Notably, GBS is the leading cause of meningitis in the neonatal period (Brouwer *et al.*, 2010; Thigpen *et al.*, 2011). Although advances in intensive care management and antibiotic therapy have changed GBS meningitis from a uniformly fatal disease to a frequently curable one, the overall outcome remains unfavourable. Morbidity is high; 25–50% of surviving infants suffer neurological sequelae of varying severity, including cerebral palsy, mental retardation, blindness, deafness or seizures.

The pathogenesis of neonatal GBS infection begins with the asymptomatic colonization of the female genital tract. Approximately 20–30% of healthy women are colonized with GBS on their vaginal or rectal mucosa, and 50–70% of infants born to these women will themselves become colonized with the bacterium (Baker and Edwards, 2001). For the purposes of epidemiological classification, neonatal GBS infections are traditionally divided among two forms: early-onset disease (EoD) and late-onset disease (LoD). Early-onset infections are described to occur through the first 7 days of life, but in fact have a median onset of only 6–8 h of life, presenting acutely with pneumonia and respiratory failure complicated by bloodstream infection and septicaemia. GBS EoD cases result from ascending infection of the bacterium through the placental membranes to initiate infection *in utero*, or, alternatively, by aspiration of infected vaginal fluids during the birth process. Premature, low-birth-weight infants are at increased risk of developing early-onset infection, with GBS placental infection itself often the critical factor triggering premature labour. In contrast, GBS LoD occurs in infants up to 7 months of age, with more indolent symptom progression related to bacteraemia, absence of lung involvement and a high incidence (~50%) of meningitis (Baker and Edwards, 2001). Universal screening of pregnant women at 35–37 weeks gestation and intrapartum antibiotic prophylaxis has resulted in a decline in early-onset GBS invasive disease in the USA (Phares *et al.*, 2008; Van Dyke *et al.*, 2009). However, this treatment has not eliminated the incidence of GBS meningitis, and concern has

*kdoran@mail.sdsu.edu

been raised about concurrent increases in non-GBS early-onset bacterial infections, especially in pre-term infants as a result of increased antibiotic use (Stoll *et al.*, 2002a,b). Furthermore, the occurrence of GBS meningitis in older children or adults is more commonly appreciated, with an approximate 4% increase in total number of cases reported between 1997 and 2007 in the USA (Thigpen *et al.*, 2011). No vaccination strategies are currently in place to prevent GBS infections, but if ultimately achieved they would be anticipated to reduce the number of meningitis cases (Thigpen *et al.*, 2011). Here we review the current understanding of the pathogenesis of GBS meningitis, highlighting important bacterial virulence factors and host interactions that promote disease progression.

9.2 Pathophysiology of GBS Meningitis

The pathophysiology of GBS meningitis varies according to age of onset. In EoD, autopsy studies demonstrate little or no evidence of leptomeningeal inflammation, despite the presence of abundant bacteria, vascular thrombosis and parenchymal haemorrhage (Quirante *et al.*, 1974). By contrast, infants with LoD usually have diffuse purulent arachnoiditis with prominent involvement of the base of the brain (Berman and Banker, 1966). Similar age-related differences in central nervous system (CNS) pathology are evident in the infant rat model of invasive disease (Ferrieri *et al.*, 1980). These histopathological differences reflect underdevelopment of the host immunological response in the immediate neonatal period, with a higher proportion of deaths resulting from overwhelming septicaemia. Clinical and neuropathological studies have documented the clear association between bacterial meningitis and brain oedema formation, increased intracranial pressure (ICP), seizure activity, arterial and venous cerebral vascular insults, and other neurological sequelae (Scheld *et al.*, 2002).

To produce meningitis, blood-borne GBS must typically penetrate the blood–brain barrier (BBB) and/or the blood–cerebrospinal fluid barrier (BCSFB). For the purposes of this review, the BBB and BCSFB are interchangeable concepts with respect to vessel endothelial cell penetration by GBS. Disruption of BBB integrity is a hallmark event in the pathophysiology of bacterial meningitis. This disruption may be due to the combined effect of bacterial entry and penetration of brain microvascular endothelial cells (BMECs), direct cellular injury by bacterial cytotoxins, and/or activation of host inflammatory pathways that compromise BMEC barrier function. It is apparent that the host immune response is not only incapable of controlling infection within the CNS but also may be responsible for many adverse events during bacterial meningitis (Tunkel and Scheld, 1995). A very complex and integrated series of events involving host cytokines, chemokines, proteolytic enzymes and oxidants appears to be responsible for meningitis-induced brain dysfunction. The development of GBS meningitis progresses through phases including: (i) bloodstream survival and the development of bacteraemia; (ii) direct GBS invasion and disruption of the BBB/BCSFB; and (iii) GBS multiplication in the CSF-containing subarachnoid and ventricular spaces, which induces inflammation with associated pathophysiological alterations leading to the development of neural damage. Brain injury results mainly from cerebrovascular involvement leading to cerebral ischaemia, brain oedema, hydrocephalus and increased ICP.

9.2.1 Bloodstream survival and the development of bacteraemia

An association between sustained high-level bacteraemia and the development of GBS meningitis has been suggested in humans and in experimental models of haematogeneous meningitis (Ferrieri *et al.*, 1980; Doran *et al.*, 2002a). This observation implies that GBS bloodstream survival is an important virulence trait to avoid immune clearance by phagocytic killing by host immune cells, prior to CNS penetration. Neonates are particularly prone to invasive disease because of their quantitative or qualitative deficiencies in phagocytic cell function, specific antibody, or the classical and alternative complement pathways. In addition to these newborn host susceptibilities, GBS possess a number of virulence determinants that promote bloodstream survival by thwarting key components of effective opsonophagocytic killing such as complement (Fig. 9.1). For example, the surface-anchored GBS β-protein prevents opsonophagocytosis by binding short consensus repeats found in the middle region of factor H, a host counter-regulator of complement (Maruvada *et al.*, 2008), enabling the unbound active region to block C3b deposition on the bacterial cell surface (Jarva *et al.*, 2004). In addition, the cell-surface GBS immunogenic bacterial adhesin (BibA) binds human C3bp, promoting resistance to phagocytic killing and contributing to virulence in the mouse model (Santi *et al.*, 2007). The β-antigen of C protein binds human IgA antibody (Jerlstrom *et al.*, 1991), and non-specific deposition of IgA on the bacterial surface probably inhibits interactions with complement. Finally, a cell-surface protease, CspA, targets host fibrinogen, producing adherent fibrin-like cleavage products that coat the bacterial surface and interfere with complement-mediated opsonophagocytic clearance (Harris *et al.*, 2003).

The profile of GBS gene transcription changes dramatically during growth in human blood, resulting in an altered cell morphology and increased expression of complement regulatory proteins (Santi *et al.*, 2007; Mereghetti *et al.*, 2008). The sialylated GBS capsular polysaccharide (CPS) represents one of the most critical factors for limiting the effectiveness of host complement and phagocytic defence. Passage of GBS in animals

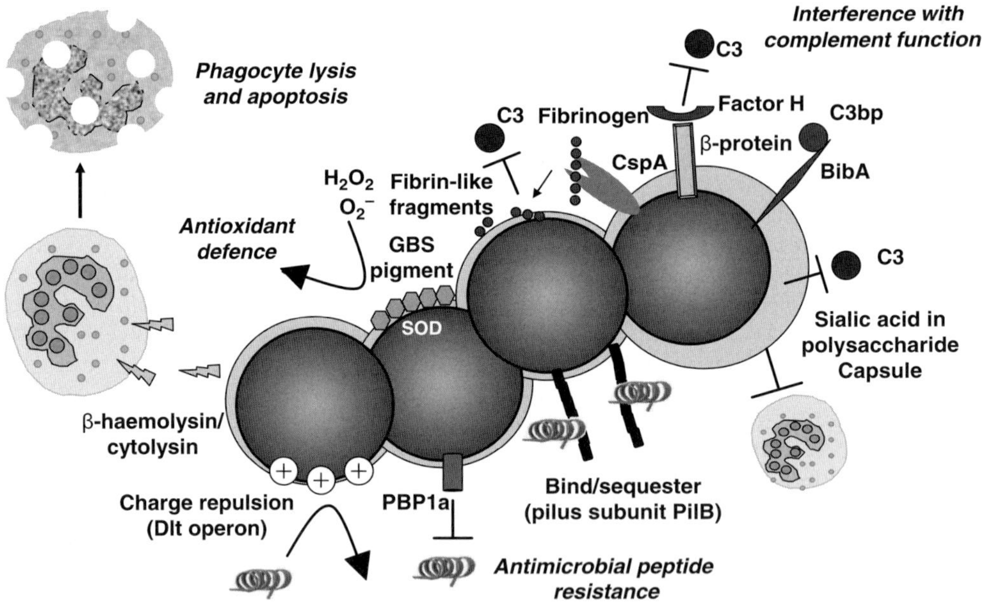

Fig. 9.1. Mechanisms of GBS immune evasion. GBS express multiple surface-exposed or secreted factors to evade host immune defences and promote bloodstream survival. The PBP1a and the PilB subunit of GBS pili contribute to antimicrobial peptide resistance. The Dlt operon is responsible for increasing incorporation of D-alanine residues in cell-wall teichoic acids, thereby reducing electronegativity and affinity for cationic antimicrobial peptides. ScpB, the sialic acid capsule, BibA, β-protein and CspA all inhibit host clearance of GBS by interfering with complement components C5a, C3 and C3bp. Superoxide dismutase (SOD) properties of the orange carotenoid pigment shield GBS from killing by phagocyte-generated reactive oxygen species. Alternatively, β-haemolysin/cytolysin can boost GBS survival by cytolytic or pro-apoptotic injury to host phagocytes.

increases capsulation, while serial *in vitro* passage leads to reduced capsule expression (Hakansson *et al.*, 1988), and strains obtained from infants with septicaemia or meningitis have increased encapsulation compared with vaginal colonizing strains (Hakansson *et al.*, 1987). Thus, it appears that GBS capsule expression is induced during bloodstream replication and repressed while on mucosal or endothelial cell surfaces, a feature common to other meningeal pathogens. Currently, ten GBS capsular serotypes have been identified (Ia, Ib, II–IX) based on the different arrangements of four monosaccharides (glucose, galactose, *N*-acetylglucosamine and sialic acid) into unique repeating units. Serotype III GBS strains have accounted for a majority of LoD and meningitis (Baker and Edwards, 2001; Tazi *et al.*, 2010), but all serotypes contain a terminal-linked sialic acid bound to galactose in an $\alpha 2 \rightarrow 3$ linkage (Cieslewicz *et al.*, 2005). The sialic acid moiety provides antiphagocytic protection by impairing deposition of opsonically active complement C3 on the bacterial surface. Isogenic GBS mutants lacking CPS or capsular sialylation are more susceptible to neutrophil killing and are less virulent in animal models of infection (Campbell *et al.*, 1991; Marques *et al.*, 1992). Furthermore, the conserved GBS terminal $\alpha 2 \rightarrow 3$ linked sialic acid capsular component is identical to a sugar epitope widely displayed on the surface of all mammalian cells. Thus, bacterial surface sialylation may have evolved to mimic host 'self' antigens, allowing GBS to avoid immune detection, manipulate phagocyte function and dampen the immune response to GBS infection (Carlin *et al.*, 2007).

When GBS are engulfed and contained within the phagosome, a rapid release of toxic reactive oxygen species (ROS) is produced through the phagocyte oxidative burst. Although GBS do not produce catalase, they are nevertheless able to resist ROS killing and survive inside macrophage phagolysosomes (Wilson and Weaver, 1985; Cornacchione *et al.*, 1998; Teixeira *et al.*, 2001). GBS possess an endogenous source of the oxygen-metabolite scavenger glutathione (Wilson and Weaver, 1985), and the GBS SodA enzyme can neutralize superoxide anions (Poyart *et al.*, 2001b). GBS also produce an orange carotenoid pigment, a property unique to GBS among haemolytic streptococci, associated with the *cyl* operon encoding the β-haemolysin/cytolysin cytotoxin (Spellerberg *et al.*, 2000). The free-radical scavenging properties of this carotenoid neutralize hydrogen peroxide, superoxide, hypochlorite and singlet oxygen, and thereby provide a shield against several elements of phagocyte ROS killing (Liu *et al.*, 2004). Other GBS factors that have been linked to survival inside phagocytic cells and/or dendritic cells include CPS (Lemire *et al.*, 2012), a pilin protein (Maisey *et al.*, 2008b) and transcriptional response regulators CovR (Cumley *et al.*, 2012) and CiaR (Quach *et al.*, 2009), which may coordinate expression of acid and stress survival genes.

Another important host defence mechanism inherent to many immune cells is the production of small cationic antimicrobial peptides (AMPs), such as cathelicidins and defensins. These peptides are attracted electrostatically to negatively charged microbial cell surfaces, followed by their self-assembly to form membrane pores or otherwise disrupt membrane integrity. GBS increase their intrinsic resistance to AMPs by incorporation of positively charged D-alanine residues into their cell wall teichoic acids, thereby reducing surface electronegative charge and affinity for the cationic peptides (Poyart *et al.*, 2001a). A surface-anchored penicillin-binding protein, PBP1a, enhances GBS resistance to cathelicidins and defensins, thereby reducing GBS susceptibility to killing by alveolar macrophages and neutrophils and promoting bacterial survival in a neonatal rat model of GBS infection (Jones *et al.*, 2007). Similarly, expression of the pilus backbone protein PilB and the action of the two-component regulator CiaR both render GBS more resistant to killing by cathelicidin AMPs (Maisey *et al.*, 2008b; Quach *et al.*, 2009).

9.2.2 GBS invasion of the BBB

Following bloodstream survival, GBS interacts directly with BBB endothelium, which can result in bacterial invasion of the BBB with subsequent infection of the CNS.

This process can result from increased permeability of the BBB and/or the direct invasion of BMECs by the pathogen. Microbial interaction with the BBB may involve crossing the brain endothelium by direct intracellular invasion and vacuole transit (transcytosis), by passage through the intercellular junctional spaces (paracytosis) or by transport inside another host cell (phagocyte-facilitated invasion). With the availability of *in vitro* tissue culture models of human (H)BMECs (Stins *et al.*, 1994; Nizet *et al.*, 1997) and animal models of GBS infection (Doran *et al.*, 2003; Tazi *et al.*, 2010), significant progress has been made in identifying and characterizing the molecular determinants that promote GBS–BBB interaction (Fig. 9.2).

Intracellular invasion (transcytosis)

GBS enter or 'invade' brain endothelium apically and exit the cell on the basolateral side, thereby crossing the BBB transcellularly (Nizet *et al.*, 1997; Lembo *et al.*, 2010). Electron microscopy has demonstrated the presence of the meningeal pathogen in membrane-bound vacuoles within HBMECs (Nizet *et al.*, 1997), suggesting the involvement of endocytic pathways as well as avoidance of lysosomal fusion for BBB traversal. Further HBMEC invasion can be blocked by inhibition of actin polymerization, suggesting that GBS trigger rearrangement of the host cytoskeleton and induce their own uptake (Nizet *et al.*, 1997). This process may be accomplished, at least in

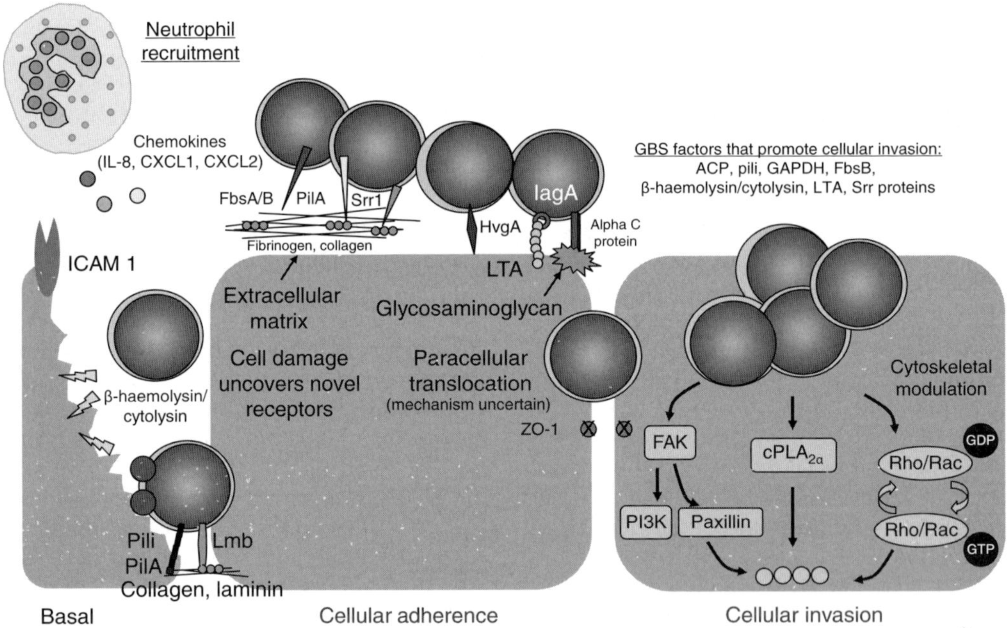

Fig. 9.2. Mechanisms of GBS penetration of the BBB. Surface-expressed proteins FbsA/B, Srr1, PilA, HvgA, lipoteichoic acid (LTA) and alpha C protein (ACP) mediate GBS binding to host cells and extracellular matrix (ECM) components, such as fibrinogen and collagen. Secreted β-haemolysin/cytolysin promotes GBS invasion, possibly by breaking down host barriers to reveal novel receptors on the basement membrane, such as laminin and collagen, as well as promoting neutrophil influx that contributes to barrier disruption. GBS also use glyceraldehyde 3-phosphate dehydrogenase (GAPDH) to activate host plasminogen and degrade the ECM. Intracellular GBS invasion is enhanced by bacterial-dependent cytoskeletal rearrangements triggered by host PI3K/AKT- and FAK-signalling pathways and the Rho family of GTPases. Alternatively, GBS can also disrupt tight junction complexes to cross the barrier by a paracellular route. Several GBS adhesins, including FbsB, pili, LTA and ACP, also contribute to cellular invasion.

part, by tyrosine phosphorylation of focal adhesion kinase (FAK), which occurs upon GBS infection. Phosphorylation of FAK induces its association with PI3K and paxillin, an actin filament adaptor protein (Shin *et al.*, 2006), and is required for efficient invasion of HBMECs by GBS. GBS-infected HBMECs also exhibit increased levels of activated Rho family members RhoA and Rac1. Rho family GTPase inhibitors and dominant-negative expression of RhoA and Rac1 are effective in blocking GBS invasion (Shin and Kim, 2006).

To elucidate the GBS determinants involved in the pathogenesis of meningitis, many groups have focused on the characterization of GBS isolates responsible for CNS disease. Clinical isolates of serotype III GBS, which are over-represented in LoD, appear to belong to two distinct evolutionary clusters (Musser *et al.*, 1989), which have now been shown through multilocus sequence typing to represent a limited number of clonal complexes (Jones *et al.*, 2003). Of these clones, sequence type (ST)-17 is strongly associated with neonatal meningitis and has been designated as the hypervirulent clone (Lamy *et al.*, 2006). Screening of a GBS ST-17 mutant library revealed a unique requirement for the novel 'invasion associated gene', *iagA*, in BBB penetration by GBS (Doran *et al.*, 2005). Decreased invasion of HBMECs by the GBS Δ*iagA* mutant *in vitro* was correlated with a reduced risk for development of meningitis and markedly diminished lethality *in vivo*. Deletion of *iagA* did not affect other key steps in the pathogenesis of GBS meningitis, including bloodstream survival, HBMEC adherence and intracellular survival. Thus, the *iagA*-encoded phenotype of GBS has a specific function in promoting HBMEC uptake of the pathogen. The *iagA* gene encodes an enzyme for the biosynthesis of diglucosyldiacylglycerol, a membrane glycolipid that functions as an anchor for lipoteichoic acid (LTA), indicating that proper LTA anchoring is important to facilitate penetration of the BBB by GBS (Doran *et al.*, 2005). The host cell receptor for GBS LTA that mediates these interactions has yet to be identified. While it is known that LTA is a molecule recognized by Toll-like receptor (TLR) 2, the data strongly suggest that the attenuated phenotype of the Δ*iagA* mutant is not dependent on TLR2 (Doran *et al.*, 2005). The evidence that the LTA surface polymer mediates unique host cell interactions is consistent with early epidemiological studies. Clinical isolates of GBS from infants with EoD or LoD possess higher quantities of cell-associated LTA than strains isolated from mucosal surfaces of asymptomatically colonized infants (Nealon and Mattingly, 1983). Furthermore, longer LTA polymer length is characteristic of isolates from carriers with invasive GBS disease compared with asymptomatic carriers. LTA is common to all GBS sero- and sequence types, but it remains to be determined if ST-17 clones contain longer or structurally distinct LTA polymers, which may account for their increased virulence.

More recently, the availability of GBS genome sequences has enabled the identification of genes restricted to the ST-17 lineage (Tettelin *et al.*, 2005; Brochet *et al.*, 2006). Mosaic variants were identified at a single genomic locus encoding a cell wall-anchored protein, with two main variants displaying 38% overall amino acid identity, namely BibA (Santi *et al.*, 2007), and a second gene to be strictly specific to the ST-17 clone (Lamy *et al.*, 2006). This gene, now called hypervirulent GBS adhesin (HvgA), was shown to be required for GBS hypervirulence (Tazi *et al.*, 2010). GBS strains that express HvgA are more efficient in gut colonization and in crossing the intestinal–blood barrier and BBB in neonates, including choroid plexus epithelial cells and brain microvascular endothelium (Tazi *et al.*, 2010). Furthermore, heterologous expression of HvgA in non-adhesive bacteria conferred the ability to adhere to intestinal barrier and BBB-constituting cells.

Serotypes Ia, Ib and V are also commonly isolated from neonates, children and adult patients with meningitis (Phares *et al.*, 2008), suggesting that other GBS determinants prevalent among these serotypes are also relevant for the pathogenesis of meningitis. Proteins targeted for cell surface expression in GBS are predicted to share a C-terminal sequence (L/IPXTG) for sortase recognition and anchoring to the Gram-positive cell wall. Several cell wall-anchored proteins promoting GBS BBB penetration have been identified and characterized. In a paradigm-shifting study, it was discovered that GBS express surface-associated pili (Lauer *et al.*, 2005). Among the sequenced GBS genomes, two genetic loci encoding pili have been identified, pilus island (PI)-1 and PI-2, the second existing in one of two variants (PI-2a and PI-2b), and not all genomes contain both loci (Rosini *et al.*, 2006). GBS PI-2a includes the genes encoding PilB, an LP(x)TG-motif-containing protein that polymerizes to form a pilus backbone, and accessory pilus proteins PilA and PilC that are incorporated in the pilus (Dramsi *et al.*, 2006). Both PilA and PilB promote adherence to and invasion of brain endothelium, respectively (Maisey *et al.*, 2007), and PilA has been implicated in BBB penetration *in vivo* using a mouse model of haematogenous GBS meningitis (Banerjee *et al.*, 2011). Analysis of the PilA protein sequence revealed an integrin I-like domain resembling the A3 domain of human von Willebrand factor, a molecule known to interact with collagens. PilA also binds the extracellular matrix (ECM) component collagen, and collagen binding enhanced GBS attachment as well as uptake into HBMECs in a dose-dependent manner (Banerjee *et al.*, 2011). The PilA-collagen complex engages α2-β1 integrins on brain endothelium to promote bacterial attachment and pro-inflammatory chemokine release. As a result, increased neutrophil infiltration was correlated with increased BBB permeability and higher levels of bacterial CNS penetration *in vivo*. This study reveals the deleterious role of the neutrophil response to the development of GBS meningitis, and indicates that the GBS PilA–BBB interaction is an important molecular event that contributes to disease progression and a detrimental outcome for the host. In addition to PilA binding collagen, other GBS factors interact with various ECM proteins and constituents to promote bacterial–BBB interactions. Recently, the GBS surface-anchored alpha C protein (APC) was shown to interact directly with glucosaminoglycans (GAGs) on brain endothelium, and promote the establishment of GBS meningitis (Chang *et al.*, 2011). Impaired host GAG expression diminished GBS penetration in the CNS in both murine and *Drosophila* models of GBS infection. GBS interactions with other ECM components also have been described. GBS mutants lacking the cell wall-anchored fibrinogen-binding protein FbsA (Schubert *et al.*, 2004), and the laminin-binding protein Lmb (Spellerberg *et al.*, 1999), have reduced ability to adhere to or invade HBMECs *in vitro* (Tenenbaum *et al.*, 2005, 2007). Many GBS strains harbour another fibrinogen-binding protein, FbsB (Gutekunst *et al.*, 2004), which is secreted and structurally unrelated to FbsA. Interestingly, the expression level of FbsA and FbsB in ST-17 strains correlated to an increased fibrinogen-binding capacity that may contribute to the hypervirulence of this lineage (Al Safadi *et al.*, 2011). The GBS genome encodes homologues to fibronectin-binding proteins that contribute to adherence, invasion and meningeal inflammation in other streptococcal pathogens (Pracht *et al.*, 2005). Whether or not the proteins function in a similar way in GBS remains to be determined.

Fibrinogen is present in the CNS following BBB disruption and vascular damage. Furthermore, the interaction of fibrinogen with integrins and non-integrin receptors expressed on cells of the haematopoietic, immune and nervous systems can induce signalling pathways that regulate inflammation and neurodegenerative functions involved in CNS disease. Interestingly, recent studies suggest that adherence to fibrinogen may be a general property of GBS (Dramsi *et al.*, 2012; Seo *et al.*, 2012) to promote bloodstream survival and host cell interactions. An important determinant recently implicated in fibrinogen binding and BBB interaction are the GBS serine rich repeat (Srr) glycoproteins (van Sorge *et al.*, 2009; Seo *et al.*, 2012). Srr proteins have a highly conserved domain organization, including a long and specialized signal sequence, two extensive Srr regions that undergo glycosylation, and a typical LP(X)TG cell wall anchoring motif. GBS strains carry one of two *srr* gene alleles, designated *srr1* (Samen *et al.*, 2007) and *srr2* (Seifert *et al.*,

2006), which are similar in architecture but show only limited homology (< 20% identity). Expression of the Srr-2 protein seems to be restricted to serotype III and ST-17 strains (Seifert *et al.*, 2006). Targeted mutagenesis of a GBS Δ*srr1* mutant resulted in a marked reduction in HMBEC adherence and invasion (van Sorge *et al.*, 2009). The *srr1* genes in GBS serotypes Ia, Ib and V, as well as *srr2* in the serotype III ST-17 clone, each contributed to HBMEC invasion *in vitro*, and Srr-1 promoted BBB penetration and the development of GBS meningitis in a mouse model of haematogenous meningitis (van Sorge *et al.*, 2009). Srr-1 contributes to GBS attachment to HBMECs via the direct interaction of its binding region (BR) with human fibrinogen (Seo *et al.*, 2012). Studies using recombinant Srr1-BR established a direct protein interaction with the amino acid sequence 283–410 of the fibrinogen Aα chain. Structural predictions indicated that the conformation of Srr1-BR resembles that of other related bacterial proteins that bind to fibrinogen through a 'dock, lock and latch' (DLL) mechanism (Ponnuraj *et al.*, 2003). The DLL mechanism results when fibrinogen engages a binding cleft between two domains, N2 and N3. At the ligand 'dock', the flexible C-terminal extension of the N3 domain (the 'latch') changes conformation, so that it 'locks' the ligand in place, and forms a β-strand complex with the N2 domain. Deletion of the predicted latch domain of Srr1-BR abolished the interaction of Srr1-BR with fibrinogen. In addition, a mutant GBS strain lacking the Srr-1 latch domain exhibited reduced binding to HBMECs, and was significantly attenuated in an *in vivo* model of meningitis (Seo *et al.*, 2012). Further studies are required to determine if similar mechanisms for fibrinogen binding and disease progression occur in Srr-2-encoding strains.

Intercellular invasion (paracytosis)

The host integrins, ECM components and glycosaminoglycans involved in GBS–BBB interactions all preferentially localize to the basolateral surface of polarized endothelium. Thus, GBS may interact with these factors once present in the CNS to amplify the host response and disease progression. Alternatively, early molecular interactions of GBS with the BBB and subsequent barrier disruption may alter cellular polarity. It has been demonstrated that GBS is capable of intercellular transit across an epithelial cell barrier, where the bacterium co-localized with junctional protein complexes (Soriani *et al.*, 2006). Recent data also indicate that GBS infection disrupts tight junctional complexes in brain endothelium (Kim *et al.*, 2012). An overall reduction in the distribution of the primary BBB tight junction protein, zona occludin (ZO)-1, was observed by immunofluorescence during GBS infection. Further evidence demonstrated a decrease in protein levels of ZO-1 and additional tight junction protein, occludin, following GBS infection compared with the uninfected control (Kim *et al.*, 2012). Whether these interactions act to disrupt tight junctional complexes in brain endothelium and result in a non-polarized distribution of proteins on the BBB plasma membrane, and/or promote GBS intercellular transit across the BBB, remains to be investigated.

Host factors involved in arachidonic acid metabolism also contribute to penetration of the BBB by GBS (Maruvada *et al.*, 2011). Pharmacological inhibition and gene deletion demonstrated that host cytosolic phospholipase $A_2\alpha$ (cPLA$_2\alpha$) contributes to type III GBS invasion of HBMEC monolayers and penetration into the brain *in vivo*. The mechanism probably involves lipoxygenated metabolites of arachidonic acid, specifically cysteinyl leukotrienes released by cPLA$_2\alpha$ as well as protein kinase Cα (PKCα). GBS penetration into the CNS in cPLA$_2\alpha^{-/-}$ mice was significantly lower than the penetration of wild-type mice. However, the magnitudes of bacteraemia were similar between cPLA$_2\alpha^{-/-}$ and wild-type mice, suggesting that decreased penetration was not the result of decreased levels of blood-borne bacteria. Interestingly, cPLA$_2\alpha$ deletion did not affect GBS penetration into non-brain organs, such as the kidneys and spleen, as similar numbers of bacterial counts were recovered from cPLA$_2\alpha^{-/-}$ and wild-type mice (Maruvada *et al.*, 2011). The basis for this selective role of host $cPLA_2\alpha$ in GBS neurotropism is unknown.

GBS disruption of the BBB

The host inflammatory response to GBS contributes significantly to the pathogenesis of meningitis and CNS injury. A vascular distribution of cortical lesions in neonatal rats with GBS meningitis indicates that disturbances of cerebral blood flow contribute to neuronal damage (Kim *et al.*, 1995). Inflammation of individual brain vessels can lead to focal lesions, whereas diffuse alterations of cerebral blood flow cause generalized hypoxic/ischaemic injury and cerebral oedema (Kim *et al.*, 1995). GBS induces nitric oxide (NO) in brain endothelial cells (Glibetic *et al.*, 2001) and in microglial cells, resulting in neuronal destruction (Lehnardt *et al.*, 2006). Furthermore, arteriolar dysfunction is associated with the presence of oxygen free radicals thought to be a by-product of infiltrating neutrophils (McKnight *et al.*, 1992). Intraventricular inoculation of newborn piglets with GBS results in an early sharp rise in CSF tumour necrosis factor-α (TNF-α) levels, followed shortly by prostaglandin release and subarachnoid inflammation (Ling *et al.*, 1995). In the neonatal rat model of meningitis, TNF-α production by astrocytes, microglia and infiltrating leucocytes contributes to apoptosis of hippocampal neurons (Bogdan *et al.*, 1997) and further increases in BBB permeability (Kim *et al.*, 1997). Recent studies have verified the levels of cytokine/chemokine, myeloperoxidase (MPO) activity, oxidative stress and disruption of the BBB in the hippocampus and cortex of neonate Wistar rats, following GBS meningitis (Barichello *et al.*, 2011). In the neonate brain, the hippocampus, mainly, produced higher levels of cytokine/chemokine in the early phase of infection, while MPO activity remained elevated at 4 days post-infection in both brain structures (Barichello *et al.*, 2011). Interestingly, in the neonatal rat, simultaneous intracisternal administration of dexamethasone with GBS challenge markedly reduced the magnitude of subarachnoid inflammation, vasculopathy and neuronal injury (Kim *et al.*, 1995).

It is clear that the GBS β-haemolysin/cytolysin (β-h/c) toxin contributes much to the observed disease pathology. Haemolysin expression has been shown to directly damage brain endothelial cells (Nizet *et al.*, 1997), leptomeninges (meningioma cells) and astrocytes (Alkuwaity *et al.*, 2012) and primary neurons (Reiss *et al.*, 2011). Infection with wild-type GBS and $\beta\text{-h/c}^+$ cell-free extracts induced cell death, whereas challenge with β-h/c-deficient ($\beta\text{-h/c}^-$) mutant strains and $\beta\text{-h/c}^-$ extracts did not. Notably, astrocytes were more sensitive to the cytotoxic effects of infection than meningioma cells (Alkuwaity *et al.*, 2012). In neurons, cell-free extracts of GBS β-h/c toxin induced apoptosis in a time- and concentration-dependent fashion; electron microscopy of the neurons showed condensation, shrinkage and partial fragmentation of cells and nuclei as well as damage to mitochondria (Reiss *et al.*, 2011). In these studies, GBS β-h/c-induced cell death could not be prevented by caspase inhibitors, nor was caspase activity detected in neurons, consistent with observations in other cell types including macrophages. Haemolysin expression has also been shown to promote the development of meningitis *in vivo* (Doran *et al.*, 2003; Lembo *et al.*, 2010). In a murine model of haematogenous meningitis, mice infected with $\beta\text{-h/c}^-$ mutants exhibited lower mortality and decreased brain bacterial counts compared with mice infected with the corresponding wild-type GBS strains (Doran *et al.*, 2003). Similarly, mutants that lack the negative repressor of β-h/c, CovR (for control of virulence), exhibited high levels of toxin expression and an increased ability to penetrate the BBB *in vivo* (Lembo *et al.*, 2010). Multiple studies have demonstrated that the lipid dipalmitoyl-phosphatidylcholine (DPPC) provides protection against β-h/c-mediated injury in various host cells (Nizet *et al.*, 1996; Doran *et al.*, 2002b; Hensler *et al.*, 2008; Alkuwaity *et al.*, 2012). DPPC might preserve the host cell membrane by providing phospholipid replacement during pore formation and/or by direct neutralization by binding to toxin itself. The therapeutic potential of surfactant phospholipids in GBS meningitis requires further study.

9.3 GBS Activation of a CNS Inflammatory Response

The first comprehensive microarray analysis of the BBB endothelium transcriptional response to a pathogen was examined during GBS infection, revealing the induction of a specific set of 80 genes, which function together to orchestrate neutrophil recruitment, activation and enhanced survival (Doran *et al.*, 2003). The most highly induced genes, interleukin (IL)-8, CXCL1 and CXCL2, all belong to the CXC chemokine family, which acts mainly on cells of neutrophil lineage. IL-8 is the most potent chemotactic factor for neutrophils because it has a high affinity for both of the chemokine receptors (CXCR1 and CXCR2) expressed on neutrophils, and it further stimulates neutrophil respiratory burst, degranulation and adherence to endothelial cells. These chemokines have been isolated from the CSF of patients with bacterial meningitis, and IL-8 may be an important biomarker to differentiate acute bacterial meningitis from aseptic meningitis (Pinto Junior *et al.*, 2011). Other GBS-induced HBMEC genes related specifically to CNS neutrophil recruitment were ICAM-1, which when upregulated leads to the enhanced adhesion of neutrophils to the brain endothelium, and granulocyte–macrophage colony-stimulating factor (GM–CSF), which increases neutrophil migration across brain endothelium. Absent during GBS infection of HBMECs was the induction of strong pro-inflammatory cytokines, such as TNF-α or IL-1. These data suggest that the BBB represents much more than a physical barrier to GBS, and also performs a sentinel function by recognizing the threat of infection and initiating a CNS-protective innate immune response. In the case of blood-borne bacteria, a specific BMEC gene expression programme for neutrophil recruitment and activation is generated, with the absence of the concurrent production of broader spectrum cytokines (e.g. TNF-α, IL-1) that could provoke a wider or unchecked pattern of inflammatory activation potentially harmful to critical CNS structures. However, the timing and magnitude of the neutrophil recruitment response is critical for the outcome of infection. Continued exposure and invasion of the pathogen may result in over-activation of BBB endothelium, leading to increased inflammation that may compromise BBB integrity or cause neuronal damage.

Several GBS factors have been implicated in promoting BBB activation. Infection of HBMECs with a GBS strain lacking β-h/c toxin markedly reduced expression of genes involved in the immune response, while an unencapsulated strain generally induced similar or greater expression levels for the same subset of genes (Doran *et al.*, 2003). Neutrophil migration across polar HBMEC monolayers was stimulated by GBS and its β-h/c through a process involving IL-8 and ICAM-1. Furthermore, cell-free bacterial supernatants containing β-h/c activity induced IL-8 release, thus identifying this toxin as a principal provocative factor for BBB activation (Doran *et al.*, 2003). In more recent studies, additional microarray experiments have demonstrated that the similar gene profile in HBMECs is effected by CovR regulation, which can result in high β-h/c expression (Lembo *et al.*, 2010) and PilA expression (Banerjee *et al.*, 2011). Infection of HBMECs *in vitro* with multiple PilA-deficient GBS strains resulted in less IL-8 protein secretion compared with the respective wild-type parental strains, and treatment of HBMECs with recombinant PilA protein induced IL-8 transcription, suggesting that PilA is both necessary and sufficient to activate the BBB response (Banerjee *et al.*, 2011). Infection *in vivo* with the PilA-deficient strain resulted in delayed mortality, decreased neutrophil infiltration and bacterial CNS dissemination, and less expression of KC, the murine homologue of IL-8 (Banerjee *et al.*, 2011). These results indicate that GBS PilA directly promotes IL-8 secretion and functional neutrophil signalling pathways *in vivo*, resulting in neutrophil recruitment during active GBS infection, which may function in tandem or concurrently with the β-h/c toxin to promote disease progression. These findings also demonstrate an association between leucocyte trafficking and BBB permeability and increased GBS penetration of the CNS, suggesting that polymorphonuclear leucocyte (PMN)-mediated damage of the BBB has a significant role in the pathogenesis of GBS meningitis.

9.4 Conclusions

Advances in microbial genetics, tissue culture systems and small-animal challenge models have enhanced our understanding of the molecular pathogenesis of GBS meningitis and the host response to this potentially life-threatening infection. New model systems using zebrafish (Patterson *et al.*, 2012) and *Drosophila* (Baron *et al.*, 2009; Chang *et al.*, 2011) promise the contribution of host genetics to enrich our understanding of host–GBS interactions. Comparative genomic and systems-level bioinformatics studies have revealed strain evolution associated with hypervirulence and CNS disease potential, including specific candidate gene and regulatory systems that promote bloodstream survival, HBMEC interactions and activation of host inflammatory responses. Genomics has led to the development of reverse and structural vaccinology technologies for vaccine discovery, including a type 2a pilus (BP-2a)-based GBS experimental vaccine (Nuccitelli *et al.*, 2011). In addition, genomics has led to the discovery of component proteins and virulence factors as potential vaccine targets. Enhanced understanding of the molecular basis of GBS meningitis may highlight novel bacterial and host molecules as therapeutic or immuno-prophylactic targets against this dangerous infectious disease condition of the neonate.

Acknowledgements

The authors thank their respective laboratory members and researchers whose work has not been discussed in detail or reviewed elsewhere. Work on the BBB and GBS meningitis in K.S. Doran's laboratory is supported by funding from the NIH/NINDS (grant no RO1NS051247).

References

Al Safadi, R., Mereghetti, L., Salloum, M., Lartigue, M.F., Virlogeux-Payant, I., Quentin, R. and Rosenau, A. (2011) Two-component system RgfA/C activates the *fbsB* gene encoding major fibrinogen-binding protein in highly virulent CC17 clone Group B *Streptococcus. PLoS One* 6, e14658.

Alkuwaity, K., Taylor, A., Heckels, J.E., Doran, K.S. and Christodoulides, M. (2012) Group B *Streptococcus* interactions with human meningeal cells and astrocytes in vitro. *PLoS One* 7, e42660.

Baker, C.J. and Edwards, M.S. (2001) *Infectious Diseases of the Fetus and Newborn Infant.* W.B. Saunders, Philadelphia, PA.

Banerjee, A., Kim, B.J., Carmona, E.M., Cutting, A.S., Gurney, M.A., Carlos, C., Feuer, R., Prasadarao, N.V. and Doran, K.S. (2011) Bacterial pili exploit integrin machinery to promote immune activation and efficient blood–brain barrier penetration. *Nature Communications* 2, 462.

Barichello, T., Lemos, J.C., Generoso, J.S., Cipriano, A.L., Milioli, G.L., Marcelino, D.M., Vuolo, F., Petronilho, F., Dal-Pizzol, F., Vilela, M.C. and Teixeira, A.L. (2011) Oxidative stress, cytokine/chemokine and disruption of blood–brain barrier in neonate rats after meningitis by *Streptococcus agalactiae. Neurochemical Research* 36, 1922–1930.

Baron, M.J., Wong, S.L., Nybakken, K., Carey, V.J. and Madoff, L.C. (2009) Host glycosaminoglycan confers susceptibility to bacterial infection in *Drosophila melanogaster. Infection and Immunity* 77, 860–866.

Berman, P.H. and Banker, B.Q. (1966) Neonatal meningitis. A clinical and pathological study of 29 cases. *Pediatrics* 38, 6–24.

Bogdan, I., Leib, S.L., Bergeron, M., Chow, L. and Tauber, M.G. (1997) Tumor necrosis factor-α contributes to apoptosis in hippocampal neurons during experimental group B streptococcal meningitis. *Journal of Infectious Diseases* 176, 693–697.

Brochet, M., Couve, E., Zouine, M., Vallaeys, T., Rusniok, C., Lamy, M.C., Buchrieser, C., Trieu-Cuot, P., Kunst, F., Poyart, C. and Glaser, P. (2006) Genomic diversity and evolution within the species *Streptococcus agalactiae. Microbes and Infection* 8, 1227–1243.

Brouwer, M.C., Tunkel, A.R. and van de Beek, D. (2010) Epidemiology, diagnosis, and antimicrobial treatment of acute bacterial meningitis. *Clinical Microbiology Reviews* 23, 467–492.

Campbell, J.R., Baker, C.J. and Edwards, M.S. (1991) Deposition and degradation of C3 on type III group B streptococci. *Infection and Immunity* 59, 1978–1983.

Carlin, A.F., Lewis, A.L., Varki, A. and Nizet, V. (2007) Group B streptococcal capsular sialic acids interact with siglecs (immunoglobulin-like lectins) on human leukocytes. *Journal of Bacteriology* 189, 1231–1237.

Chang, Y.C., Wang, Z., Flax, L.A., Xu, D., Esko, J.D., Nizet, V. and Baron, M.J. (2011) Glycosaminoglycan binding facilitates entry of a bacterial pathogen into central nervous systems. *PLoS Pathogens* 7, e1002082.

Cieslewicz, M.J., Chaffin, D., Glusman, G., Kasper, D., Madan, A., Rodrigues, S., Fahey, J., Wessels, M.R. and Rubens, C.E. (2005) Structural and genetic diversity of Group B *Streptococcus* capsular polysaccharides. *Infection and Immunity* 73, 3096–3103.

Cornacchione, P., Scaringi, L., Fettucciari, K., Rosati, E., Sabatini, R., Orefici, G., von Hunolstein, C., Modesti, A., Modica, A., Minelli, F. and Marconi, P. (1998) Group B streptococci persist inside macrophages. *Immunology* 93, 86–95.

Cumley, N.J., Smith, L.M., Anthony, M. and May, R.C. (2012) The CovS/CovR acid response regulator is required for intracellular survival of Group B *Streptococcus* in macrophages. *Infection and Immunity* 80, 1650–1661.

Doran, K.S., Benoit, V.M., Gertz, R.E., Beall, B. and Nizet, V. (2002a) Late-onset group B streptococcal infection in identical twins: insight to disease pathogenesis. *Journal of Perinatology* 22, 326–330.

Doran, K.S., Chang, J.C., Benoit, V.M., Eckmann, L. and Nizet, V. (2002b) Group B streptococcal β-hemolysin/cytolysin promotes invasion of human lung epithelial cells and the release of interleukin-8. *Journal of Infectious Diseases* 185, 196–203.

Doran, K.S., Liu, G.Y. and Nizet, V. (2003) Group B streptococcal β-hemolysin/cytolysin activates neutrophil signaling pathways in brain endothelium and contributes to development of meningitis. *Journal of Clinical Investigation* 112, 736–744.

Doran, K.S., Engelson, E.J., Khosravi, A., Maisey, H.C., Fedtke, I., Equils, O., Michelsen, K.S., Arditi, M., Peschel, A. and Nizet, V. (2005) Blood–brain barrier invasion by Group B *Streptococcus* depends upon proper cell-surface anchoring of lipoteichoic acid. *Journal of Clinical Investigation* 115, 2499–2507.

Dramsi, S., Caliot, E., Bonne, I., Guadagnini, S., Prevost, M.C., Kojadinovic, M., Lalioui, L., Poyart, C. and Trieu-Cuot, P. (2006) Assembly and role of pili in group B streptococci. *Molecular Microbiology* 60, 1401–1413.

Dramsi, S., Morello, E., Poyart, C. and Trieu-Cuot, P. (2012) Epidemiologically and clinically relevant Group B *Streptococcus* isolates do not bind collagen but display enhanced binding to human fibrinogen. *Microbes and Infection* 14, 1044–1048.

Ferrieri, P., Burke, B. and Nelson, J. (1980) Production of bacteremia and meningitis in infant rats with group B streptococcal serotypes. *Infection and Immunity* 27, 1023–1032.

Glibetic, M., Samlalsingh-Parker, J., Raykova, V., Ofenstein, J. and Aranda, J.V. (2001) Group B Streptococci and inducible nitric oxide synthase: modulation by nuclear factor kappa B and ibuprofen. *Seminars in Perinatology* 25, 65–69.

Gutekunst, H., Eikmanns, B.J. and Reinscheid, D.J. (2004) The novel fibrinogen-binding protein FbsB promotes *Streptococcus agalactiae* invasion into epithelial cells. *Infection and Immunity* 72, 3495–3504.

Hakansson, S., Holm, S.E. and Wagner, M. (1987) Density profile of group B streptococci, type III, and its possible relation to enhanced virulence. *Journal of Clinical Microbiology* 25, 714–718.

Hakansson, S., Bergholm, A.M., Holm, S.E., Wagner, B. and Wagner, M. (1988) Properties of high and low density subpopulations of group B streptococci: enhanced virulence of the low density variant. *Microbial Pathogenesis* 5, 345–355.

Harris, T.O., Shelver, D.W., Bohnsack, J.F. and Rubens, C.E. (2003) A novel streptococcal surface protease promotes virulence, resistance to opsonophagocytosis, and cleavage of human fibrinogen. *Journal of Clinical Investigation* 111, 61–70.

Hensler, M.E., Miyamoto, S. and Nizet, V. (2008) Group B streptococcal β-hemolysin/cytolysin directly impairs cardiomyocyte viability and function. *PLoS One* 3, e2446.

Jarva, H., Hellwage, J., Jokiranta, T.S., Lehtinen, M.J., Zipfel, P.F. and Meri, S. (2004) The group B streptococcal β and pneumococcal Hic proteins are structurally related immune evasion molecules that bind the complement inhibitor factor H in an analogous fashion. *Journal of Immunology* 172, 3111–3118.

Jerlstrom, P.G., Chhatwal, G.S. and Timmis, K.N. (1991) The IgA-binding β antigen of the c protein complex of Group B streptococci: sequence determination of its gene and detection of two binding regions. *Molecular Microbiology* 5, 843–849.

Jones, A.L., Mertz, R.H., Carl, D.J. and Rubens, C.E. (2007) A streptococcal penicillin-binding protein is critical for resisting innate airway defenses in the neonatal lung. *Journal of Immunology* 179, 3196–3202.

Jones, N., Bohnsack, J.F., Takahashi, S., Oliver, K.A., Chan, M.S., Kunst, F., Glaser, P., Rusniok,

C., Crook, D.W., Harding, R.M., Bisharat, N. and Spratt, B.G. (2003) Multilocus sequence typing system for group B *Streptococcus*. *Journal of Clinical Microbiology* 41, 2530–2536.

Kim, B.J., Mu, R., Banerjee, A. and Doran, K.S. (2012) Regulation of tight junction complexes in brain endothelium by *Streptococcus agalactiae*. In: 4th International Conference on Gram-Positive Pathogens, 7–12 October 2012, Omaha, NE, USA.

Kim, K.S., Wass, C.A. and Cross, A.S. (1997) Blood–brain barrier permeability during the development of experimental bacterial meningitis in the rat. *Experimental Neurology* 145, 253–257.

Kim, Y.S., Sheldon, R.A., Elliott, B.R., Liu, Q., Ferriero, D.M. and Tauber, M.G. (1995) Brain injury in experimental neonatal meningitis due to group B streptococci. *Journal of Neuropathology and Experimental Neurology* 54, 531–539.

Lamy, M.C., Dramsi, S., Billoet, A., Reglier-Poupet, H., Tazi, A., Raymond, J., Guerin, F., Couve, E., Kunst, F., Glaser, P., Trieu-Cuot, P. and Poyart, C. (2006) Rapid detection of the 'highly virulent' group B *Streptococcus* ST-17 clone. *Microbes and Infection* 8, 1714–1722.

Lauer, P., Rinaudo, C.D., Soriani, M., Margarit, I., Maione, D., Rosini, R., Taddei, A.R., Mora, M., Rappuoli, R., Grandi, G. and Telford, J.L. (2005) Genome analysis reveals pili in Group B *Streptococcus*. *Science* 309, 105.

Lehnardt, S., Henneke, P., Lien, E., Kasper, D.L., Volpe, J.J., Bechmann, I., Nitsch, R., Weber, J.R., Golenbock, D.T. and Vartanian, T. (2006) A mechanism for neurodegeneration induced by group B streptococci through activation of the TLR2/MyD88 pathway in microglia. *Journal of Immunology* 177, 583–592.

Lembo, A., Gurney, M.A., Burnside, K., Banerjee, A., de los Reyes, M., Connelly, J.E., Lin, W.J., Jewell, K.A., Vo, A., Renken, C.W., Doran, K.S. and Rajagopal, L. (2010) Regulation of CovR expression in Group B *Streptococcus* impacts blood–brain barrier penetration. *Molecular Microbiology* 77, 431–443.

Lemire, P., Houde, M., Lecours, M.P., Fittipaldi, N. and Segura, M. (2012) Role of capsular polysaccharide in Group B *Streptococcccus* interactions with dendritic cells. *Microbes and Infection* 14, 1064–1076.

Ling, E.W., Noya, F.J., Ricard, G., Beharry, K., Mills, E.L. and Aranda, J.V. (1995) Biochemical mediators of meningeal inflammatory response to group B *Streptococcus* in the newborn piglet model. *Pediatric Research* 38, 981–987.

Liu, G.Y., Doran, K.S., Lawrence, T., Turkson, N., Puliti, M., Tissi, L. and Nizet, V. (2004) Sword and shield: linked group B streptococcal β-hemolysin/cytolysin and carotenoid pigment function to subvert host phagocyte defense. *Proceedings of the National Academy of Sciences USA* 101, 14491–14496.

Maisey, H.C., Hensler, M., Nizet, V. and Doran, K.S. (2007) Group B *streptococcal* pilus proteins contribute to adherence to and invasion of brain microvascular endothelial cells. *Journal of Bacteriology* 189, 1464–1467.

Maisey, H.C., Doran, K.S. and Nizet, V. (2008a) Recent advances in understanding the molecular basis of group B *Streptococcus* virulence. *Expert Reviews in Molecular Medicine* 10, e27.

Maisey, H.C., Quach, D., Hensler, M.E., Liu, G.Y., Gallo, R.L., Nizet, V. and Doran, K.S. (2008b) A group B streptococcal pilus protein promotes phagocyte resistance and systemic virulence. *FASEB Journal* 22, 1715–1724.

Marques, M.B., Kasper, D.L., Pangburn, M.K. and Wessels, M.R. (1992) Prevention of C3 deposition by capsular polysaccharide is a virulence mechanism of type III group B streptococci. *Infection and Immunity* 60, 3986–3993.

Maruvada, R., Blom, A.M. and Prasadarao, N.V. (2008) Effects of complement regulators bound to *Escherichia coli* K1 and Group B *Streptococcus* on the interaction with host cells. *Immunology* 124, 265–276.

Maruvada, R., Zhu, L., Pearce, D., Sapirstein, A. and Kim, K.S. (2011) Host cytosolic phospholipase $A_2\alpha$ contributes to group B *Streptococcus* penetration of the blood-brain barrier. *Infection and Immunity* 79, 4088–4093.

McKnight, A.A., Keyes, W.G., Hudak, M.L. and Jones, M.D. Jr (1992) Oxygen free radicals and the cerebral arteriolar response to group B streptococci. *Pediatric Research* 31, 640–644.

Mereghetti, L., Sitkiewicz, I., Green, N.M. and Musser, J.M. (2008) Extensive adaptive changes occur in the transcriptome of *Streptococcus agalactiae* (Group B *Streptococcus*) in response to incubation with human blood. *PLoS One* 3, e3143.

Musser, J.M., Mattingly, S.J., Quentin, R., Goudeau, A. and Selander, R.K. (1989) Identification of a high-virulence clone of type III *Streptococcus agalactiae* (group B *Streptococcus*) causing invasive neonatal disease. *Proceedings of the National Academy of Sciences USA* 86, 4731–4735.

Nealon, T.J. and Mattingly, S.J. (1983) Association of elevated levels of cellular lipoteichoic acids of group B streptococci with human neonatal disease. *Infection and Immunity* 39, 1243–1251.

Nizet, V., Gibson, R.L., Chi, E.Y., Framson, P.E., Hulse, M. and Rubens, C.E. (1996) Group B streptococcal beta-hemolysin expression is associated with injury of lung epithelial cells. *Infection and Immunity* 64, 3818–3826.

Nizet, V., Kim, K.S., Stins, M., Jonas, M., Chi, E.Y., Nguyen, D. and Rubens, C.E. (1997) Invasion of brain microvascular endothelial cells by group B streptococci. *Infection and Immunity* 65, 5074–5081.

Nuccitelli, A., Cozzi, R., Gourlay, L.J., Donnarumma, D., Necchi, F., Norais, N., Telford, J.L., Rappuoli, R., Bolognesi, M., Maione, D., Grandi, G. and Rinaudo, C. (2011) Structure-based approach to rationally design a chimeric protein for an effective vaccine against Group B *Streptococcus* infections. *Proceedings of the National Academy of Sciences USA* 108, 10278–10283.

Patterson, H., Saralahti, A., Parikka, M., Dramsi, S., Trieu-Cuot, P., Poyart, C., Rounioja, S. and Ramet, M. (2012) Adult zebrafish model of bacterial meningitis in *Streptococcus agalactiae* infection. *Developmental and Comparative Immunology* 38, 447–455.

Phares, C.R., *et al.* (2008) Epidemiology of invasive group B streptococcal disease in the United States, 1999–2005. *Journal of the American Medical Association* 299, 2056–2065.

Pinto Junior, V.L., Rebelo, M.C., Gomes, R.N., Assis, E.F., Castro-Faria-Neto, H.C. and Boia, M.N. (2011) IL-6 and IL-8 in cerebrospinal fluid from patients with aseptic meningitis and bacterial meningitis: their potential role as a marker for differential diagnosis. *Brazilian Journal of Infectious Diseases* 15, 156–158.

Ponnuraj, K., Bowden, M.G., Davis, S., Gurusiddappa, S., Moore, D., Choe, D., Xu, Y., Hook, M. and Narayana, S.V. (2003) A 'dock, lock, and latch' structural model for a staphylococcal adhesin binding to fibrinogen. *Cell* 115, 217–228.

Poyart, C., Lamy, M.C., Boumaila, C., Fiedler, F. and Trieu-Cuot, P. (2001a) Regulation of D-alanyl-lipoteichoic acid biosynthesis in *Streptococcus agalactiae* involves a novel two-component regulatory system. *Journal of Bacteriology* 183, 6324–6334.

Poyart, C., Pellegrini, E., Gaillot, O., Boumaila, C., Baptista, M. and Trieu-Cuot, P. (2001b) Contribution of Mn-cofactored superoxide dismutase (SodA) to the virulence of *Streptococcus agalactiae. Infection and Immunity* 69, 5098–5106.

Pracht, D., Elm, C., Gerber, J., Bergmann, S., Rohde, M., Seiler, M., Kim, K.S., Jenkinson, H.F., Nau, R. and Hammerschmidt, S. (2005) PavA of *Streptococcus pneumoniae* modulates adherence, invasion, and meningeal inflammation. *Infection and Immunity* 73, 2680–2689.

Quach, D., van Sorge, N.M., Kristian, S.A., Bryan, J.D., Shelver, D.W. and Doran, K.S. (2009) The CiaR response regulator in group B *Streptococcus* promotes intracellular survival and resistance to innate immune defenses. *Journal of Bacteriology* 191, 2023–2032.

Quirante, J., Ceballos, R. and Cassady, G. (1974) Group B β-hemolytic streptococcal infection in the newborn. I. Early onset infection. *American Journal of Diseases of Children* 128, 659–665.

Reiss, A., Braun, J.S., Jager, K., Freyer, D., Laube, G., Buhrer, C., Felderhoff-Muser, U., Stadelmann, C., Nizet, V. and Weber, J.R. (2011) Bacterial pore-forming cytolysins induce neuronal damage in a rat model of neonatal meningitis. *Journal of Infectious Diseases* 203, 393–400.

Rosini, R., *et al.* (2006) Identification of novel genomic islands coding for antigenic pilus-like structures in *Streptococcus agalactiae. Molecular Microbiology* 61, 126–141.

Samen, U., Eikmanns, B.J., Reinscheid, D.J. and Borges, F. (2007) The surface protein Srr-1 of *Streptococcus agalactiae* binds human keratin 4 and promotes adherence to epithelial HEp-2 cells. *Infection and Immunity* 75, 5405–5414.

Santi, I., Scarselli, M., Mariani, M., Pezzicoli, A., Masignani, V., Taddei, A., Grandi, G., Telford, J.L. and Soriani, M. (2007) BibA: a novel immunogenic bacterial adhesin contributing to group B *Streptococcus* survival in human blood. *Molecular Microbiology* 63, 754–767.

Scheld, W.M., Koedel, U., Nathan, B. and Pfister, H.W. (2002) Pathophysiology of bacterial meningitis: mechanism(s) of neuronal injury. *Journal of Infectious Diseases* 186 Suppl. 2, S225–S233.

Schubert, A., Zakikhany, K., Pietrocola, G., Meinke, A., Speziale, P., Eikmanns, B.J. and Reinscheid, D.J. (2004) The fibrinogen receptor FbsA promotes adherence of *Streptococcus agalactiae* to human epithelial cells. *Infection and Immunity* 72, 6197–6205.

Seifert, K.N., Adderson, E.E., Whiting, A.A., Bohnsack, J.F., Crowley, P.J. and Brady, L.J. (2006) A unique serine-rich repeat protein (Srr-2) and novel surface antigen (ε) associated with a virulent lineage of serotype III *Streptococcus agalactiae. Microbiology* 152, 1029–1040.

Seo, H.S., Mu, R., Kim, B.J., Doran, K.S. and Sullam, P.M. (2012) Binding of glycoprotein Srr1 of *Streptococcus agalactiae* to fibrinogen promotes attachment to brain endothelium and the development of meningitis. *PLoS Pathogens* 8, e1002947.

Shin, S. and Kim, K.S. (2006) RhoA and Rac1 contribute to type III group B streptococcal invasion of human brain microvascular endothelial cells. *Biochemical and Biophysical Research Communications* 345, 538–542.

Shin, S., Paul-Satyaseela, M., Lee, J.S., Romer, L.H. and Kim, K.S. (2006) Focal adhesion kinase is involved in type III group B streptococcal invasion of human brain microvascular endothelial cells. *Microbial Pathogenesis* 41, 168–173.

Soriani, M., Santi, I., Taddei, A., Rappuoli, R., Grandi, G. and Telford, J.L. (2006) Group B *Streptococcus* crosses human epithelial cells by a paracellular route. *Journal of Infectious Diseases* 193, 241–250.

Spellerberg, B., Rozdzinski, E., Martin, S., Weber-Heynemann, J., Schnitzler, N., Lutticken, R. and Podbielski, A. (1999) Lmb, a protein with similarities to the LraI adhesin family, mediates attachment of *Streptococcus agalactiae* to human laminin. *Infection and Immunity* 67, 871–878.

Spellerberg, B., Martin, S., Brandt, C. and Lutticken, R. (2000) The *cyl* genes of *Streptococcus agalactiae* are involved in the production of pigment. *FEMS Microbiology Letters* 188, 125–128.

Stins, M.F., Prasadarao, N.V., Ibric, L., Wass, C.A., Luckett, P. and Kim, K.S. (1994) Binding characteristics of S fimbriated *Escherichia coli* to isolated brain microvascular endothelial cells. *American Journal of Pathology* 145, 1228–1236.

Stoll, B.J., *et al.* (2002a) Changes in pathogens causing early-onset sepsis in very-low-birth-weight infants. *New England Journal of Medicine* 347, 240–247.

Stoll, B.J., *et al.* (2002b) Late-onset sepsis in very low birth weight neonates: the experience of the NICHD Neonatal Research Network. *Pediatrics* 110, 285–291.

Tazi, A., *et al.* (2010) The surface protein HvgA mediates group B *Streptococcus* hypervirulence and meningeal tropism in neonates. *Journal of Experimental Medicine* 207, 2313–2322.

Teixeira, C.F., Azevedo, N.L., Carvalho, T.M., Fuentes, J. and Nagao, P.E. (2001) Cytochemical study of *Streptococcus agalactiae* and macrophage interaction. *Microscopy Research and Technique* 54, 254–259.

Tenenbaum, T., Bloier, C., Adam, R., Reinscheid, D.J. and Schroten, H. (2005) Adherence to and invasion of human brain microvascular endothelial cells are promoted by fibrinogen-binding protein FbsA of *Streptococcus agalactiae*. *Infection and Immunity* 73, 4404–4409.

Tenenbaum, T., Spellerberg, B., Adam, R., Vogel, M., Kim, K.S. and Schroten, H. (2007) *Streptococcus agalactiae* invasion of human brain microvascular endothelial cells is promoted by the laminin-binding protein Lmb. *Microbes and Infection* 9, 714–720.

Tettelin, H., *et al.* (2005) Genome analysis of multiple pathogenic isolates of *Streptococcus agalactiae*: implications for the microbial 'pan-genome'. *Proceedings of the National Academy of Sciences USA* 102, 13950–13955.

Thigpen, M.C., *et al.* (2011) Bacterial meningitis in the United States, 1998–2007. *New England Journal of Medicine* 364, 2016–2025.

Tunkel, A.R. and Scheld, W.M. (1995) Acute bacterial meningitis. *Lancet* 346, 1675–1680.

Van Dyke, M.K., *et al.* (2009) Evaluation of universal antenatal screening for group B *Streptococcus*. *New England Journal of Medicine* 360, 2626–2636.

van Sorge, N.M., Quach, D., Gurney, M.A., Sullam, P.M., Nizet, V. and Doran, K.S. (2009) The group B streptococcal serine-rich repeat 1 glycoprotein mediates penetration of the blood–brain barrier. *Journal of Infectious Diseases* 199, 1479–1487.

Wilson, C.B. and Weaver, W.M. (1985) Comparative susceptibility of group B streptococci and *Staphylococcus aureus* to killing by oxygen metabolites. *Journal of Infectious Diseases* 152, 323–329.

10 Chronic Meningitis

Erich Schmutzhard* and Raimund Helbok†
Medical University Hospital Innsbruck, Innsbruck, Austria

10.1 Introduction

Chronic meningitis is defined, quite arbitrarily, as the persistence of clinical signs and symptoms of meningitis for more than 4 weeks or, even better, as a syndrome of meningeal inflammation based upon clinical features and cerebrospinal fluid (CSF) findings (Cho and Venna, 2010). Both infective and non-infective causes may lead to this clinical entity of a chronic meningitis syndrome (Helbok *et al.*, 2009). In contrast to chronic meningitis, recurrent meningitis is a syndrome where clinical episodes of meningitis are separated by asymptomatic periods, including normalization of CSF (Ginsberg and Kidd, 2008).

This chapter deals exclusively with common infectious causes of chronic meningitis in the immunocompetent patient, citing particular examples of bacterial, fungal and helminthic causes (Table 10.1). The non-infectious causes (Table 10.2), chronic meningitis in the immunocompromised patient, rare infectious causes of chronic meningitis (Table 10.3), chronic encephalitis, chronic space occupying inflammatory lesions (cysts, granuloma formation, etc.), chronic meningovascular syndromes and other chronic autoimmune systemic and isolated encephalitic diseases (e.g. NMDA-receptor antibody-, VGKC antibody-, AMPA-receptor antibody- and GAD antibody-associated encephalitides, Hashimoto encephalopathy, systemic lupus erythematosus, Wegener granulomatosis, etc.), are all outside the scope of this review.

In every patient with chronic meningitis the diagnostic workup should be as structured as possible, including a goal-oriented anamnestic and clinical evaluation (Tables 10.4 and 10.5). The important neurological signs and symptoms, which may help to guide the clinician in the diagnostic workup, are given in Table 10.6. An extensive laboratory workup is needed in every patient with chronic meningitis, including repetitive lumbar punctures as well as meningeal (or parenchymal) biopsies. If extracerebral or extracranial pathological changes are found (Table 10.7), interdisciplinary workup of such a patient, including biopsy from the respective organ, is essential and is the basis of good clinical and scientific practice. If the cause is not found and the signs and symptoms persist and deteriorate, repetitive spinal taps might increase the diagnostic yield; if not, then a

*erich.schmutzhard@i-med.ac.at
†raimund.helbok@uki.at

Table 10.1. Common infectious causes of chronic meningitis. (Adapted from Helbok *et al.*, 2009.)

Bacteria	*Mycobacterium tuberculosis*
	Treponema pallidum
	Parameningeal infectious causes
Viruses	Cytomegalovirus: in immunocompromised patients
	Herpes simplex virus type II: Mollaret meningitis: usually recurrent/relapsing meningitis
Fungi	*Cryptococcus neoformans*: in patients with travel history to tropical countries as well as in immunocompromised patients
	Candida: in immunocompromised patients, patients with longstanding intensive care unit history
Helminths	*Cysticercus cellulosae* (racemose form): travel history, history of exposure

Table 10.2. Non-infective causes of chronic meningitis. (Adapted from Gripshover and Ellner, 1997; Ginsberg and Kidd, 2008; and Helbok *et al.*, 2009.)

Uveo-mengitic syndromes	Sarcoidosis
	Behçet's disease
	Wegener's granulomatosis
	Vogt–Koyanagi–Harada syndrome
	Sjögren's syndrome
	Systemic lupus erythematosus
	Other vasculitides
Hypertrophic pachymeningitis	
Drugs	Non-steroidal anti-inflammatory drugs
	Antimicrobial agents
	Intravenous immunoglobulin
	Immunosuppressants
	Allopurinol
	Vaccination
	Intrathecally administered agents
	Chemical meningitis
Malignant meningitis	Carcinomatous meningitis
	Lymphomatous meningitis
	Leukaemic meningitis
Miscellaneous	Hereditary auto-inflammatory periodic fever syndromes
	Cholesterol embolization syndrome
	Fabry's disease
	Subarachnoid haemorrhage
	HaNDL
	Migraine[a]
	No cause found[b]

[a]Migraine may be associated with a CSF lymphocytosis, which can be chronic, but clearly this should be a diagnosis of exclusion.

[b]In up to one-third of cases.

HaNDL, transient headache with neurological deficit and CSF lymphocytosis.

Table 10.3. Rare infectious causes of chronic meningitis. (Adapted from Gripshover and Ellner, 1997; Ginsberg and Kidd, 2008; and Helbok *et al.*, 2009.)

Bacteria	*Borrelia* spp.	–
	Listeria monocytogenes	–
	Parameningeal focus	–
	Pasteurella tularensis	–
	Brucella spp.	Travel history
	Leptospira spp.	Exposure
	Actinomyces spp.	Immunocompromised state
	Nocardia spp.	Immunocompromised state
Viruses	Lymphocytic choriomeningitis virus	In children
	Epstein–Barr virus-associated lymphoma	In immunocompromised state
Protozoa	*Trypanosoma brucei*	Travel history (Africa): quickly turning into encephalitis
Fungi	*Zygomycetes* spp.	–
	Pseudallescheria boydii	–
	Sporothrix schenckii	–
	Coccidioides spp.	Travel history: to the Americas
	Histoplasma spp.	Travel history: South America, sub-Saharan Africa
	Blastomyces spp.	Travel history to sub-Saharan Africa
	Aspergillus spp.	Immunocompromised state
	Zygomycetes	History of diabetes mellitus
Helminths	*Echinococcus granulosus*	Cyst formation
	Toxocara spp.	Larva migrans, including chronic (eosinophilic) meningitis
	Angiostrongylus spp.	Travel history, eosinophilic meningitis
	Gnathostoma spinigerum	Travel history, eosinophilic meningitis and encephalitis, myelitis, etc.
	Schistosoma spp.	Travel history, frequently plexus lumbus sacralis lesion
	Paragonimus spp.	Cyst formation
	Fasciola hepatica	Exposure

meningeal biopsy needs to be considered. Only then, and in case this meningeal biopsy does not yield a positive result or help to find the cause, respectively, might the administration of steroids with or without immunosuppressive therapeutic agents be considered.

10.2 Tuberculous Meningitis

Mycobacterium tuberculosis complex, i.e. *Mycobacterium tuberculosis, Mycobacterium bovis* and *Mycobacterium africanum,* and non-tuberculous mycobacteria or atypical mycobacteria, e.g. *Mycobacterium avium* complex, *Mycobacterium kansasii, Mycobacterium scrofulaceum, Mycobacterium xenopi, Mycobacterium genavense, Mycobacterium gordonae, Mycobacterium marinum, Mycobacterium fortuitum* and *Mycobacterium chelonei,* can cause human disease (Zuger and Lowy, 1997). All mycobacteria potentially can invade the central nervous system (CNS): *M. tuberculosis* complex cause chronic meningitis, intracranial tuberculoma and, in rare cases, tuberculous abscesses, whereas the non-tuberculous mycobacteria only cause disease in immunocompromised individuals (in particular AIDS with very low CD4 counts) and invade the CNS infrequently, causing meningitis or meningoencephalitis. Some non-tuberculous mycobacteria may be associated with foreign bodies, abscess formation and prior traumatic brain injury or CNS surgery. Nevertheless, even in severely immunocompromised patients, *M. tuberculosis* is the most commonly isolated

Table 10.4. Pathogenic agents and their type of CNS involvement. (Adapted from Gripshover and Ellner, 1997; del Brutto, 2006; Schmutzhard, 2006a,b; Ginsberg and Kidd, 2008; Helbok *et al.*, 2009; and Yorgancilar *et al.*, 2012.)

	Meningitis	Neurologic focal lesion (granuloma, cyst, abscess, vasculitis)	Meningo-encephalitis
Viruses			
Lymphocytic choriomeningitidis (L)	++	–	+
Mumps (L)	++	–	(+)
Herpes simplex (L+N)/Mollaret's meningitis (HSV II)	(+)	+	++
Herpes zoster (L)	++	++	++
Cytomegalovirus (L+N)	+	–	++
Arboviruses (L)	++	–	++
Echoviruses (L)	++	–	+
Measles (L)	(+)	–	–
Bacteria			
Mycobacterium tuberculosis (L+N+E)	+++	++	(+)
Brucella spp. (L+N)	++	++	–
Pasteurella tularensis (L)	+	+	+
Treponema pallidum (L+E)	+++	++	–
Borrelia spp. (L)	+++	(+)	(+)
Leptospira spp. (L)	+	(+)	(+)
Nocardia spp. (L+N)	(+)	++	–
Actinomyces spp. (L+N)	(+)	(+)	–
Listeria monocytogenes (L+N)	++	(+)	+
Subacute bacterial endocarditis (mainly streptococci) (L+N)	(+)	++	+
Parameningeal infectious focus (L+N)	++	+++	++
Fungi			
Cryptococcus neoformans (L)	+++	+	–
Coccidioides spp. (L+N+E)	+++	+	–
Histoplasma spp. (L+N)	+	++	–
Blastomyces spp. (L+N)	+	++	–
Candida spp. (L+N)	++	++	–
Aspergillus spp. (L+N)	(+)	+++	–
Zygomycetes spp. (L+N)	++	++	–
Pseudallescheria boydii (L+N)	++	++	–
Sporothrix schenckii (L+N)	++	–	–
Protozoa			
Toxoplasma gondii (L+N+E)	(+)	+++	+
Trypanosoma brucei spp. (L)	+	(+)	+++
Trypanosoma cruzi (L)	+	+	+
Acanthamoeba spp. (L+N)	(+)	++	+
Entamoeba histolytica	(+)	++	–

Continued

Table 10.4. Continued

	Meningitis	Neurologic focal lesion (granuloma, cyst, abscess, vasculitis)	Meningo-encephalitis
Helminths			
Cysticercus cellulosae (L+E)	+	+++	++
Echinococcus granulosus (L+E)	–	++	–
Schistosoma spp. (L+E)	(+)	++	+
Fasciola hepatica (L+E)	+	++	(+)
Paragonimus spp. (L+E)	+	++	(+)
Toxocara spp. (L+E)	+	++	+
Angiostrongylus spp. (E)	++	(+)	–
Gnathostoma spinigerum (E)	++	++	++
Trichinella spiralis (L+E)	+	+	+++

This table lists the organisms according to the type of CNS involvement in chronic CNS infection and inflammation, respectively.
E: mainly eosinophilic pleocytosis in CSF; L: mainly lymphocytic pleocytosis in CSF; N: mainly granulocytic (neutrophils) pleocytosis in CSF; (+) very rare; + rare; ++ moderately frequent; +++ frequent; – not known.

Table 10.5. Goal-oriented anamnestic and clinical evaluation in a patient with chronic meningitis. (Adapted from Helbok *et al.*, 2009.)

Disease or pathogen	Exposure
Tuberculosis	Contact with pulmonary tuberculosis, history of tuberculosis, positive tuberculin skin test, genital ulcera, sexual contact
Syphilis Borreliosis Brucellosis (unpasteurized milk, contact with cows, pigs, sheep, goats) Listeriosis (milk) Cysticercosis (pig) Leptospirosis (rats) Lymphocytic choriomeningitis-virus (rodents)	Tick bite, erythema chronicum migrans Contact with animals and animal products (immunocompetent)
HIV, HTLV-1, -2, syphilis	Sexual contact, intravenous drug abuse
Candida spp.	Long-term intensive care measures
Coccidioides immitis	Laboratory technician or worker
Drug-induced aseptic meningitis	Non-steroidal anti-inflammatory agents, trimethoprim/sulfamethoxazol, sulfonamides, ciprofloxacin, isoniacid, metronidazole, penicillin, cytosin/arabinosid, azathioprine, carbamazepine, 7S-immunoglobulins

HIV, human immunodeficiency virus; HTLV-1, -2, human T-lymphotropic virus type 1 and type 2.

Table 10.6. Neurological signs and symptoms in chronic meningitis. (Adapted from Gripshover and Ellner, 1997; Ginsberg and Kidd, 2008; and Helbok *et al.*, 2009.)

Neurological evaluation	Pathology
Cranial nerve deficit (III, IV, VI, VII, VIII, XI)	Tuberculosis (VI, II, IV), syphilis (VI, VIII, XI), borreliosis (VII), sarcoidosis (VII), fungi vasculitis (e.g. Wegener's granulomatosis)
Radicular pain	Borreliosis, spinal tuberculosis, carcinomatous meningitis
Spinal cord symptoms	Tuberculosis, syphilis, rare: brucellosis, HIV, VZV
Focal neurological deficit	Septic emboli in bacterial endocarditis, arbovirus encephalitis
Granuloma	Tuberculoma; cryptococcoma; granuloma (aspergillosis, toxoplasmosis, rare: *Toxocara* spp., *Angiostrongylus cantonensis*, *Acanthamoeba* spp.); abscess (brucellosis, nocardiosis, *Actinomyces* infection, aspergillosis)
Cerebral ischaemia	Tuberculosis, endocarditis, rare: fungi, syphilis
Dementia	Creutzfeldt–Jakob disease, frontal brain abscess

VZV: varicella zoster virus.

Table 10.7. Systemic/multi-organ involvement in chronic meningitis. (Adapted from Gripshover and Ellner, 1997; Hildebrand and Aoun, 2003; Helbok *et al.*, 2006, 2009; Ginsberg and Kidd, 2008; de Broucker and Martinez-Almoyna, 2011; and Yorgancilar *et al.*, 2012.)

Dermatological evaluation	Oral and genital ulcers	Behçet's disease
	Erythema	SLE, borreliosis
	Erythema nodosum	Sarcoidosis
	Exanthema, skin lesions	HIV, VZV, EBV, CMV, HSV
	(+ HIV)	Polyomavirus JC
Ophthalmological evaluation	Uveiits, iridocyclitis	Behçet's disease, sarcoidosis
	Xerophthalmy, xerostomy	Sjögren syndrome
	Poliosis	Vogt–Koyanagi–Harada syndrome
	Chemosis	Leptospirosis
	Retinitis	CMV
Urological evaluation	Haematuria	Schistosomiasis
Rheumatological evaluation	Arthritis	Borreliosis, tuberculosis, brucellosis, Behçet's disease
Internal evaluation	Lymphadenopathy, hepatosplenomegaly	Tuberculosis, brucellosis, sarcoidosis, cancer
ENT evaluation	Parameningeal focus	Otitis, mastoiditis, sinusitis

SLE: systemic lupus erythematosus; EBV: Epstein–Barr virus; CMV: cytomegalovirus; HSV: herpes simplex virus; ENT: eaer, nose and throat.

mycobacterial organism. *M. tuberculosis* is an obligate intracellular aerobic bacillus, whose entire genome has been sequenced; the organism exhibits antigenic variation, which is one possible explanation for the chronicity of disease (Garcia-Monco, 2006; Galimi, 2011). The pathophysiology of tuberculous meningitis is reviewed in the chapter by Thwaites (Chapter 11, this volume).

10.2.1 Clinical signs, symptoms and diagnostic features

Tuberculous meningitis is usually a chronic meningitis, presenting with a prodromal period of up to 4 weeks (or longer) of non-specific symptoms, e.g. malaise, subfebrile temperatures, fatigue, etc. After this prodromal period, headache and vomiting with a wide range of impairment of mental status and neck stiffness ensues. The mycobacteria and the tubercles spreading mainly into the basal subarachnoid space (SAS) lead to cranial nerve palsy in more than 25% of patients, inflammatory invasion of basal intracranial arteries leading to stroke and stroke-like syndromes, and blocking of the CSF flow leading to hydrocephalus (Thwaites *et al.*, 2002; Garcia-Monco, 2006; Garg, 2010; Sharma *et al.*, 2011; Hristea and Olaru, 2012; Vibha *et al.*, 2012). Thus, in a patient with clinical signs and symptoms of chronic meningitis, the triad – or any of these three clinical entities – consisting of hydrocephalus, stroke and cranial nerve neuropathy is almost confirmatory for tuberculous meningitis (Pasco, 2012).

The CSF shows a mild to moderate lymphocytic pleocytosis, a clearly increased protein content and borderline low glucose levels (Garcia-Monco, 2006). In severely immunosuppressed patients in whom mycobacteria can multiply at a much higher rate, glucose levels are low to very low (Garg and Sinha, 2011; George *et al.*, 2012). Initially, the CSF may show a neutrophilic predominance; however, within a few days the lymphocytic pleocytosis is a major hallmark of tuberculous meningitis. In a few cases, mixed pleocytosis might persist. This might also happen in patients who respond appropriately to anti-tuberculous antimicrobial chemotherapy; in some cases, this 'therapeutic paradox' has been regarded as virtually pathognomonic of tuberculous meningitis (Garcia-Monco, 2006).

Neuroimaging usually reveals enhancement of the basal meninges, including enhancing granulomatous lesions (Fig. 10.1). Hydrocephalus can easily be observed by neuroimaging and ischaemic infarctions reflect the arteritic involvement (Javaud *et al.*, 2011; Misra *et al.*, 2011; Kalita *et al.*, 2012; Singh *et al.*, 2012). Tuberculous meningitis is often complicated by hyponatremia, and regular laboratory check-ups are necessary (Garcia-Monco, 2006). In any patient presenting with subacute or chronic meningitis (with or without additional neurological findings), and laboratory diagnosis being frequently unspecific or even negative, a high level of suspicion is required. In CSF acid-fast stains (Ziehl–Neelsen or Kinyoun) that are only positive in up to 25% of patients with tuberculous meningitis, cultures of the CSF may take up to 8 weeks for a full and unequivocal identification and are only positive in around 50%. This range can be enhanced by repetitive CSF cultures, reaching up to 85% after the fifth CSF culture (Chen *et al.*, 2012; Kirwan *et al.*, 2012). Newer diagnostic methods, including radiometric assays, rapid broth systems (Chen *et al.*, 2012), measurement of CSF adenosine deaminase levels (Sun *et al.*, 2012), polymerase chain reaction (PCR) techniques (Takahashi *et al.*, 2012) and a propagated T-cell interferon-γ release assay (TIGRA) (Principi and Esposito, 2012) may increase diagnostic capacity.

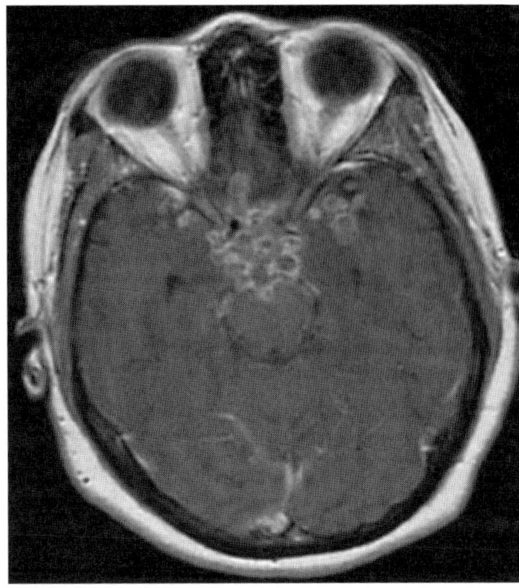

Fig. 10.1. Chronic basal granulomatous meningitis (MR, T1, i.v. gadolinium enhancement).

10.2.2 Therapy

In many patients with suspected tuberculous meningitis, a definite diagnosis is difficult, delayed or late. It is recommended to start empirical therapy as early as possible, a fact that has reduced morbidity and mortality. Figure 10.2 shows the algorithm recommended for diagnosing and treating a patient with chronic meningitis.

The anti-tuberculous drugs have been divided into first-line (rifampicin, isoniazid, ethambutol, pyrazinamide and streptomycin) and second-line drugs (paraminosalicylic acid, ethionamide, cycloserine, other aminoglycosides, quinolones, linezolide and, in rare cases, also macrolides) (Garg, 2010; van der Harst and Luijckx, 2011; Vibha *et al.*, 2012). All anti-tuberculous drugs have a wide range of potentially life-threatening side effects. The optimal therapy combination differs

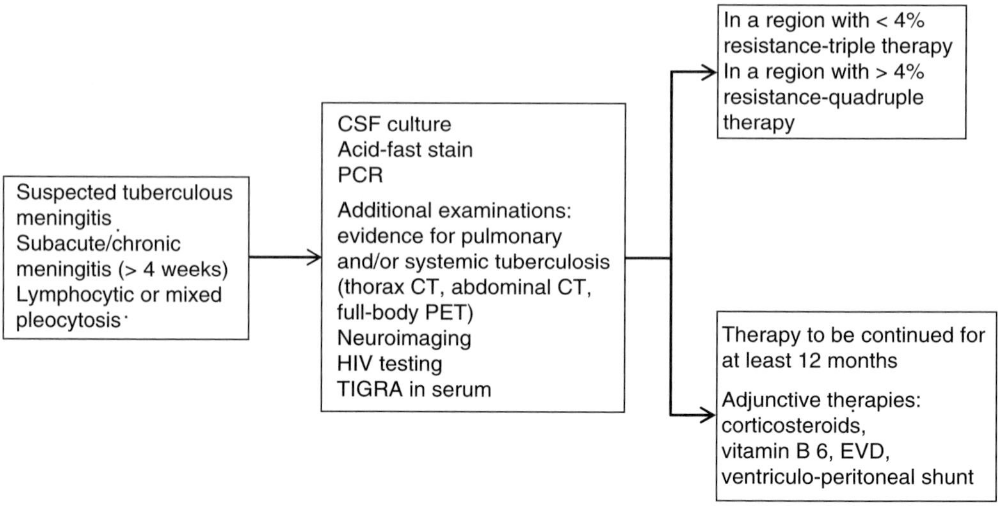

Fig. 10.2. Recommended algorithm for diagnosing and treating a patient with chronic meningitis. CT, computed tomography; EVD, external ventricular drain; PET, positron tomography.

from region to region and needs to be adapted according to the clinical findings, and, in particular, local resistance patterns. The minimum is a combination therapy of three drugs, i.e. isoniazid, rifampizin and pyrazinamide for a minimum of 2–3 months followed by isoniazide and rifampicin for another 9–12 months. In the case of positive PCR, acid-fast stain and culture from the CSF, therapy needs to be continued for a minimum of 6 months after the respective examination has turned negative.

Resistance to various anti-tuberculous drugs has become a real problem, mainly for southern Africa, Russia/Ukraine, Central Asia, the Dominican Republic and Argentina. Occasionally, up to seven drugs – including all second-line drugs, in particular quinolones – are needed (Garcia-Monco, 2006; Garg and Sinha, 2011; Vinnard *et al.*, 2011). CNS tuberculosis is particularly difficult to control in HIV-infected patients. Protease inhibitors and non-nucleoside reverse transcriptase inhibitors (and others) may interact with anti-tuberculous drugs leading to subtherapeutic blood levels of anti-retroviral agents and toxic drug levels, e.g. of rifampicin. This means that instead of rifampicin, rifabutin might be the drug of choice. HIV patients frequently have several organs involved, including the intestine, causing malabsorption even of anti-tuberculous drugs; therefore, close drug monitoring is highly recommended (Garg and Sinha, 2011; Dau *et al.*, 2012). Surgery for hydrocephalus and/or intracranial tuberculoma is indicated in the case of increased intracranial pressure (ICP) and if the tuberculoma does not decrease in size within 3 months (Figaji and Fieggen, 2013; Lin *et al.*, 2012). Dexamethasone improves the outcome in HIV-negative patients with tuberculous meningitis (Torok *et al.*, 2011).

10.3 Fungal Meningitis

Several fungi can cause meningitis in humans. Yeasts (*Cryptococcus neoformans* and *Candida* spp.), dimorphic fungi (*Histoplasma capsulatum, Coccidioides immitis, Paracoccidioides brasiliensis* and *Blastomyces dermatitidis*), filamentous fungi (*Zygomycetes* and *Aspergillus* spp.) and dematiaceous moulds have all been implicated in CNS infection, in particular subacute/chronic meningitis (Schmutzhard, 2006a). The most common fungal meningitis is caused by *C. neoformans*, especially in regions of high HIV I (II) seroprevalence (Bamba *et al.*, 2012). Besides meningitis, CNS cryptococcosis may present as encephalitis or cryptococcoma (intracranial/cerebral space-occupying granuloma) (Schmutzhard, 2006a). Cryptococcal meningitis occurs in 8–40% of patients with HIV infection (AIDS). Each year up to 1 million cases of cryptococcal meningitis occur in the AIDS population on a worldwide basis with up to 600,000 deaths (Desalermos *et al.*, 2012).

10.3.1 *Cryptococcus neoformans* meningitis

Two *Cryptococcus* spp. cause human infections: *C. neoformans* (serotypes A and D) and *Cryptococcus gattii* (serotypes B and C), the former being commonly associated with bird droppings (particularly pigeon) and having global distribution, and the latter frequently diagnosed in tropical or subtropical regions and having been shown to be associated with certain tree species, notably *Eucalyptus* spp.

Pathophysiology including molecular mechanisms

Cryptococcus spores are produced when cryptococci reproduce sexually. Such spores or desiccated yeasts are thought to be the initial infectious particles, which eventually are inhaled by human hosts. These spores colonize the respiratory tract, leading to a dormant form of colonization usually referred to as latent infection. In most instances, only impairment or compromise of host immunity can lead to reactivation of the latent form and eventually cause haematogenous dissemination leading to systemic infection (Liu *et al.*, 2012). In the immunocompetent person, cryptococci are contained in the lung by a combination of cell-mediated and innate as well as antibody-related immunity. Complement-mediated phagocytosis is thought to be the primary initial defence against cryptococcal infection: however, cytokines such as tumour necrosis factor (TNF)-α, interferon-γ and interleukin $(IL)^{+}$-18, as well as $CD4^{+}$ and $CD8^{+}$ T-cells and, possibly, antibodies directed towards the fungal capsule, constitute further host defence mechanisms against fungal invasion (Feldmesser and Casadevall, 1997; Huffnagle and Lipscomb, 1998). Only if this complex host immune system fails to contain the fungus, mainly within the alveolar compartment of the lungs, can cryptococci spread – haematogenously – to other organs, including myocardium, bones, the urinary tract and, in particular, into the CNS (Liu *et al.*, 2012).

When phagocytic cells fail to kill the yeast, i.e. when the host defence mechanisms are compromised, the fungi can replicate inside macrophages to form cryptococcal phagosomes leading eventually to the burst of host macrophages to release these fungi (Liu *et al.*, 2012). Conversely, cryptococci can also exit macrophages by extrusion without lysis. Cryptococci are facultative intracellular organisms, and survival and replication within phagocytes in the blood is a critical virulence attribute, as extracellular cryptococci are normally cleared from the blood by host defences (Chang *et al.*, 2004).

Surprisingly little is known about the cryptococcal adhesins that mediate fungal attachment to human respiratory tract epithelia, to blood vessel endothelia or to cells of the immune system and brain. Moreover, the mechanisms by which cryptococci enter the CSF from the blood are not entirely known, but they do share some similarities with mechanisms described for bacterial meningeal pathogens. The organism reaches the blood–brain barrier/blood–CSF barrier (BBB/BCSFB) via the blood and they have been hypothesized to cross the barrier by a transcellular route, a paracellular route and/or via a 'Trojan horse mechanism' as yeast cells internalized within macrophages (Liu *et al.*, 2012). These routes are not likely to be mutually exclusive, and entry into the CSF may occur by these pathways simultaneously. Evidence for transcellular passage comes from experimental mouse models as well as from cases of human meningitis (Chretien *et al.*, 2002) and the portal of entry appears to be the cerebral capillaries in the SAS and not the choroid plexus (Charlier *et al.*, 2005). Cryptococci have been observed entering human brain microvascular endothelial cells (HBMECs), inducing host cytoskeletal changes, e.g. actin microfilament activity regulation by host protein kinase Cα and microvillus formation, similar to many bacterial pathogens (Jong *et al.*, 2008a). Invasion is not accompanied by endothelial cell death and appears to involve host lipid-raft associated molecules such as GM1, CD44 and DYRK3 kinase (Jong *et al.*, 2008b; Huang *et al.*, 2011). In contrast to intracellular passage through HBMECs, there is evidence to show that cryptococci can also penetrate vessel endothelia by the paracellular route, which was demonstrated by a disruption of the intercellular junction protein occludin during HBMEC monolayer infection (Chen *et al.*, 2003). Phagocytes play a critical role in *Cryptococcus* dissemination, and circumstantial evidence for the Trojan horse mechanism of SAS invasion comes from the observation of yeast cells in close association with macrophages in the meningeal vasculature (Chretien *et al.*, 2002). More direct evidence comes from animal studies, in which mice infected with macrophages containing internalized cryptococci had higher levels of yeast cells intracranially compared with mice infected with free cryptococci (Charlier *et al.*, 2009).

The virulence factors important for dissemination in the host and penetration of the BBB/BCSFB are not entirely known, but some details are summarized in Table 10.8. After having crossed the barrier, cryptococci rapidly replicate within the SAS, causing meningeal irritation and inflammation, although the virulence factors that initiate meningitis are not understood.

Table 10.8. Known *Cryptococcus* virulence factors. (Based on the review of Liu *et al.*, 2012.)

Cryptococcus virulence factor	Role in cryptococcal pathogenesis
Calcineurin pathway Protein kinase C1-activated MAP kinase pathways	Tolerance to mammalian oxidative and nitrosative stresses and body temperature
Polysaccharide capsule	Resists phagocytosis
Polysaccharide glucuronoxylomannan	Interferes with T-cell function, disrupts cell-mediated immunity
Cell-wall phenolic melanin	Protects organism from oxidation
Laccase	Enzyme required for virulence
Hyaluronic acid	Interacts with host CD44 on endothelium; aids penetration of BBB/BCSFB
Inositol phosphoryl ceramide synthase 1 (Ipc1) Anti-phagocytic protein 1 (App1)	Both required for regulating *Cryptococcus* phagocytosis and dissemination
Inositol phosphosphingolipid phospholipase C1 (Isc1)	Breaks down inositol sphingolipids and necessary for survival in activated macrophages
Phospholipase B1 (PlB1)	Multifunctional enzyme activities: facilitates adherence to lung epithelium, establishes interstitial lung infection, intra-macrophage survival and replication; bloodstream dissemination to CNS
Mating type	α cells show enhanced dissemination to the CNS, whereas giant/titan cells are inefficient at dissemination
Urease	Production of NH_3 by urease induces local endothelial cell damage, enabling *Cryptococcus* penetration into the CNS
Inositol transporters	Inositol is abundant in the CNS and can be utilized by *Cryptococcus* as a carbon source. Inositol increases the rate of fungal penetration of BBB/BCSFB in *in vitro* models. Cryptococci have been observed in close association with inositol-rich microglia
Regulatory factors Sterol regulatory element-binding protein (Sre1) Copper-dependent transcription factor 1 (Cuf1)	Sre1 is important for adaptation and growth in the CSF. Cuf1 is important for dissemination to the brain, as copper acquisition may be important for pathogenesis

Neurological signs and symptoms

In many cases, the initial colonization or even infection of the lungs remains unnoticed, until haematogenous dissemination ensues. Patients frequently present with the 'chronic meningitis syndrome'. Clinical findings are often non-specific and neurological findings even more so (Schmutzhard, 2006a). The patient presents with general malaise, fever, headache, vomiting and lethargy progressing to confusion, finally presenting with impaired consciousness and neurological deficits. Vomiting and neck stiffness indicate the meningeal irritation and increased ICP, which is likely to develop when the disease progresses. During this stage, cranial nerve palsies, seizures and progressive impairment of consciousness may be observed. In general, cryptococcal meningitis presents as subacute or chronic meningitis, and very rarely as acute meningitis. Signs and symptoms fluctuate over time, erroneously indicating improvement, which, however, is not persistent. Whereas in the immunocompetent individual, the course of disease may be extremely protracted and only meticulous repeated observations and CSF studies may lead to a diagnosis, in the immunocompromised patient the signs and symptoms may develop within a few days, mimicking acute meningitis syndrome (Schmutzhard, 2006a).

Diagnosis of cryptococcal meningitis

CSF findings in cryptococcal meningitis are well known. A mononuclear pleocytosis (up to 500 cells/mm^3) is usually found, polymorphonuclear leucocytes (PMNLS) being usually below 50%. In patients receiving high-dose corticosteroids or suffering from AIDS, a normal CSF may even be found, although cryptococcal meningitis may be highly active at this point in time. Protein is usually elevated and CSF glucose mildly decreased or normal. In cryptococcal meningitis, CSF cultures are positive in up to 75%. In AIDS patients, usually showing a higher number of causative agents in the CSF, over 90% may have positive CSF culture (Jackson and van der Horst, 2012). Diagnosis can be made by measuring cryptococcal antigen in serum as well as CSF (99% sensitivity if the titres are >1 : 2048) (Jarvis *et al.*, 2011), Indian ink staining, the cheapest technique and relatively easy to perform (75% sensitivity), and fungal culture, with 90% sensitivity (Jackson and van der Horst, 2012). Further diagnostic tests include neuroimaging and electrophysiology, both being of limited diagnostic value. Cerebral computed tomography (cCT) may be normal in up to 50% of proven cases. However, neuroimaging (cCT or cerebral magnetic resonance tomography) is indicated if a mass lesion or increased ICP, including hydrocephalus, or basal accentuation of meningitis is suspected.

Treatment/therapeutic management

Untreated cryptococcal meningitis is uniformly fatal (Mathiesen *et al.*, 2012). The introduction of amphotericin B improved this ominous prognosis, curing cryptococcal meningitis patients in more than 50%. Reduced doses of amphotericin B administered in combination with flucytosine have been shown to be as effective as amphotericin B alone, and without the toxicity related to high doses of amphotericin B. The drug combination routinely sterilizes the CSF within 2 weeks and allows treatment to be shortened to a total of 6 weeks. Follow-up studies show that more than 80% of patients with cryptococcal meningitis are cured or definitely improve with this recommended combination therapeutic regimen (Sloan *et al.*, 2009).

Raised ICP is quite common in cryptococcal meningitis, occurring in more than 50% of patients and requiring therapeutic techniques to reduce ICP, including repeated lumbar puncture, extraventricular drain insertion and/or ventriculo-peritoneal shunting. Osmotherapy or corticosteroids have an unproven effect on increased ICP (Jackson and van der Horst, 2012). Mannitol, acetozolamide and corticosteroids have also been tried. Repeated lumbar puncture, mannitol, acetozolamide, corticosteroids and immunotherapy have effects that are at best unproven (Desalermos *et al.*, 2012; Jarvis *et al.*, 2012). In individual cases, intraventricular or intrathecal application of amphotericin B has been employed successfully in cases with poor prognosis. Although intrathecal application allows a reduction of systemic doses and therefore reduces side effects, it may produce intracranial complications, ranging from arachnoiditis to acute secondary bacterial infection. Cryptococcomas in the brain parenchyma are rather rare, in small and/or multiple granulomata, and antifungal chemotherapy alone is generally successful. In surgically accessible areas, large cryptococcoma may be surgically removed.

10.3.2 *Coccidioides immitis*

This fungus is found within strictly limited areas in the south-western USA and Central and South America (Blair, 2009). Because of travel into and out of these areas, coccidioidomycoses and coccidial meningitis may be seen outside the organism's natural geographic boundaries. As in cryptococcosis, infection begins with inhalation of conidia, which establish a primary pulmonary infection (Davis and Porter, 2005). The vast majority of patients remains asymptomatic, and only 0.1% present as subacute or chronic meningitis, usually occurring within months of primary infection. Although sometimes stipulated, the link between immunosuppression and meningitis is much less conclusive than it is for cryptococcosis, with only a small majority of cases having a known underlying immunosuppressive disease. Whether immunosuppression may increase the risk of dissemination after primary lung infection is not known.

C. immitis is a highly infectious (laboratory infections) bimorphic fungus that normally inhabits dry, acid soil. In coccidioidal meningitis, the majority of patients shows CSF eosinophilia (even >10 cells/mm^3). The significance of this eosinophilic cellular response and the mechanisms involved are not known.

Diagnosis is established on history, clinical grounds and CSF pathology. If the CSF shows eosinophilia, the likelihood of *C. immitis*-associated meningitis is very high. *C. immitis* can be cultured, but, as with other dimorphic fungi, culture identification may take weeks (Schmutzhard, 2006a). Elevated complement fixation antibodies are the hallmark of disseminated *C. immitis* infection. Patients with coccidioidal meningitis may have rather low serum complement fixation antibody titres, whereas CSF titres are increased in meningitis. The CSF titre parallels the course of meningeal disease and can be used as a basis for both diagnosis and treatment monitoring (Williams, 2007; Vucicevic *et al.*, 2010).

Coccidioidal meningitis remains a serious illness with high morbidity and mortality. In the past decade, the management of coccidioidal meningitis has shown an almost complete change to azole-based therapy from the previous standard of intrathecal amphotericin B (Stevens and Shatsky, 2001). Although recommended as first-line therapy, azole-based therapies are not curative and do not necessarily prevent complications associated with the disease. The most recent recommendation is to start with fluconazole (>800 mg/day) according to the Infectious Disease Society of America 'Guidelines for the treatment of coccidioidal meningitis' (http://www.idsociety.org/Index.aspx). However, some patients who appear to be failing with high-dose fluconazole can be treated, with partial success, with voriconazole. Drug interactions between voriconazole and anti-retroviral agents, in the case of HIV-positive patients, render the use of voriconazole even more difficult in such patients (Mathisen *et al.*, 2010). Posaconazole has excellent *in vitro* activity against *C. immitis*; however, CSF penetration is extremely poor and therefore it is currently not considered for treatment of coccidioidal meningitis. In rare cases, the combination of fluconazole with posaconazole has been successfully employed. However, in those cases in which the entire spectrum of azoles has failed, intrathecal application of amphotericin B is still a second-line treatment option (Stevens and Shatsky, 2001). A combination therapy with liposomal amphotericin B and azole should be considered, in particular with severe disease or clinical relapse (Vinh, 2011).

Hydrocephalus requires a shunt placement or an external ventricular drainage (Arsura *et al.*, 2005). In rare cases, accompanying vasculitis may complicate the course: the management of such a vasculitic complication leading to ischaemic stroke remains unclear and should be carried out according to an accepted stroke protocol. It remains unclear whether corticosteroids may be beneficial in such cases.

With regard to the duration of therapy, recommendations are extremely variable. The clinical condition, CSF leucocyte count and decreasing CSF antibody titres, considered to be a good prognostic sign, might guide the decision to continue or to stop antifungal therapy. After cessation of antifungal therapy, high vigilance is essential in order to detect early signs of relapsing meningitis. In immunosuppressed patients, lifelong antifungal therapy is necessary.

10.3.3 Prognosis of chronic fungal meningitis

The prognosis of fungal meningitis depends on the early diagnosis, early treatment and control of complications and of any underlying disease (Table 10.9).

In the rare case of *Candida* meningitis (status post (s.p.) critical care management, longtime antibacterial chemotherapy) amphotericin B in combination with flucytosine or azole therapy (fluconazole) has reduced mortality to 10–20% (Horn *et al.*, 2009). Prognostic factors for *Candida* meningitis are the time that elapsed after start of symptoms (if greater than 2 weeks), the initial CSF glucose levels being below 35 mg/100 ml and the development of intracranial hypertension and focal neurological signs and symptoms (O'Brien *et al.*, 2011). More than half of patients with coccidioidal meningitis will survive, but these survivors are at high risk of relapse. Such patients require antifungal suppressive therapy and a patient with coccidioidal meningitis is considered cured only after he/she has survived for a minimum of 5 years without relapse. Unfavourable outcome is predicated by hydrocephalus (Arsura *et al.*, 2005), an underlying disease and a high complement fixation antibody titre in the CSF at the end of therapy. The disappearance of complement fixation antibodies in CSF at the end of therapy suggests a favourable outcome.

Table 10.9. Prognosis of chronic cryptococcal meningitis. (Adapted from Mathiesen *et al.*, 2012.)

Factors influencing		
Poor prognosis in patients	Relapse of cryptococcal meningitis	Favourable response
Initial positive CSF India ink test Very high CSF opening pressure Low CSF leucocytes Cryptococci isolated from extracranial sites Absence of anti-cryptococcal antibodies Initial CSF or serum cryptococcal antigen titre > 1:32 Preceding corticosteroid therapy or lymphoreticular malignancy	Abnormal CSF glucose during more than 4 weeks of therapy Low initial CSF leucocytes Cryptococci isolated from extraneural sites Absent anti-cryptococcal antibodies Post-treatment CSF or serum cryptococcal antigen titres > 1:8 No significant decrease in CSF and serum antigen titres during therapy and accompanying daily corticosteroid therapy during or after completion of therapy	Headache is an initial symptom Mental status is normal CSF leucocyte count is high

Patients with concomitant cancer or HIV infection rarely survive cryptococcal meningitis for more than 2 (to 5) years after onset of the fungal infection.

10.4 Neurosyphilis

The incidence of *Treponema pallidum* neurosyphilis has been on the decline throughout recent decades, after extremely high incidence peaks in the first half of the 20th century. However, since the advent of HIV and even more so in recent years also in immunocompetent persons, an increasing incidence and prevalence has been observed, at least in some parts of the world (Marra, 2009). The pathogenesis and pathophysiology of neurosyphilis and meningeal involvement is reviewed in the chapter by Ang (Chapter 12, this volume).

10.4.1 Clinical signs and symptoms

Syphilitic meningitis as defined by meningism, including headache and stiff neck, is frequently associated with cranial nerve involvement and the presence of CSF abnormalities (Chang *et al.*, 2011). An accompanying syphilitic vasculitis may lead to stroke-like episodes, and blood vessels of any size might be involved, thus leading to the respective focal neurological signs and symptoms, ranging from lacunar stroke syndromes to territorial infarctions. Tabes dorsalis and general paresis (progressive paralysis = dementia paralytica) are very rarely seen and are not covered in this chapter (Jantzen *et al.*, 2012).

10.4.2 Diagnosis and treatment

Diagnosis of neurosyphilis may be complicated in elderly patients who have cerebrovascular risk factors and present with ischaemic stroke. In a recent study from Thailand, 2.5% of stroke patients were eventually diagnosed with symptomatic neurosyphilis (= meningovascular syphilis) (Dharmasaroja and Dharmasaroja, 2012). Diagnosis of neurosyphilis is by a reactive serum treponemal test and CSF examination, which shows lymphocytic or mononuclear pleocytosis and elevated protein concentration (Roos, 2006).

Serological tests for syphilis are divided into two categories: treponemal and non-treponemal (Harding and Ghanem, 2012). Treponemal tests are more specific than non-treponemal tests and become positive early in the course of infection, 3–4 weeks after infection, at about the same time as the appearance of the chancre (Roos, 2006), and remain positive for life. Treponemal tests detect specific antibody to *T. pallidum* antigen and include the fluorescent treponemal antibody absorption test (FTA-ABS) and *T. pallidum* microhaemagglutination assay (MHA-TP) (Ghanem and Workowski, 2011; Peng *et al.*, 2011; Harding and Ghanem, 2012). However, they can be falsely positive in Lyme disease, non-venereal treponematoses, genital herpes simplex virus infection, pregnancy, systemic lupus erythematosus, alcoholic cirrhosis, scleroderma and mixed connective tissue disease (Roos, 2006; Naesens *et al.*, 2011). Non-treponemal tests detect antibodies to lipids found on the membranes of *T. pallidum*, using antigens such as cardiolipin or cholesterol. Such non-treponemal tests include the Venereal Disease Research Laboratory (VDRL) and rapid plasma reagin test; these tests take longer to become positive (up to 6 weeks after inoculation), they are highest during the secondary and latency stages of syphilis, and these tests tend to fall after adequate treatment, becoming eventually negative within 1 year of successful treatment (Roos, 2006).

The recommended therapy for neurosyphilis is 18–24 million units of penicillin G intravenously daily (3–4 million units every 4 h) for a minimum of 10 days (usually 2 weeks). This regimen is followed by 2.4 million units of benzathine penicillin G intramuscularly, once a week for 3 weeks. Treatment success is determined by a decrease in the non-treponemal serological titre (VDRL) over 6–12 months. The CSF should be examined at 6-monthly intervals for a minimum of 2 years and VDRL non-reactive titres should be observed within 2 years of completing the appropriate antimicrobial chemotherapy. An increase in the CSF VDRL titre, a failure of the CSF pleocytosis to resolve, or an increase in the cell count in the CSF suggests either persistent infection or re-infection and requires immediate re-initiation of treatment (Roos, 2006; Marra, 2009; Blank *et al.*, 2011; Ghanem and Workowski, 2011).

10.5 Neurocysticercosis

(Neuro)cysticercosis occurs when eggs from contaminated food are ingested or through contact with faeces of *Taenia solium* carriers (e.g. pigs), thus causing the human to become an intermediate host of *Taenia solium*. Neurocysticercosis is widespread, the most frequent single cause of symptomatic epilepsy in tropical and subtropical areas in Latin America, sub-Saharan Africa and South and South-East Asia, and rarely presents as a chronic meningitis (Carabin *et al.*, 2011).

10.5.1 Pathogenesis and pathology

Cysticerci are vesicles containing an invaginated scolex, frequently located in brain parenchyma, the ventricular system and/or spinal cord, and, rarely, in the SAS (Fleury *et al.*, 2011; Kelesidis and Tsiodras, 2012; Sinha and Sharma, 2012). The single parenchymal cyst is in most cases less than 20 mm in diameter, but ventricular cysts may be larger. Subarachnoidal cysts are most commonly located in the Sylvian fissure or in the basal cisterns, leading to chronic irritation within the SAS, clinically presenting as chronic meningitis (Carabin *et al.*, 2011; Fleury *et al.*, 2011). Ventricular cysticercal cysts may lead to acute restructive hydrocephalus (Matushita *et al.*, 2011) and spinal cysticerci are usually found within the spinal SAS, leading to extramedullary space-occupying lesions. CNS cysticerci remain viable for years, eliciting anything from no inflammatory changes in the surrounding tissue to acute and prompt complex immune reaction resulting in encephalitis, meningitis, brain oedema and even acute space-occupying presentation (Moskowitz and Mendelsohn, 2010). Vasculitis, ependymitis and cranial nerve involvement are seen in rare cases (Manuel Marquez and Arauz, 2012).

10.5.2 Clinical manifestations

The most common manifestation of neurocysticercosis is symptomatic epilepsy, in particular when seizures present for the first time in adulthood. If cysticercal cysts are located in the basal cisterns or in the Sylvian fissure, the clinical presentation is indistinguishable from chronic meningitis, including cranial nerve involvement. Headache, vomiting, cranial neuropathy and, in rare cases, hydrocephalus are the hallmarks in this chronic meningitis type of (racemose) subarachnoidal neurocysticercosis (Kelesidis and Tsiodras, 2012; Manuel Marquez and Arauz, 2012).

10.5.3 Diagnosis and therapy

Neuroimaging is essential in diagnosing neurocysticercosis (Cardenas *et al.*, 2010), including the chronic meningitis type (Verma and Lalla, 2012). Calcifications are easily seen in cerebral CT: in addition, cyst formation, and especially the presence of cysts in the basal cisterns, is clearly visible in magnetic resonance imaging (Verma and Lalla, 2012). In case of doubt, the intrathecal application of contrast medium may add to the diagnostic yield (Fig. 10.3). Recently, the value of

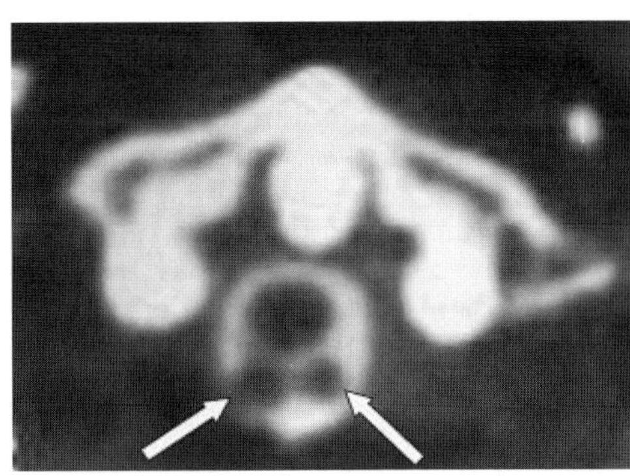

Fig. 10.3. Post myelography CT (level C1). Multiple small cystic lesions (indicated by arrows) in a patient with the clinical syndrome of chronic meningitis and very mild CSF eosinophilia, but intrathecal production of *Cysticercus cellulosae* antibodies.

immunological antigen testing in the CSF has also been shown to be a clear indicator of active neurocysticercosis (Esquivel-Velazquez *et al.*, 2011). CSF eosinophilia is seen only in rare cases, and the meningitic form of subarachnoidal cysticercosis may be more frequently associated with eosinophilia in the usually mildly pleocytotic CSF. Active neurocysticercosis is best treated by a combination of the anti-helminthic drugs praziquantel (50 mg/kg/day for 15 days, with the daily dosage divided into three) and albendazole (15 mg/kg/day for 1 month) (Garcia *et al.*, 2011).

10.5.4 Other helminths

In South-East Asia, parts of Latin America and sub-Saharan Africa, a few cases of chronic meningitis have been reported to be caused by *larvae migrantes viscerales*, in particular *Angiostrongylus cantonensis*, *Angiostrongylus costaricensis* and *Gnathostoma spinigerum*. The hallmark of these meningitides is a high level of eosinophilia in the CSF. Serological testing or, in rare cases, direct proof of the migrant larva are the diagnostic mainstays. Albendazole (400–800 mg/day for 3 weeks) or thiabendazole is the appropriate anti-helminthic drug (Graeff-Teixeira *et al.*, 2009; Ramirez-Avila *et al.*, 2009; Wang *et al.*, 2012).

10.6 Conclusions

Infective causes of chronic meningitis include several bacteria, viruses, fungi and helminths. Untreated, chronic meningitis is associated with high mortality. These infections are difficult to treat and the pathophysiology of neuroinfection is still poorly understood for many of these pathogens. Understanding the molecular and cellular basis of these infections is essential for the development of new therapies and experimental vaccines.

References

Arsura, E.L., Johnson, R., Penrose, J., Stewart, K., Kilgore, W., Reddy, C.M. and Bobba, R.K. (2005) Neuroimaging as a guide to predict outcomes for patients with coccidioidal meningitis. *Clinical Infectious Diseases* 40, 624–627.

Bamba, S., Lortholary, O., Sawadogo, A., Millogo, A., Guiguemde, R.T. and Bretagne, S. (2012) Decreasing incidence of cryptococcal meningitis in West Africa in the era of highly active antiretroviral therapy. *AIDS* 26, 1039–1041.

Blair, J.E. (2009) Coccidioidal meningitis: update on epidemiology, clinical features, diagnosis, and management. *Current Infectious Disease Reports* 11, 289–295.

Blank, L.J., Rompalo, A.M., Erbelding, E.J., Zenilman, J.M. and Ghanem, K.G. (2011) Treatment of syphilis in HIV-infected subjects: a systematic review of the literature. *Sexually Transmitted Infections* 87, 9–16.

Carabin, H., Ndimubanzi, P.C., Budke, C.M., Hai, N., Qian, Y., Cowan, L.D., Stoner, J.A., Rainwater, E. and Dickey, M. (2011) Clinical manifestations associated with neurocysticercosis: a systematic review. *PLoS Neglected Tropical Diseases* 5, e1152.

Cardenas, G., Jung, H., Rios, C., Fleury, A. and Luis Soto-Hernandez, J. (2010) Severe cysticercal meningitis: clinical and imaging characteristics. *American Journal of Tropical Medicine and Hygiene* 82, 121–125.

Chang, C.C., Leslie, D.E., Spelman, D., Chua, K., Fairley, C.K., Street, A., Crowe, S.M. and Hoy, J.F. (2011) Symptomatic and asymptomatic early neurosyphilis in HIV-infected men who have sex with men: a retrospective case series from 2000 to 2007. *Sexual Health* 8, 207–213.

Chang, Y.C., Stins, M.F., McCaffery, M.J., Miller, G.F., Pare, D.R., Dam, T., Paul-Satyasee, M., Kim, K.S. and Kwon-Chung, K.J. (2004) Cryptococcal yeast cells invade the central nervous system via transcellular penetration of the blood–brain barrier. *Infection and Immunity* 72, 4985–4995.

Charlier, C., Chretien, F., Baudrimont, M., Mordelet, E., Lortholary, O. and Dromer, F. (2005) Capsule structure changes associated with *Cryptococcus neoformans* crossing of the blood–brain barrier. *American Journal of Pathology* 166, 421–432.

Charlier, C., Nielsen, K., Daou, S., Brigitte, M., Chretien, F. and Dromer, F. (2009) Evidence of a role for monocytes in dissemination and brain invasion by *Cryptococcus neoformans*. *Infection and Immunity* 77, 120–127.

Chen, S.H.M., Stins, M.F., Huang, S.H., Chen, Y.H., Kwon-Chung, K.J., Chang, Y., Kim, K.S., Suzuki, K. and Jong, A.Y. (2003) *Cryptococcus neoformans* induces alterations in the cytoskeleton of human brain microvascular endothelial cells. *Journal of Medical Microbiology* 52, 961–970.

Chen, P., *et al.* (2012) A highly efficient Ziehl-Neelsen stain: identifying *de novo* intracellular *Mycobacterium tuberculosis* and improving detection of extracellular *M. tuberculosis* in cerebrospinal fluid. *Journal of Clinical Microbiology* 50, 1166–1170.

Cho, T.A. and Venna, N. (2010) Management of acute, recurrent, and chronic meningitides in adults. *Neurologic Clinics* 28, 1061–1088.

Chretien, F., Lortholary, O., Kansau, I., Neuville, S., Gray, F. and Dromer, F. (2002) Pathogenesis of cerebral *Cryptococcus neoformans* infection after fungemia. *Journal of Infectious Diseases* 186, 522–530.

Dau, Q.T., Toeroek, M., Nguyen Thi, B.Y., Nguyen, D.B., Nguyen Thi, N.L., Vo, S.K., Nguyen, V.V, Nguyen, H.D., Day, J., Farrar, J., Wolbers, M. and Caws, M. (2012) Influence of anti-tuberculosis drug resistance and *Mycobacterium tuberculosis* lineage on outcome in HIV-associated tuberculous meningitis. *Antimicrobial Agents and Chemotherapy* 56, 3074–3079.

Davis L.E. and Porter B.S. (2005) Central nervous system *Coccidioides immitis* infections. *Current Treatment Options in Neurology* 7, 157–165.

de Broucker, T. and Martinez-Almoyna, L. (2011) Chronic meningitis: differential diagnosis. *Revue de Medecine Interne* 32, 159–172.

del Brutto, O.H. (2006) Helminthic infections of the nervous system. In: Noseworthy J.H. (ed.) *Neurological Therapeutics: Principles and Practice*, 2nd edn. Informa Health Care, Abingdon, pp. 1133–1152.

Desalermos, A., Kourkoumpetis, T.K. and Mylonakis, E. (2012) Update on the epidemiology and management of cryptococcal meningitis. *Expert Opinion on Pharmacotherapy* 13, 783–789.

Dharmasaroja, P. and Dharmasaroja, P. (2012) Serum and cerebrospinal fluid profiles for syphilis in Thai patients with acute ischaemic stroke. *International Journal of STD & AIDS* 23, 340–345.

Esquivel-Velazquez, M., Ostoa-Saloma, P., Morales-Montor, J., Hernandez-Bello, R. and Larralde, C. (2011) Immunodiagnosis of neurocysticercosis: ways to focus on the challenge. *Journal of Biomedicine and Biotechnology* 2011, 516042.

Feldmesser, M. and Casadevall, A. (1997) Effect of serum IgG1 to *Cryptococcus neoformans* glucuronoxylomannan on murine pulmonary infection. *Journal of Immunology* 158, 790–799.

Figaji, A.A. and Fieggen, A.G. (2013) Endoscopic challenges and applications in tuberculous meningitis. *World Neurosurgery* 79, S24.e9–e14.

Fleury, A., Carrillo-Mezo, R., Flisser, A., Sciutto, E. and Corona, T. (2011) Subarachnoid basal neurocysticercosis: a focus on the most severe form of the disease. *Expert Review of Anti-Infective Therapy* 9, 123–133.

Galimi, R. (2011) Extrapulmonary tuberculosis: tuberculous meningitis new developments. *European Review for Medical and Pharmacological Sciences* 15, 365–386.

Garcia, H.H., Gonzalez, A.E. and Gilman, R.H. (2011) Cysticercosis of the central nervous system: how should it be managed? *Current Opinion in Infectious Diseases* 24, 423–427.

Garcia-Monco, J.C. (2006) Tuberculosis and other mycobacterial infections. In: Noseworthy, J.H. (ed.) *Neurological Therapeutics: Principles and Practice*, 2nd edn. Informa Health Care, Abingdon, pp.1011–1020.

Garg, R. (2010) Tuberculous meningitis. *Acta Neurologica Scandinavica* 122, 75–90.

Garg, R.K. and Sinha, M.K. (2011) Tuberculous meningitis in patients infected with human immunodeficiency virus. *Journal of Neurology* 258, 3–13.

George, E.L., Iype, T., Cherian, A., Chandy, S., Kumar, A., Balakrishnan, A. and Vijayakumar, K. (2012) Predictors of mortality in patients with meningeal tuberculosis. *Neurology India* 60, 18–22.

Ghanem, K.G. and Workowski, K.A. (2011) Management of adult syphilis. *Clinical Infectious Diseases* 53, S110–S128.

Ginsberg, L. and Kidd, D. (2008) Chronic and recurrent meningitis. *Practical Neurology* 8, 348–361.

Graeff-Teixeira, C., Aramburu da Silva, A.C. and Yoshimura, K. (2009) Update on eosinophilic meningoencephalitis and its clinical relevance. *Clinical Microbiology Reviews* 22, 322–348.

Gripshover B.M. and Ellner J.J. (1997) Chronic meningitis. In: Scheld, W.M.,Whitley, R.J. and Durack D.T. (eds) *Infections of the Central Nervous System*, 2nd edn. Lippincott–Raven Publishers, Philadelphia, PA, pp. 881–898.

Harding, A.S. and Ghanem, K.G. (2012) The performance of cerebrospinal fluid treponemal-specific antibody tests in neurosyphilis: a systematic review. *Sexually Transmitted Diseases* 39, 291–297.

Helbok, R., Pongpakdee, S., Yenjun, S., Dent, W., Beer, R., Lackner, P., Bunyaratvej, P., Prasert, B., Vejjajiva, A. and Schmutzhard, E. (2006) Chronic meningitis in Thailand – clinical characteristics, laboratory data and outcome in patients with specific reference to tuberculosis and cryptococcosis. *Neuroepidemiology* 26, 37–44.

Helbok, R., Broessner, G., Pfausler, B. and Schmutzhard, E. (2009) Chronic meningitis. *Journal of Neurology* 256, 168–175.

Hildebrand, J. and Aoun, M. (2003) Chronic meningitis: still a diagnostic challenge. *Journal of Neurology* 250, 653–660.

Horn, D.L., Neofytos, D., Anaissie, E.J., Fishman, J.A., Steinbach, W.J., Olyaei, A.J., Marr, K.A., Pfaller, M.A., Chang, C.H. and Webster, K.M. (2009) Epidemiology and outcomes of candidemia in 2019 patients: data from the Prospective Antifungal Therapy Alliance Registry. *Clinical Infectious Diseases* 48, 1695–1703.

Hristea, A. and Olaru, I.D. (2012) Applying a consensus case definition to patients with confirmed tuberculous meningitis. *International Journal of Infectious Diseases* 16, e758–e759.

Huang, S.H., Long, M., Wu, C.H., Kwon-Chung, K.J., Chang, Y.C., Chi, F., Lee, S. and Jong, A. (2011) Invasion of *Cryptococcus neoformans* into human brain microvascular endothelial cells is mediated through the lipid rafts–endocytic pathway via the dual specificity tyrosine phosphorylation-regulated kinase 3 (DYRK3). *Journal of Biological Chemistry* 286, 34761–34769.

Huffnagle, G.B. and Lipscomb, M.F. (1998) Cells and cytokines in pulmonary cryptococcosis. *Research in Immunology* 149, 387–396.

Jackson, A. and van der Horst, C. (2012) New insights in the prevention, diagnosis, and treatment of cryptococcal meningitis. *Current HIV/AIDS Reports* 9, 267–277.

Jantzen, S.U., Ferrea, S., Langebner, T., Gaebel, W., Griese, M., Arendt, G. and Dihne, M. (2012) Late-stage neurosyphilis presenting with severe neuropsychiatric deficits: diagnosis, therapy, and course of three patients. *Journal of Neurology* 259, 720–728.

Jarvis, J.N., Percival, A., Bauman, S., Pelfrey, J., Meintjes, G., Williams, G., Longley, N., Harrison, T.S. and Kozel, T.R. (2011) Evaluation of a novel point-of-care cryptococcal antigen test on serum, plasma, and urine from patients with HIV-associated cryptococcal meningitis. *Clinical Infectious Diseases* 53, 1019–1023.

Jarvis, J.N., Meintjes, G., Rebe, K., Williams, G.N., Bicanic, T., Williams, A., Schutz, C., Bekker, L.G., Wood, R. and Harrison, T.S. (2012) Adjunctive interferon-γ immunotherapy for the treatment of HIV-associated cryptococcal meningitis: a randomized controlled trial. *AIDS* 26, 1105–1113.

Javaud, N., Certal, R.D.S., Stirnemann, J., Morin, A.S., Chamouard, J.M., Augier, A., Bouchaud, O., Carpentier, A., Dhote, R., Dumas, J.L., Fantin, B. and Fain, O. (2011) Tuberculous cerebral vasculitis: retrospective study of 10 cases. *European Journal of Internal Medicine* 22, E99–E104.

Jong, A., Wu, C.H., Prasadarao, N.V., Kwon-Chung, K.J., Chang, Y.C., Ouyang, Y., Shackleford, G.M. and Huang, S.H. (2008a) Invasion of *Cryptococcus neoformans* into human brain microvascular endothelial cells requires protein kinase C-α activation. *Cellular Microbiology* 10, 1854–1865.

Jong, A., Wu, C.H., Shackleford, G.M., Kwon-Chung, K.J., Chang, Y.C., Chen, H.M., Ouyang, Y. and Huang, S.H. (2008b) Involvement of human CD44 during *Cryptococcus neoformans* infection of brain microvascular endothelial cells. *Cellular Microbiology* 10, 1313–1326.

Kalita, J., Prasad, S., Maurya, P.K., Kumar, S. and Misra, U.K. (2012) MR angiography in tuberculous meningitis. *Acta Radiologica* 53, 324–329.

Kelesidis, T. and Tsiodras, S. (2012) Extra-parenchymal neurocysticercosis in the United States. *American Journal of the Medical Sciences* 344, 79–82.

Kirwan, D.E., Cardenas, M.K. and Gilman, R.H. (2012) Rapid implementation of new TB diagnostic tests: is it too soon for a global roll-out of Xpert MTB/RIF? *American Journal of Tropical Medicine and Hygiene* 87, 197–201.

Lin, J., Zhou, H., Zhang, N., Yin, B. and Sheng, H.S. (2012) Effects of the implantation of Ommaya reservoir in children with tuberculous meningitis hydrocephalus: a preliminary study. *Childs Nervous System* 28, 1003–1008.

Liu, T.B., Perlin, D.S. and Xye, C. (2012) Molecular mechanisms of cryptococcal meningitis. *Virulence* 3, 173–181.

Manuel Marquez, J. and Arauz, A. (2012) Cerebrovascular complications of neuro-cysticercosis. *Neurologist* 18, 17–22.

Marra, C.M. (2009) Update on neurosyphilis. *Current Infectious Disease Reports* 11, 127–134.

Mathiesen, I.H.M., Knudsen, J.D., Gerstoft, J., Cowan, S. and Benfield, T. (2012) Outcome of HIV-1-associated cryptococcal meningitis, Denmark 1988–2008. *Scandinavian Journal of Infectious Diseases* 44, 197–200.

Mathisen, G., Shelub, A., Truong, J. and Wigen, C. (2010) Coccidioidal meningitis clinical presentation and management in the fluconazole era. *Medicine (Baltimore)* 89, 251–284.

Matushita, H., Gomes Pinto, F.C., Cardeal, D.D. and Teixeira, M.J. (2011) Hydrocephalus in neurocysticercosis. *Child's Nervous System* 27, 1709–1721.

Misra, U.K., Kalita, J. and Maurya, P.K. (2011) Stroke in tuberculous meningitis. *Journal of the Neurological Sciences* 303, 22–30.

Moskowitz, J. and Mendelsohn, G. (2010) Neurocysticercosis. *Archives of Pathology and Laboratory Medicine* 134, 1560–1563.

Naesens, R., Vermeiren, S., Van Schaeren, J. and Jeurissen, A. (2011) False positive Lyme serology due to syphilis: report of 6 cases and review of the literature. *Acta Clinica Belgica* 66, 58–59.

O'Brien, D., Stevens, N.T., Lim, C.H., O'Brien, D.F., Smyth, E., Fitzpatrick, F. and Humphreys, H. (2011) *Candida* infection of the central nervous system following neurosurgery: a 12-year review. *Acta Neurochirurgica* 153, 1347–1350.

Pasco, P.M. (2012) Diagnostic features of tuberculous meningitis: a cross-sectional study. *BMC Research Notes* 5, 49.

Peng, R.R., Wang, A.L., Li, J., Tucker, J.D., Yin, Y.P. and Chen, X.S. (2011) Molecular typing of *Treponema pallidum*: a systematic review and meta-analysis. *PLoS Neglected Tropical Diseases* 5, e1273.

Principi, N. and Esposito, S. (2012) Diagnosis and therapy of tuberculous meningitis in children. *Tuberculosis* 92, 377–383.

Ramirez-Avila, L., Slome, S., Schuster, F.L., Gavali, S., Schantz, P.M., Sejvar, J. and Glaser, C.A. (2009) Eosinophilic meningitis due to *Angiostrongylus* and *Gnathostoma* species. *Clinical Infectious Diseases* 48, 322–327.

Roos K.J. (2006) Neurosyphilis. In: Noseworthy J.H. (ed.) *Neurological Therapeutics: Principles and Practice*, 2nd edn. Informa Health Care, Abingdon, pp. 1020–1024.

Schmutzhard, E. (2006a) Fungal infections In: Noseworthy J.H. (ed). *Neurological Therapeutics: Principles and Practice*, 2nd edn. Informa Health Care, Abingdon, pp. 1085–1115.

Schmutzhard, E. (2006b) Protozoal infections. In: Noseworthy J.H. (ed.) *Neurological Therapeutics: Principles and Practice*, 2nd edn. Informa Health Care, Abingdon, pp. 1116–1132.

Sharma, P., Garg, R.K., Verma, R., Singh, M.K. and Shukla, R. (2011) Incidence, predictors and prognostic value of cranial nerve involvement in patients with tuberculous meningitis: a retrospective evaluation. *European Journal of Internal Medicine* 22, 289–295.

Singh, B., Garg, R.K., Singh, M.K., Verma, R., Malhotra, H.S., Jain, A., Singh, R., Kohli, N., Phadke, R.V., Shukla, R. and Parihar, A. (2012) Computed tomography angiography in patients with tuberculous meningitis. *Journal of Infection* 64, 565–572.

Sinha, S. and Sharma, B.S. (2012) Intraventricular neurocysticercosis: a review of current status and management issues. *British Journal of Neurosurgery* 26, 305–309.

Sloan, D.J., Dedicoat, M.J. and Lalloo, D.G. (2009) Treatment of cryptococcal meningitis in resource limited settings. *Current Opinion in Infectious Diseases* 22, 455–463.

Stevens, D.A. and Shatsky, S.A. (2001) Intrathecal amphotericin in the management of coccidioidal meningitis. *Seminars in Respiratory Infections* 16, 263–269.

Sun, Q., Sha, W., Xiao, H.P., Tian, Q. and Zhu, H. (2012) Evaluation of cerebrospinal fluid adenosine deaminase activity for the differential diagnosis of tuberculous and non-tuberculous meningitis. *American Journal of the Medical Sciences* 344, 116–121.

Takahashi, T., Tamura, M. and Takasu, T. (2012) The PCR-based diagnosis of central nervous system tuberculosis: up to date. *Tuberculosis Research and Treatment* 2012, 831292.[query – this reference doesn't look right but couldn't find on internet]

Thwaites, G.E., Chau, T.T.H., Stepniewska, K., Phu, N.H., Chuong, L.V., Sinh, D.X., White, N.J., Parry, C.M. and Farrar, J.J. (2002) Diagnosis of adult tuberculous meningitis by use of clinical and laboratory features. *Lancet* 360, 1287–1292.

Torok, M.E., Nguyen, D.B., Tran, T.H.C., Nguyen, T.B.Y., Thwaites, G.E., Hoang, T.Q., Nguyen, H.D., Tran, T.H., Nguyen, T.C., Hoang, H.T.T., Wolbers, M. and Farrar, J.J. (2011) Dexamethasone and long-term outcome of tuberculous meningitis in Vietnamese adults and adolescents. *PloS One* 6, e27821.

van der Harst, J. and Luijckx, G. (2011) Treatment of central nervous system tuberculosis infections and neurological complications of tuberculosis treatment. *Current Pharmaceutical Design* 17, 2940–2947.

Verma, R. and Lalla, R. (2012) Why MRI of brain is superior to CT in multiple neurocysticercosis? *BMJ Case Reports*. DOI: 10.1136/bcr.03.2012.6046. Epub ahead of print.

Vibha, D., Bhatia, R., Prasad, K., Srivastava, M.V., Tripathi, M., Kumar, G. and Singh, M.B. (2012) Validation of diagnostic algorithm to differentiate between tuberculous meningitis and acute bacterial meningitis. *Clinical Neurology and Neurosurgery* 114, 639–644.

Vinh, D.C. (2011) Coccidioidal meningitis: disseminated disease in patients without HIV/AIDS. *Medicine (Baltimore)* 90, 87.

Vinnard, C., Winston, C.A., Wileyto, E.P., MacGregor, R.R. and Bisson, G.P. (2011)

Multidrug resistant tuberculous meningitis in the United States, 1993–2005. *Journal of Infection* 63, 240–242.

Vucicevic, D., Blair, J.E., Binnicker, M.J., McCullough, A.E., Kusne, S., Vikram, H.R., Parish, J.M. and Wengenack, N.L. (2010) The utility of *Coccidioides* polymerase chain reaction testing in the clinical setting. *Mycopathologia* 170, 345–351.

Wang, Q.P., Wu, Z.D., Wei, J., Owen, R. and Lun, Z.R. (2012) Human *Angiostrongylus cantonensis*: an update. *European Journal of Clinical Microbiology & Infectious Diseases* 31, 389–395.

Williams, P.L. (2007) Coccidioidal meningitis. *Coccidioidomycosis: Sixth International Symposium* 1111, 377–384.

Yorgancilar, E., Yildirim, M., Gun, R., Bakir, S., Tekin, R., Gocmez, C., Meric, F. and Topcu, I. (2012) Complications of chronic suppurative otitis media: a retrospective review. *European Archives of Oto-Rhino-Laryngology* 270, 69–76.

Zuger, A. and Lowy, F.D. (1997) Tuberculosis. In: Scheld W.M., Whitley R.J. and Durack D.T. (eds) *Infections of the Central Nervous System*, 2nd edn. Lippincott-Raven Publishers, Philadelphia, PA, pp. 417–443.

11 The Pathophysiology of Tuberculous Meningitis

Guy Thwaites*
Kings College, London, UK

11.1 Introduction

Tuberculosis is caused by members of the *Mycobacterium tuberculosis* complex of bacteria. The complex is formed by several closely related subspecies that have plagued human and animal populations for thousands of years. The human-adapted species, which cause tuberculosis, include *Mycobacterium tuberculosis, Mycobacterium africanum, Mycobacterium bovis* and *Mycobacterium canettii; M. africanum* causes up to one-quarter of tuberculosis cases in some parts of West Africa and *M. canettii* is a rare cause of tuberculosis in people from the Horn of Africa. This chapter, however, will deal exclusively with *M. tuberculosis*, which causes the majority of tuberculosis globally and is responsible for nearly all disease involving the central nervous system (CNS).

The World Health Organization estimated that in 2010 there were 8.8 million new cases of tuberculosis worldwide and 1.45 million deaths from the infection (World Health Organization, 2011). *M. tuberculosis* is transmitted by individuals with pulmonary disease; their coughing expels droplets of respiratory secretions containing the bacteria into the surrounding air, which can be inhaled to infect others. Once inhaled, the bacteria are engulfed by pulmonary alveolar macrophages, initiating a struggle between bacteria and host that can last a lifetime, with a panoply of potential outcomes. In a few individuals, the innate, and probably genetically determined, antimicrobial activity of macrophages will kill all the inhaled bacteria and terminate the infection. In the majority, the bacteria survive and replicate, infecting other macrophages recruited to the site of infection. The burgeoning infection is characterized by granulomatous inflammation, which, in the majority, controls the infection and leads to prolonged asymptomatic infection or 'latent' tuberculosis. Approximately one-third of the world's population (3 billion people) are believed to have latent tuberculosis: 10% of individuals with latent tuberculosis develop active tuberculosis in their lifetime and this figure rises to more than 50% if they have untreated human immunodeficiency virus (HIV). In a small proportion of people, usually the very young or immunosuppressed, the infection is never controlled and primary progressive disease occurs, characterized by severe lung

*guy.thwaites@btinternet.com

disease and haematogenous dissemination to other organs, particularly the brain, with high case fatality.

Tuberculosis most commonly affects the lung, but the most devastating clinical consequences of the disease result from the ability of *M. tuberculosis* to disseminate from the lung to other organs and, in particular, the brain. CNS tuberculosis represents around 1% of all cases of the disease, but is disproportionately important because it kills or maims nearly half of those affected, despite the best available treatment. It takes two major forms: tuberculous meningitis and cerebral tuberculomas. Tuberculous meningitis causes progressive confusion and coma, with death if treatment is not started sufficiently quickly. Tuberculomas are well-defined, granulomatous, space-occupying lesions, which can occur anywhere in the CNS. Their clinical manifestations depend upon their anatomical location, but an isolated seizure (epileptic fit) is the commonest presentation. Tuberculomas are not immediately life-threatening unless they rupture and release bacteria into the subarachnoid space (SAS) to cause tuberculous meningitis.

The clinical features of tuberculous meningitis are variable and non-specific. The cardinal features are progressively worsening headache, fever and vomiting over days to weeks (Thwaites and Tran, 2005). The insidious onset sets the disease apart from meningitis caused by pyogenic bacteria, which usually presents over 1 or 2 days.

The neurological manifestations of tuberculous meningitis are numerous and varied. Their nature and diversity can be predicted from the site of disease and its pathogenesis. Basal meningeal inflammation and fibrotic adhesions can result in cranial nerve palsies, or constriction of the vessels resulting in cerebral infarction (stroke). Infarcts occur in approximately 30% of cases, commonly in the internal capsule and basal ganglia, causing a range of problems from paralysis to movement disorders. Obstruction of cerebrospinal fluid (CSF) flow leads to raised intracranial pressure, hydrocephalus and reduced conscious level. Seizures occur in around 30% of children and less than 5% of adults with tuberculous meningitis, and may be caused by hydrocephalus, infarction, tuberculoma, oedema and low plasma sodium concentrations (hyponatraemia) due to inappropriate anti-diuretic hormone secretion. Approximately 10% of those with tuberculous meningitis will have concomitant spinal cord involvement, which is frequently overlooked and commonly leads to permanent paralysis of limbs.

The key to understanding the pathogenesis of tuberculosis is the granuloma, which is the basic unit of pathology for all forms of the disease (Flynn *et al.*, 2011). The classical microscopic description is of macrophages and occasional neutrophils surrounding a central necrotic core. Circumscribing the macrophages is a cuff of lymphocytes (both T- and B-cells), which are contained within a rim of fibroblasts. *M. tuberculosis* is found within the macrophages or the central necrotic debris, an environment considered to be hypoxic. Tuberculous granulomas are extremely heterogenous, with their size, structure, cellular consistency and location of bacteria changing independently over time, especially during anti-tuberculosis chemotherapy (Barry *et al.*, 2009). Granuloma size varies from 1 mm to >2 cm, the largest being clearly visible macroscopically (and often radiographically) as nodules.

11.2 The Pathogenesis of Tuberculous Meningitis

In this chapter, the following questions will be addressed: How does *M. tuberculosis* travel from lung to brain? What is the role of the granuloma in *M. tuberculosis* dissemination? How does *M. tuberculosis* invade the CNS? Are some strains of *M. tuberculosis* more likely to cause CNS tuberculosis than others? How does the host response influence the pathogenesis of tuberculous meningitis?

11.2.1 How does *Mycobacterium tuberculosis* travel from lung to brain?

The pioneering investigations of Arnold Rich and Howard McCordock remain central to our current understanding of the pathogenesis of tuberculous meningitis (Rich and McCordock, 1933). They began with the simple clinical observation that not all patients with miliary tuberculosis (haematogenously disseminated disease of multiple organs) developed tuberculous meningitis. By then, it had been shown that the blood of patients with miliary tuberculosis frequently contained viable bacteria and, as a consequence, most authorities believed that tuberculous meningitis was the result of the direct and simultaneous invasion of the meninges by blood-borne *M. tuberculosis*. The strong association between miliary tuberculosis and the development of meningitis lent support to this view, but the observation that the association was not invariable led Rich and McCordock to question the contemporary model of disease pathogenesis. First, they showed that the intravenous injection of virulent *M. tuberculosis* into numerous rabbits and guinea pigs did not result in immediate meningitis in any of the animals. Secondly, by meticulous post-mortem examinations they found foci of infection (granulomas) in communication with the SAS in 77 of 82 people with fatal tuberculous meningitis (not all the brain could be examined in the five without these lesions). These granulomas, now called Rich foci, were found predominantly within the brain parenchyma, rather than the meninges, and were believed to develop during a preceding bacteraemia. Meningitis occurred once mycobacteria contained within these lesions were released into the SAS, an event that might happen months or years after the initial bacteraemia. Thus, the two-step model of tuberculous meningitis pathogenesis was conceived and it has remained largely unchallenged ever since.

The ability of *M. tuberculosis* to disseminate within blood appears to be a key component of tuberculosis pathogenesis (Krishnan *et al.*, 2010). The trafficking of bacteria from the initial site of infection – the pulmonary alveolus – to regional lymph nodes, blood and elsewhere has two conflicting consequences. First, it facilitates the presentation of *M. tuberculosis* antigens within the regional lymph nodes, essential for the development of a protective T-cell-mediated immune response. Secondly, it results in the dissemination of bacteria from the lung to other organs and can lead to extra-pulmonary disease (Krishnan *et al.*, 2010). Studies in mice have indicated that haematogenous dissemination occurs early in the infection, before it has been controlled by the adaptive immune response (Chackerian *et al.*, 2002). In humans, this explains why those with impaired T-cell responses (e.g. untreated HIV infection) are particularly susceptible to disseminated disease and why those whose T-cell response has been primed with BCG vaccination are protected against miliary tuberculosis and meningitis. In addition, polymorphisms in innate immune response genes, e.g. Toll-like receptor (TLR) 2 (Thuong *et al.*, 2007), have been associated with the development of tuberculous meningitis.

The mechanisms by which *M. tuberculosis* leaves the lungs remain speculative. The first obstacle to the bacilli is the alveolar epithelium, which may be breached by direct invasion and lysis of epithelial cells, translocation across epithelial cells or by travelling within professional phagocytes (Fig. 11.1). It is evident, at least *in vitro*, that *M. tuberculosis* is able to replicate and undergo cell–cell spreading through cultured monolayers (Byrd *et al.*, 1998; Castro-Garza *et al.*, 2002). A number of studies have suggested that cell–cell spread is enhanced by the ability of *M. tuberculosis* to replicate within epithelial cells and ultimately lyse them, thus enabling neighbouring cells to become infected (McDonough and Kress, 1995; Dobos *et al.*, 2000). Two proteins produced by *M. tuberculosis* have been strongly linked to the lysis of both macrophages and pneumocytes: early secretory antigenic target 6 kDa (ESAT-6) and culture filtrate protein 10 kDa (CFP-10), encoded by genes *Rv3874* and *Rv3875* of the RD1 gene cluster (Gao *et al.*, 2004; Kinhikar *et al.*, 2010). In addition, ESAT-6 can bind laminin on the basolateral surface of alveolar epithelial cells and lyse both type 1 and 2 pneumocytes (Kinhikar *et al.*, 2010).

There is some evidence for an alternative, non-lytic pathway of intercellular spread of *M. tuberculosis*. Studies using the amoeba *Dictyostelium* as a model of a basic innate immune cell have found that *M. tuberculosis*

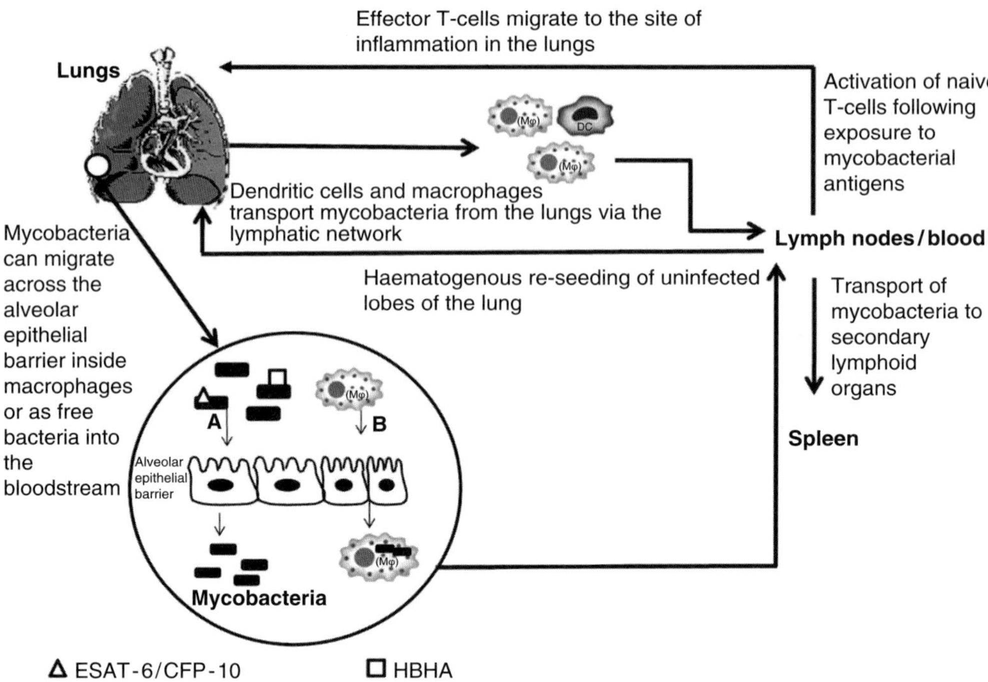

Fig. 11.1. Extrapulmonary dissemination of *M. tuberculosis.* Haematogenous dissemination is the critical first step in the development of tuberculous meningitis. Following infection, *M. tuberculosis* migrates from the primary site of infection in the lungs to the lymph nodes and bloodstream. Bacteria can cross the alveolar epithelial barrier by direct invasion and lysis of epithelial cells (A) or by travelling within professional phagocytes (B). Bacterial factors, heparin-binding haemagglutinin adhesin (HBHA) and products of the ESX-1 secretion pathway (ESAT-6/CFP-10) aid in the translocation of bacteria across the alveolar epithelium. Dissemination of the bacteria is also critical to the development of cell-mediated immunity and control of bacterial growth. Mϕ, macrophage. (Reprinted from Krishnan *et al.*, 2010, with permission from Elsevier.)

and *Mycobacterium marinum* were able to exit the cells without lysis via an F-actin-rich structure called the ejectosome, an activity dependent upon GTPase activity (Hagedorn *et al.*, 2009). However, bacteria were only able to exit by this route if they were able to escape the endosomal vacuole, a process that, again, appeared dependent upon the RD1 locus of *M. tuberculosis*. Whether phagolysosomal escape is an important component of *M. tuberculosis* cellular pathogenesis, or an artefact of *in vitro* infection models, remains controversial. However, *M. bovis* BCG and RD1 mutants of *M. tuberculosis* fail to enter the cytosol of infected human monocyte dendritic cells, whereas RD1-complemented bacteria are able to leave the phagolysosome (van Well *et al.*, 2007).

Currently, the strongest evidence for the role of alveolar epithelial involvement in *M. tuberculosis* dissemination comes from studies of the bacterial factors involved in epithelial cell adhesion (Pethe *et al.*, 2001). Heparin-binding haemagglutinin adhesin (HBHA) enables mycobacteria to bind to sulfated glycoconjugates on epithelial cells (Locht *et al.*, 2006). Experiments in mice performed with both *M. bovis* BCG and *M. tuberculosis* demonstrated that, following pulmonary infection, HBHA-disrupted strains showed a 30–200-fold decrease in the number of bacteria recovered from the spleen, in comparison with the parental strain. Fewer bacteria disseminated from the lungs to the spleen if the bacteria were coated with anti-HBHA antibodies before infection.

Furthermore, gold particles coupled with recombinant HBHA traversed a polarized epithelial cell layer without affecting the cellular tight junctions (Menozzi *et al.*, 2006). These observations strongly support a role for HBHA in the endocytosis of *M. tuberculosis* and transcytosis across an epithelial cell layer, with subsequent entry into the bloodstream.

While the interactions between *M. tuberculosis* and alveolar epithelial cells appear to be important for the initial steps in bacterial dissemination, there is strong evidence that professional phagocytic cells are responsible for the trafficking of bacteria to distant sites. Indeed, studies using an *in vitro* model of human alveolar epithelial and endothelial cells found that mononuclear phagocytes that the efficiency of bacterial translocation across the alveolar wall (Bermudez *et al.*, 2002). But it is not just macrophages that may carry *M. tuberculosis*. Dendritic cells infected with *M. tuberculosis* play a crucial role in the priming of interferon-γ producing T-cells and the cell-mediated response to the infection (Tascon *et al.*, 2000). Given that they transport antigens from the periphery to secondary lymphoid organs for the priming of the adaptive immune system, they may also disseminate viable bacteria. Dendritic cells phagocytose mycobacteria and provide a favourable environment for intracellular survival and growth (Bodnar *et al.*, 2001), particularly as they are less efficient at killing mycobacteria than macrophages (Henderson *et al.*, 1997). Cellular trafficking studies in mice revealed that dendritic cells were the primary infected subset of professional phagocytic cells in the lungs and mediastinal lymph nodes of *M. bovis*-infected mice (Humphreys *et al.*, 2006). Around 80% of *M. tuberculosis* following aerosol infection was associated with myeloid dendritic cells ($CD11c^{high}/CD11b^{high}$) in the lymph nodes, but these cells were poor stimulators of T-cells in comparison with resident lymph node dendritic cells, which expressed low or negligible levels of CD11b (Wolf *et al.*, 2007). The interaction between dendritic cell-specific intercellular adhesion molecule-3 grabbing non-integrin (DC-SIGN), a c-type lectin receptor, and mannosylated lipoarabinomannan (ManLAM) of *M. tuberculosis* may modify the environment of the dendritic cell, allowing the bacteria to escape the normal immune surveillance mechanisms of the host (van Kooyk *et al.*, 2003).

11.2.2 What is the role of the granuloma in *M. tuberculosis* dissemination?

For much of the last 100 years, the granuloma has been seen as benefiting the host, walling off mycobacteria from surrounding tissues and so limiting its ability to spread and cause disease (Flynn *et al.*, 2011). Macrophages are the principal cell in the formation of granulomas and a key player in the control of mycobacterial infection. The ability of *M. tuberculosis* to replicate and survive within macrophages has long been known (Houben *et al.*, 2006). Studying the formation and dynamics of tuberculous granulomas in humans is extremely difficult. However, various animal models have been used to better understand the interactions between *M. tuberculosis* and the host's immune cells leading to granuloma formation. Important new insights have recently been obtained using zebrafish embryos infected with *M. marinum*, a mycobacterium that shares some key virulence determinants with *M. tuberculosis* (most notably the RD1 virulence locus) and induces granulomatous inflammation in fish (Clay *et al.*, 2007; Davis and Ramakrishnan, 2009; Volkman *et al.*, 2010). Uniquely, the model enables both macrophages and bacteria to be tracked *in vivo* as granulomas are formed following infection. Contrary to prior assumptions, the model suggests granulomas facilitate early mycobacterial growth and dissemination: uninfected macrophages are actively recruited to granulomas, where they are productively infected and then disseminate to infect surrounding tissues. These findings suggest that, in early infection, before the induction of T-cell-mediated immunity, mycobacteria subvert the host's granulomatous response to augment their own replication and dissemination. These investigations provide compelling evidence for the dynamic role of macrophages and granulomas in early mycobacterial dissemination and challenge

Rich and McCordock's model of tuberculous meningitis pathogenesis. Their model depends upon the traditional notion of a static, protective granuloma (the Rich focus) forming a physical and temporal barrier between bacteria in blood and infection of the SAS. These new observations suggest the interactions between bacteria in blood, the Rich focus and the SAS may be more dynamic than previously thought.

11.2.3 How does *M. tuberculosis* invade the CNS?

One of the key events preceding the development of tuberculous meningitis is the breach of the blood–brain barrier (BBB)/blood–cerebrospinal fluid barrier (BCSFB) by *M. tuberculosis*. The mechanisms by which the bacteria cross this interface is not well characterized and a summary of the *M. tuberculosis* genes currently implicated in CNS invasion and survival is provided in Table 11.1. Using an *in vitro* model of human brain microvascular endothelial cells, Jain and others demonstrated that *M. tuberculosis* was able to invade and traverse the cell monolayers by an active process involving actin cytoskeletal rearrangements (Jain *et al.*, 2006). The efficiency of traversal across these monolayers was an attribute of pathogenic mycobacteria, as opposed to the less pathogenic *Mycobacterium smegmatis*. The investigators also performed microarrays to determine which *M. tuberculosis* genes were upregulated during the early stages of BBB invasion. The expression of 33 genes increased at least eightfold, and 18 of them belonged to a set of genes (*Rv0960–Rv1001*) that was previously shown to be upregulated during mouse lung infection – the so-called '*in vivo*-expressed genomic island' (iVEGI) (Talaat *et al.*, 2004). The majority of these genes are absent in non-pathogenic mycobacteria and are involved in cell-wall biosynthesis and lipid metabolism. To further investigate the role of these genes in BBB invasion, isogenic transposon mutants of all 33 upregulated genes were constructed and their phenotype examined in the BBB model. Bacteria with mutations in four of the genes (*Rv0980c*, *Rv0987*, *Rv0989c* and *Rv1801*) had reduced ability to invade the BBB; three of them (*Rv0980c*, *Rv0987* and *Rv0989c*) belonged to the iVEGI gene group (Table 11.1).

Table 11.1. *M. tuberculosis* genes implicated in BBB invasion.

Strain H37Rv gene number	Gene name	Probable function	Evidence supporting role in BBB invasion: effect of transposon mutagenesis
Rv0311	–	Hypothetical protein	Attenuates survival in mouse brain
Rv0805	–	Cyclic nucleotide phosphodiesterase	Attenuates invasion and survival in mouse brain
Rv0931c	*pknD*	Serine–threonine protein kinase; involved in signal transduction	Attenuates survival in mouse brain; *pknD* required for brain endothelial invasion
Rv0980c	*PE-PGRS18*	PE-PGRS family protein	Reduces ability to invade *in vitro* BBB model
Rv0986	–	ATP-binding cassette (ABC) transporter (part of a three-gene operon comprising *Rv0986–Rv 0988*)	Attenuates invasion and survival in mouse brain and reduces capacity to invade macrophages and endothelial cells
Rv0987	–	ABC transporter	Reduces ability to invade *in vitro* BBB model
Rv0989c	*grcC2*	Supplier of polyprenyl diphosphate	Reduces ability to invade *in vitro* BBB model
Rv1801	*PPE29*	PPE family protein	Reduces ability to invade *in vitro* BBB model

M. tuberculosis brain invasion has been investigated with *in vivo* models. The mouse has long been used to study tuberculosis pathogenesis, although it has some major limitations as a model. Especially pertinent is that mice do not develop meningitis, despite *M. tuberculosis* disseminating to the brain following intravenous injection. This problem has been overcome by one group, who showed that inducible nitric oxide synthase (iNOS) knock-out mice developed florid cerebral pathology similar to that observed in humans with tuberculous meningitis (Olin *et al.*, 2008). However, Be and colleagues contend that, although the mouse cannot be used to study meningitis, it can be used to study brain invasion (Be *et al.*, 2008). Thus, to discover bacterial factors responsible for BBB invasion, they compared the ability of the *M. tuberculosis* laboratory strain H37Rv, the clinical strain CDC1551 and 28 transposon mutants of CDC1551 to invade and survive within the mouse brain. They found five mutants that grew normally in the lungs, but failed to invade or survive within the brain, suggesting a specific role for these genes in CNS invasion (Table 11.1). Two of the strains had mutations in the *M. tuberculosis* genes *Rv0805* and *Rv0986*, which encode a phosphodiesterase and an ATP-binding cassette (ABC) transporter, respectively. *Rv0986* is part of a three-gene operon, *Rv0986–Rv0988*, which is upregulated during endothelial infection, but absent in non-pathogenic mycobacteria (Jain *et al.*, 2006). The genes are probably involved in cell adhesion and entry (Braibant *et al.*, 2000). Three additional mutant strains (with genes *Rv0311*, *Rv0805* and *Rv0931c* disrupted) were attenuated for survival in the mouse brain. The role of one gene in particular – *Rv0931c* (*pknD*) encoding a serine–threonine protein kinase (STPK) – appeared particularly important and has become the focus of further and ongoing investigations.

Guinea pigs have long been used as a model of tuberculosis. They are uniquely susceptible to infection with *M. tuberculosis* and develop nectrotizing granulomas, which closely resemble those found in humans. Be and colleagues used guinea pigs to screen a panel of 398 transposon mutants of *M. tuberculosis* CDC1551 (Be *et al.*, 2012) and 14 of these mutants were unable to disseminate to the guinea pig brain. Again, mutations in *pknD* (*Rv0931c*) caused the most extreme phenotype and the investigators proceeded to show that *pknD* was needed for the invasion of CNS-derived endothelial cells but not for entry into macrophages, umbilical endothelial cells or alveolar epithelial cells. Using confocal microscopy and flow cytometry, they also demonstrated that the *M. tuberculosis pknD* sensor is sufficient to trigger invasion of brain endothelia, a process that can be neutralized by specific antiserum, suggesting a novel vaccine or therapeutic target. Whether naturally occurring polymorphisms in *pknD* are responsible for strains more or less likely to cause tuberculous meningitis is unknown.

11.2.4 Are some strains of *M. tuberculosis* more likely to cause CNS tuberculosis than others?

One of the most intriguing consequences of *M. tuberculosis* infection is the diversity of possible outcomes. Various host factors – age, malnutrition and co-infection with HIV, for example – have a well-defined influence on the development of tuberculous meningitis, but the role of bacterial genetic variation on the development of disease is less clear. Fifty years ago, Mitchison and colleagues reported that strains of *M. tuberculosis* from southern India were less virulent in guinea pigs than UK strains (Mitchison *et al.*, 1960) and, more recently, others have documented a wide variation in the virulence of *M. tuberculosis* strains following infection of mice (Dunn and North, 1995; Lopez *et al.*, 2003; Dormans *et al.*, 2004) and rabbits (Bishai *et al.*, 1999). The significance of these findings to human disease, however, remains uncertain.

Intracisternal injection of mycobacteria into rabbits has provided the best model of human tuberculous meningitis and delivered substantial insights into its pathogenesis. Tsenova and colleagues used this model to evaluate the severity of disease caused by different clinical isolates (Tsenova *et al.*, 2005), comparing the outcome and pathology of rabbits intracerebrally infected with the *M. tuberculosis* clinical isolates CDC1551, HN878 and W4 (the latter two are members of the virulent W/Beijing family of *M. tuberculosis*). Compared with infection with CDC1551, brain infection with HN878 or W4 resulted in higher bacillary loads, increased dissemination of bacilli to other organs, persistently high concentrations of tumour necrosis factor-α (TNF-α), higher numbers of CSF white cells and more severe clinical manifestations. In an earlier investigation, the hypervirulence of HN878 was associated with the production of a polyketide synthase-derived phenolic glycolipid (PGL) (Reed *et al.*, 2004). Compared with the wild-type strain, an HN878 mutant with a disrupted PGL synthesis induced lower concentrations of TNF-α from macrophages and caused fewer mice to die following infection. The link between PGL production among East Asian/Beijing strains and hypervirulence has subsequently become much less clear; many related strains of this lineage do not produce PGL and its induced expression in other strains has failed to alter the virulence of the bacteria (Sinsimer *et al.*, 2008).

Nevertheless, epidemiological studies support the hypothesis that some strains of *M. tuberculosis* are more likely than others to cause tuberculous meningitis. A study in Vietnam compared the host and bacterial genotype of 187 Vietnamese adults with tuberculous meningitis and 237 Vietnamese adults with uncomplicated pulmonary tuberculosis (Caws *et al.*, 2008). Strains from the Euro-American lineage of *M. tuberculosis* were significantly less likely than those of the Indo-Oceanic or East Asian Beijing lineage to cause meningeal tuberculosis (odds ratio 0.4, 95% confidence intervals 0.2–0.8, P = 0.009), suggesting that these strains were less capable of extrapulmonary dissemination than others in the study population. Furthermore, individuals with a polymorphism in the TLR2 gene were significantly more likely to have tuberculosis caused by the East Asian/Beijing genotype than other individuals, demonstrating, for the first time, an interaction between host and bacterial genotypes and the development of tuberculosis.

A mechanistic explanation for these observations would represent a major advance in understanding the pathogenesis of disseminated tuberculosis and tuberculous meningitis, but it has so far proved elusive. Detailed characterization of selected strains from three of the major *M. tuberculosis* lineages examined in the Vietnam study (the East Asian/Beijing, Indo-Oceanic and Euro-American) in macrophages, dendritic cells and mice revealed the East Asian/Beijing and Indo-Oceanic strains induced significantly more TNF-α and interleukin (IL)-1β from macrophages than the Euro-American strains, were detectable earlier in the blood of infected mice and grew faster in the lungs (Krishnan *et al.*, 2011). Given the likely importance of mycobacterial lipids to bacterial virulence and disease pathogenesis, the investigators hypothesized that these phenotypic differences were induced by lineage-specific variation in cell envelope lipids. Whole lipid extracts from East Asian/Beijing and Indo-Oceanic strains induced higher concentrations of TNF-α from macrophages than Euro-American lipids and correlated with TNF-α production following live bacterial infections. The lipid extracts were fractionated and compared by thin layer chromatography to reveal a distinct pattern of lineage-associated profiles. A phthiotriol dimycoserosate was exclusively produced by East Asian/Beijing strains, but independent investigations have suggested that this molecule does not have a specific role in virulence (Huet *et al.*, 2009). None of the strains produced the PGL previously associated with the hypervirulent phenotype of some isolates of this lineage (Reed *et al.*, 2004), despite all Indo-Oceanic and East Asian/Beijing strains having an intact *pks1/15* gene.

However, all the Indo-Oceanic strains produced a unique phenolphthiocerol dimycoserosate lipid, which was dependent on an intact *pks15/1* for its production. Mutation of *pks15/1* in a representative Indo-Oceanic strain prevented phenolphthiocerol dimycoserosate synthesis and caused increased expression of TNF-α from infected macrophages compared with the wild type. These findings suggest that the early interactions between *M. tuberculosis* and host are determined by the lineage of the infecting strain and their bacterial cell surface-expressed lipids. This may partly explain why strains from some lineages cause more meningitis than others in Vietnam but does not provide a complete explanation for the original epidemiological observation that strains of Euro-American lineage cause less meningitis than those of the Indo-Oceanic and East Asian/Beijing lineages.

11.2.5 How does host response influence the pathogenesis of tuberculous meningitis?

Ever since tuberculosis became a treatable disease in the late 1940s, it has been recognized that the host's response to the infection is a critical determinant of outcome. First-line anti-tuberculosis agents kill more than 90% of susceptible bacteria within the first 2 weeks of therapy, but the pathology – characterized by necrotizing granulomatous inflammation – may take many months to subside. This conundrum is especially well documented for tuberculous meningitis. Anti-tuberculosis drugs sterilize the CSF within a week, yet the inflammatory response persists for many months with serious clinical consequences (Thwaites and Tran, 2005). The inflammatory response is characterized by the gross pathological changes of fibrinous basal meningeal exudate, vasculitis and the formation of tuberculomas.

Figure 11.2 summarizes the host inflammatory response before and after the start of treatment for tuberculous meningitis. The rabbit model has been especially useful in highlighting that TNF-α is a key cytokine in the pathogenesis of tuberculous meningitis. Following intracisternal injection of bacteria, the rabbits developed meningitis, characterized by CSF mononuclear leucocytosis, raised protein and high TNF-α concentrations (Tsenova *et al.*, 1998). When the rabbits were

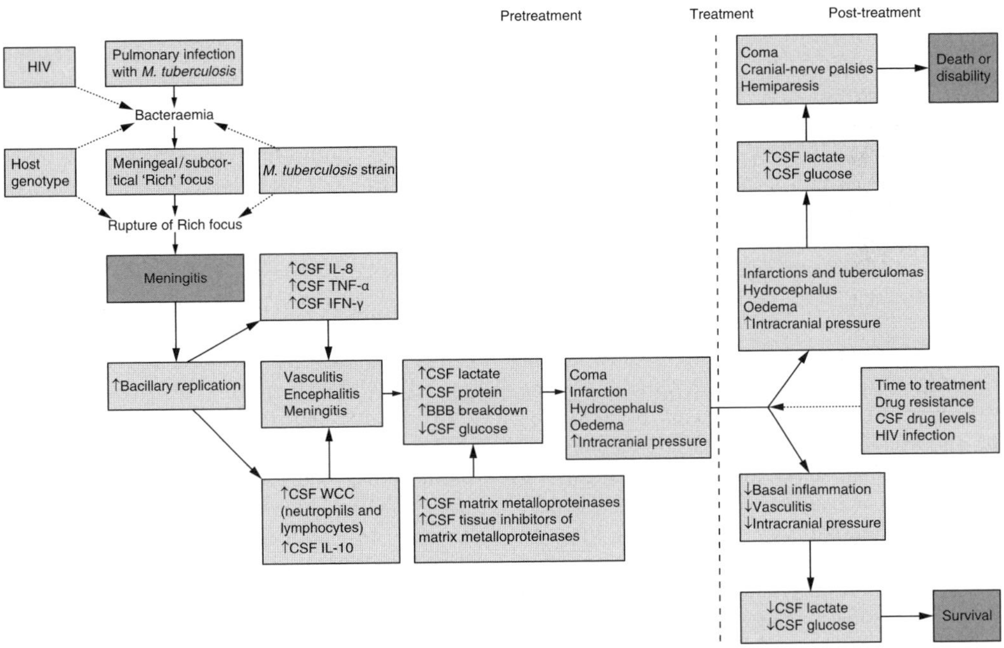

Fig. 11.2. Overview of the host intracerebral inflammatory response before and after the start of treatment for tuberculous meningitis. IL, interleukin; IL-10; IFN-γ, interferon-γ; WCC, total white cell count; BBB, blood–brain barrier. (Reprinted from Thwaites and Tran (2005), with permission from Elsevier.)

treated with anti-tuberculosis drugs, the bacteria were killed rapidly, but the pathology persisted and 50% of the animals died. When the adjunctive thalidomide, which inhibits TNF-α, was added to the treatment regimen, a marked reduction in CSF leucocyte numbers, TNF-α concentration and mortality was observed. To test whether CSF TNF-α concentrations correlated with pathology and outcome, the response of rabbits infected with various *M. bovis* strains of differing virulence was assessed (Tsenova *et al.*, 1999). The strains that caused the most severe pathology were associated with the highest CSF concentrations of TNF-α, and the greatest CSF leucocytosis, CSF protein concentration and meningeal inflammation. They then infected the rabbits with a low-virulence *M. bovis* strain and the same strain expressing the murine TNF-α gene. Expression of murine TNF-α by the bacteria rendered them more virulent than the wild type, with induction of severe meningeal inflammation with progressive clinical deterioration of the affected rabbits.

Whether TNF-α has the same role in the pathogenesis of human tuberculous meningitis remains controversial and an array of other pro- and anti-inflammatory mediators have been implicated. A study of pro- and anti-inflammatory molecules in serial blood and CSF samples from 21 adults treated for tuberculous meningitis found CSF concentrations of lactate, TNF-α, IL-8, and interferon-γ were high before treatment and then decreased rapidly once anti-tuberculosis chemotherapy was begun (Thwaites *et al.*, 2003). CSF concentrations of the anti-inflammatory cytokine IL-10 were elevated at the start of treatment and persisted for more than 2 months into treatment, as did evidence of significant BBB dysfunction. Death was associated with high initial CSF concentrations of lactate, low numbers of CSF leucocytes, in particular neutrophils, and low CSF glucose levels. CSF TNF-α concentration did not correlate with outcome in this study.

Tuberculous meningitis causes substantial and protracted BBB breakdown. The mechanisms are probably multifactorial, although the matrix metalloproteinases (MMPs), in particular, have been implicated (Price *et al.*, 2001; Thwaites *et al.*, 2003). MMPs may cause cerebral injury by disrupting the BBB, facilitating leucocyte migration and cleaving myelin proteins. Elevated CSF MMP-9 concentrations have been associated with focal neurological deficit and death in adults with tuberculous meningitis (Price *et al.*, 2001). The activity of the specific tissue inhibitors of MMPs (TIMPs) may be equally important, in particular the balance between MMP-9 and TIMP-1 (its specific inhibitor), but further work is required to delineate these relationships in greater detail and determine their precise role in pathogenesis.

Probably the strongest evidence for the importance of host immune response in the pathogenesis of tuberculous meningitis comes from the clinical studies of adjunctive anti-inflammatory agents. These studies have been based on the long-standing hypothesis that outcomes from tuberculous meningitis can be improved if the host inflammatory response is controlled while the anti-tuberculosis drugs kill the bacteria. Over the last 60 years, seven randomized controlled trials involving 1140 people with tuberculous meningitis have been performed and, when the results of these trials are combined, they show that adjunctive corticosteroids reduce the risk of death from this infection by around 30% (Prasad and Singh, 2008). How corticosteroids exert this effect is an important question, for it would pinpoint the key pathogenetic pathways and may suggest novel, more targeted therapies. However, until very recently, the mechanism by which corticosteroids improved survival from tuberculous meningitis remained elusive. Subsets of patients enrolled into the largest and most recent trial were carefully studied to determine whether corticosteroids reduced intracerebral inflammation (Simmons *et al.*, 2005; Thwaites *et al.*, 2007). CSF inflammatory indices, including a panel of cytokines and MMPs, were compared between those treated with corticosteroid or placebo, but no significant difference between the two groups was found, other than a possible reduction in CSF MMP-9 in those given corticosteroids (Green *et al.*, 2009). Likewise, comparison of the gross pathological changes of tuberculous meningitis did not reveal any significant differences between the treatment arms (Thwaites *et al.*, 2007).

However, a possible explanation for this puzzling lack of anti-inflammatory effect has recently been uncovered. Using the zebrafish model of mycobacterial infection, Tobin and others screened a large number of genetic mutants for resistance or susceptibility to mycobacterial infection (Tobin *et al.*, 2010). They found that a polymorphism in the gene encoding the leukotriene A4 hydrolase enzyme influenced tuberculosis susceptibility in both zebrafish and humans, by causing either excessive or inadequate TNF-α expression. Zebrafish at both poles of the inflammatory response (minor and major allele homozygotes) were unable to control mycobacterial replication within granulomas, whereas those fish with an intermediate TNF-α response (the heterozygotes) controlled the infection. The phenotype of the homozygous fish could be changed to that of the heterozygotes through the respective addition or inhibition of TNF-α. Furthermore, adjunctive corticosteroids were only found to benefit major allele-homozygous adult humans (hyperinflammatory) with tuberculous meningitis (Tobin *et al.*, 2012). Indeed, corticosteroid treatment of those with a hypo-inflammatory phenotype appeared to be detrimental. These findings need replication in a different population, but they provide an elegant explanation for the previous failure to find the mechanism by which corticosteroids improve survival from tuberculous meningitis in Vietnamese adults (Fig. 11.3). They also place TNF-α back at the centre of tuberculous meningitis pathogenesis and offer a more intelligent approach to future adjunctive therapy. The findings suggest that specific therapies targeted against TNF-α (e.g. with thalidomide or anti-TNF-α antibodies) may be more effective than corticosteroids and, for the first time, that host genotype may be used to predict the response to these adjunctive therapies.

11.3 Conclusions and Future Research

Tuberculous meningitis is the most dangerous form of tuberculosis, causing death or severe neurological disability in around half of all those who contract the disease. Yet, despite its severity, our understanding of the pathogenesis of the disease is rudimentary. The key events of bacteraemia, Rich focus formation and then meningitis, following the release of bacteria from the Rich focus into the SAS, have been known for more than 80 years. Likewise, the importance of granulomatous inflammation to the early control of infection in the lung and subsequent pathology in the brain has long been appreciated. However, the host and bacterial factors that influence these events are only partly and poorly elucidated.

A better understanding of the pathogenesis of tuberculous meningitis requires better animal models and innovative clinical studies. The rabbit may be the best available model of human disease, but it does not replicate the bacteraemic step in pathogenesis, and investigations are disadvantaged by the limited numbers of reagents available to assess the rabbit inflammatory response. A mouse model would overcome this latter disadvantage and there may be novel ways of gaining closer replication of human tuberculosis, possibly through manipulation of the mouse NO response (Olin *et al.*, 2008) or MMP expression (Elkington *et al.*, 2011).

A better animal model would enable finer dissection of the key cellular and molecular events in pathogenesis, but all such work should be performed with continual reference to the disease in humans. The relative rarity of tuberculous meningitis in the resource-rich world has distanced many clinical studies of the disease from recent advances in molecular biology and imaging. Characterizing the genes (both bacterial and human) and mechanisms responsible for the development and clinical consequences of tuberculous meningitis will require ambitious studies, utilizing large numbers of well-characterized patients. Meticulous clinical phenotyping will be essential to these studies and should include new imaging techniques, e.g. functional magnetic resonance imaging (MRI) and positron emission tomography (PET), to illuminate the dynamics of cerebral pathology over time. Better definition of the central pathological events by these methods will

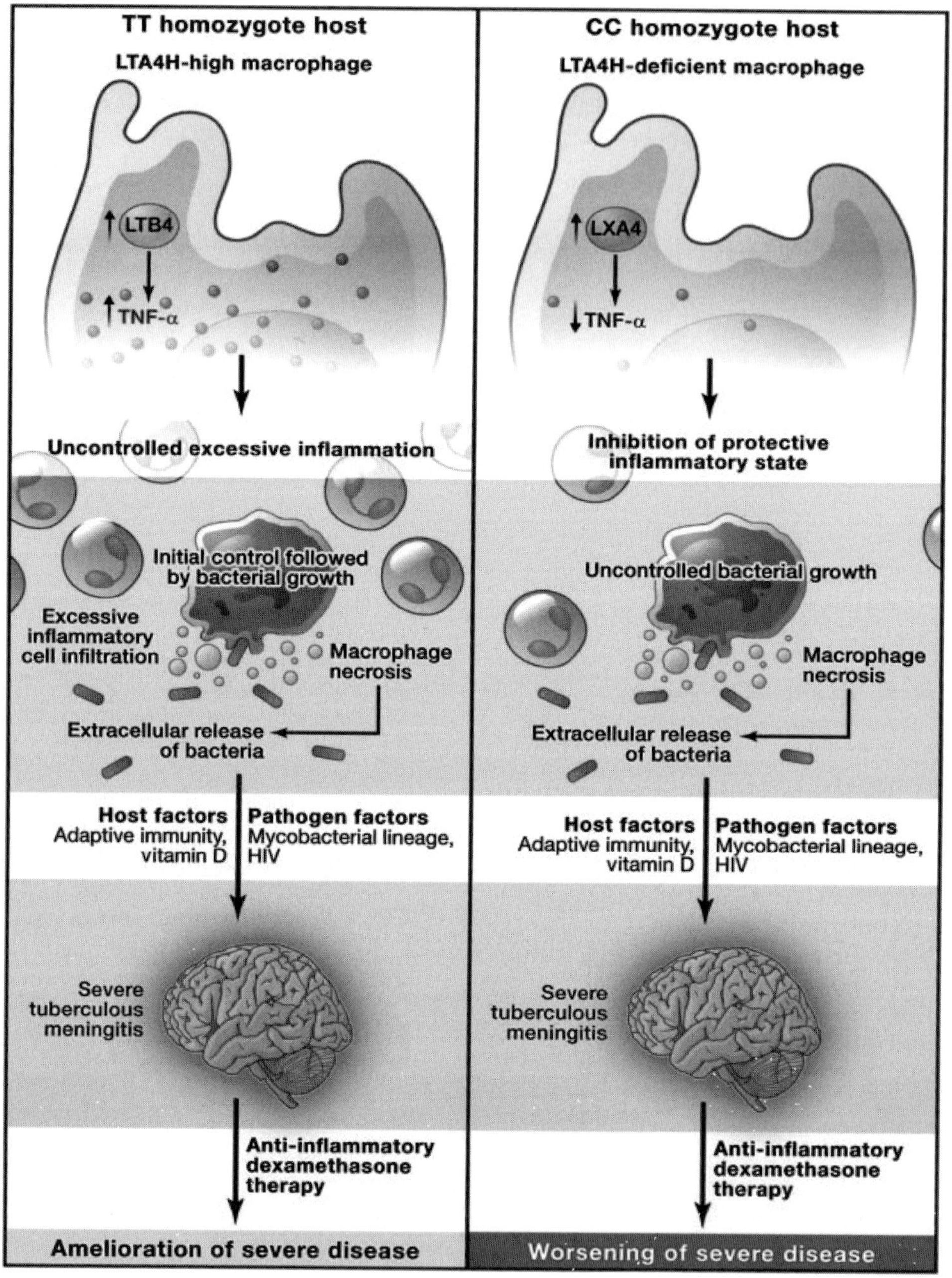

Fig. 11.3. LTA4H genotype determines the 'yin and yang' of TNF-α in the pathogenesis of tuberculous meningitis. *M. tuberculosis* disseminates from lung to brain. In a host with genetically determined high expression of LTA4H (TT homozygote, left) or deficient in LTA4H (CC homozygote, right), excess pro-inflammatory LTB4 (left) and anti-inflammatory LXA4 (right) lead to an excess or reduced levels of TNF-α, respectively. Reduced TNF-α (right) and excessive TNF-α (left) both result in macrophage necrosis and uncontrolled bacterial growth. Adjunctive dexamethasone reduces excessive inflammation in the TT homozygous (LTA4H-high) individuals and improves survival but potentially has an adverse effect in CC homozygous individuals. (Reprinted from Lalvani *et al.* (2012), with permission from Elsevier.)

allow the mechanisms that underpin them to be explored through genomic, proteomic and metabolomic approaches. Such studies would have the potential to discover novel molecular targets for better diagnostics and therapeutics; both are desperately needed for this lethal infection.

References

Barry, C.E. 3rd, Boshoff, H.I., Dartois, V., Dick, T., Ehrt, S., Flynn, J., Schnappinger, D., Wilkinson, R.J. and Young, D. (2009) The spectrum of latent tuberculosis: rethinking the biology and intervention strategies. *Nature Reviews Microbiology* 7, 845–855.

Be, N.A., Lamichhane, G., Grosset, J., Tyagi, S., Cheng, Q.J., Kim, K.S., Bishai, W.R. and Jain, S.K. (2008) Murine model to study the invasion and survival of *Mycobacterium tuberculosis* in the central nervous system. *Journal of Infectious Diseases* 198, 1520–1528.

Be, N.A., Bishai, W.R. and Jain, S.K. (2012) Role of *Mycobacterium tuberculosis pknD* in the pathogenesis of central nervous system tuberculosis. *BMC Microbioogy* 12, 7.

Bermudez, L.E., Sangari, F.J., Kolonoski, P., Petrofsky, M. and Goodman, J. (2002) The efficiency of the translocation of *Mycobacterium tuberculosis* across a bilayer of epithelial and endothelial cells as a model of the alveolar wall is a consequence of transport within mononuclear phagocytes and invasion of alveolar epithelial cells. *Infection and Immunity* 70, 140–146.

Bishai, W.R., Dannenberg, A.M., Jr, Parrish, N., Ruiz, R., Chen, P., Zook, B.C., Johnson, W., Boles, J.W. and Pitt, M.L. (1999) Virulence of *Mycobacterium tuberculosis* CDC1551 and H37Rv in rabbits evaluated by Lurie's pulmonary tubercle count method. *Infection and Immunity* 67, 4931–4934.

Bodnar, K.A., Serbina, N.V. and Flynn, J.L. (2001) Fate of *Mycobacterium tuberculosis* within murine dendritic cells. *Infection and Immunity* 69, 800–809.

Braibant, M., Gilot, P. and Content, J. (2000) The ATP binding cassette (ABC) transport systems of *Mycobacterium tuberculosis. FEMS Microbiology Reviews* 24, 449–467.

Byrd, T.F., Green, G.M., Fowlston, S.E. and Lyons, C.R. (1998) Differential growth characteristics and streptomycin susceptibility of virulent and avirulent *Mycobacterium tuberculosis* strains in a novel fibroblast-mycobacterium microcolony assay. *Infection and Immunity* 66, 5132–5139.

Castro-Garza, J., King, C.H., Swords, W.E. and Quinn, F.D. (2002) Demonstration of spread by *Mycobacterium tuberculosis* bacilli in A549 epithelial cell monolayers. *FEMS Microbiology Letters* 212, 145–149.

Caws, M., *et al.* (2008) The influence of host and bacterial genotype on the development of disseminated disease with *Mycobacterium tuberculosis. PLoS Pathogens* 4, e10000034.

Chackerian, A.A., Alt, J.M., Perera, T.V., Dascher, C.C. and Behar, S.M. (2002) Dissemination of *Mycobacterium tuberculosis* is influenced by host factors and precedes the initiation of T-cell immunity. *Infection and Immunity* 70, 4501–4509.

Clay, H., Davis, J.M., Beery, D., Huttenlocher, A., Lyons, S.E. and Ramakrishnan, L. (2007) Dichotomous role of the macrophage in early *Mycobacterium marinum* infection of the zebrafish. *Cell Host & Microbe* 2, 29–39.

Davis, J.M. and Ramakrishnan, L. (2009) The role of the granuloma in expansion and dissemination of early tuberculous infection. *Cell* 136, 37–49.

Dobos, K.M., Spotts, E.A., Quinn, F.D. and King, C.H. (2000) Necrosis of lung epithelial cells during infection with *Mycobacterium tuberculosis* is preceded by cell permeation. *Infection and Immunity* 68, 6300–6310.

Dormans, J., Burger, M., Aguilar, D., Hernandez-Pando, R., Kremer, K., Roholl, P., Arend, S.M. and van Soolingen, D. (2004) Correlation of virulence, lung pathology, bacterial load and delayed type hypersensitivity responses after infection with different *Mycobacterium tuberculosis* genotypes in a BALB/c mouse model. *Clinical and Experimental Immunology* 137, 460–468.

Dunn, P.L. and North, R.J. (1995) Virulence ranking of some *Mycobacterium tuberculosis* and *Mycobacterium bovis* strains according to their ability to multiply in the lungs, induce lung pathology, and cause mortality in mice. *Infection and Immunity* 63, 3428–3437.

Elkington, P., *et al.* (2011) MMP-1 drives immunopathology in human tuberculosis and transgenic mice. *Journal of Clinical Investigation* 121, 1827–1833.

Flynn, J.L., Chan, J. and Lin, P.L. (2011) Macrophages and control of granulomatous inflammation in tuberculosis. *Mucosal Immunology* 4, 271–278.

Gao, Q., Kripke, K., Arinc, Z., Voskuil, M. and Small, P. (2004) Comparative expression studies of a complex phenotype: cord formation in *Mycobacterium tuberculosis. Tuberculosis* 84, 188–196.

Green, J.A., Tran, C.T., Farrar, J.J., Nguyen, M.T., Nguyen, P.H., Dinh, S.X., Ho, N.D., Ly, C.V., Tran, H.T., Friedland, J.S. and Thwaites, G.E. (2009) Dexamethasone, cerebrospinal fluid matrix metalloproteinase concentrations and clinical outcomes in tuberculous meningitis. *PLoS ONE* 4, e7277.

Hagedorn, M., Rohde, K.H., Russell, D.G. and Soldati, T. (2009) Infection by tubercular mycobacteria is spread by nonlytic ejection from their amoeba hosts. *Science* 323, 1729–1733.

Henderson, R.A., Watkins, S.C. and Flynn, J.L. (1997) Activation of human dendritic cells following infection with *Mycobacterium tuberculosis*. *Journal of Immunology* 159, 635–643.

Houben, E.N., Nguyen, L. and Pieters, J. (2006) Interaction of pathogenic mycobacteria with the host immune system. *Current Opinion in Microbiology* 9, 76–85.

Huet, G., Constant, P., Malaga, W., Laneelle, M.A., Kremer, K., van Soolingen, D., Daffe, M. and Guilhot, C. (2009) A lipid profile typifies the Beijing strains of *Mycobacterium tuberculosis*: identification of a mutation responsible for a modification of the structures of phthiocerol dimycocerosates and phenolic glycolipids. *Journal of Biological Chemistry* 284, 27101–27113.

Humphreys, I.R., Stewart, G.R., Turner, D.J., Patel, J., Karamanou, D., Snelgrove, R.J. and Young, D.B. (2006) A role for dendritic cells in the dissemination of mycobacterial infection. *Microbes and Infection* 8, 1339–1346.

Jain, S.K., Paul-Satyaseela, M., Lamichhane, G., Kim, K.S. and Bishai, W.R. (2006) *Mycobacterium tuberculosis* invasion and traversal across an in vitro human blood–brain barrier as a pathogenic mechanism for central nervous system tuberculosis. *Journal of Infectious Diseases* 193, 1287–1295.

Kinhikar, A.G., Verma, I., Chandra, D., Singh, K.K., Weldingh, K., Andersen, P., Hsu, T., Jacobs, W.R., Jr and Laal, S. (2010) Potential role for ESAT6 in dissemination of *M. tuberculosis* via human lung epithelial cells. *Molecular Microbiology* 75, 92–106.

Krishnan, N., Robertson, B.D. and Thwaites, G. (2010) The mechanisms and consequences of the extra-pulmonary dissemination of *Mycobacterium tuberculosis*. *Tuberculosis* 90, 361–366.

Krishnan, N., *et al.* (2011) *Mycobacterium tuberculosis* lineage influences innate immune response and virulence and is associated with distinct cell envelope lipid profiles. *PLoS ONE* 6, e23870.

Lalvani, A., Behr, M.A. and Sridhar, S. (2012) Innate immunity to TB: a druggable balancing act. *Cell* 148, 389–391.

Locht, C., Hougardy, J.M., Rouanet, C., Place, S. and Mascart, F. (2006) Heparin-binding hemagglutinin, from an extrapulmonary dissemination factor to a powerful diagnostic and protective antigen against tuberculosis. *Tuberculosis* 86, 303–309.

Lopez, B., Aguilar, D., Orozco, H., Burger, M., Espitia, C., Ritacco, V., Barrera, L., Kremer, K., Hernandez-Pando, R., Huygen, K. and van Soolingen, D. (2003) A marked difference in pathogenesis and immune response induced by different *Mycobacterium tuberculosis* genotypes. *Clinical and Experimental Immunology* 133, 30–37.

McDonough, K.A. and Kress, Y. (1995) Cytotoxicity for lung epithelial cells is a virulence-associated phenotype of *Mycobacterium tuberculosis*. *Infection and Immunity* 63, 4802–4811.

Menozzi, F.D., Reddy, V.M., Cayet, D., Raze, D., Debrie, A.S., Dehouck, M.P., Cecchelli, R. and Locht, C. (2006) *Mycobacterium tuberculosis* heparin-binding haemagglutinin adhesin (HBHA) triggers receptor-mediated transcytosis without altering the integrity of tight junctions. *Microbes and Infection* 8, 1–9.

Mitchison, D.A., Wallace, J.G., Bhatia, A.L., Selkon, J.B., Subbaiah, T.V. and Lancaster, M.C. (1960) A comparison of the virulence in guinea-pigs of South Indian and British tubercle bacilli. *Tubercle* 41, 1–22.

Olin, M.R., Armien, A.G., Cheeran, M.C., Rock, R.B., Molitor, T.W. and Peterson, P.K. (2008) Role of nitric oxide in defense of the central nervous system against *Mycobacterium tuberculosis*. *Journal of Infectious Diseases* 198, 886–889.

Pethe, K., Alonso, S., Biet, F., Delogu, G., Brennan, M.J., Locht, C. and Menozzi, F.D. (2001) The heparin-binding haemagglutinin of *M. tuberculosis* is required for extrapulmonary dissemination. *Nature* 412, 190–194.

Prasad, K. and Singh, M.B. (2008) Corticosteroids for managing tuberculous meningitis. *Cochrane Database of Systematic Reviews* 1, CD002244.

Price, N.M., Farrar, J., Tran, T.T., Nguyen, T.H., Tran, T.H. and Friedland, J.S. (2001) Identification of a matrix-degrading phenotype in human tuberculosis in vitro and in vivo. *Journal of Immunology* 166, 4223–4230.

Reed, M.B., Domenech, P., Manca, C., Su, H., Barczak, A.K., Kreiswirth, B.N., Kaplan, G. and Barry, C.E. 3rd (2004) A glycolipid of hypervirulent tuberculosis strains that inhibits

the innate immune response. *Nature* 431, 84–87.
Rich, A.R. and McCordock, H.A. (1933) The pathogenesis of tuberculous meningitis. *Bulletin of the John Hopkins Hospital* 52, 37.
Simmons, C.P., Thwaites, G.E., Quyen, N.T., Chau, T.T., Mai, P.P., Dung, N.T., Stepniewska, K., White, N.J., Hien, T.T. and Farrar, J. (2005) The clinical benefit of adjunctive dexamethasone in tuberculous meningitis is not associated with measurable attenuation of peripheral or local immune responses. *Journal of Immunology* 175, 579–590.
Sinsimer, D., Huet, G., Manca, C., Tsenova, L., Koo, M.S., Kurepina, N., Kana, B., Mathema, B., Marras, S.A., Kreiswirth, B.N., Guilhot, C. and Kaplan, G. (2008) The phenolic glycolipid of *Mycobacterium tuberculosis* differentially modulates the early host cytokine response but does not in itself confer hypervirulence. *Infection and Immunity* 76, 3027–3036.
Talaat, A.M., Lyons, R., Howard, S.T. and Johnston, S.A. (2004) The temporal expression profile of *Mycobacterium tuberculosis* infection in mice. *Proceedings of the National Academy of Sciences USA* 101, 4602–4607.
Tascon, R.E., Soares, C.S., Ragno, S., Stavropoulos, E., Hirst, E.M. and Colston, M.J. (2000) *Mycobacterium tuberculosis*-activated dendritic cells induce protective immunity in mice. *Immunology* 99, 473–480.
Thuong, N.T., Hawn, T.R., Thwaites, G.E., Chau, T.T., Lan, N.T., Quy, H.T., Hieu, N.T., Aderem, A., Hien, T.T., Farrar, J.J. and Dunstan, S.J. (2007) A polymorphism in human TLR2 is associated with increased susceptibility to tuberculous meningitis. *Genes and Immunity* 8, 422–428.
Thwaites, G.E. and Tran, T.H. (2005) Tuberculous meningitis: many questions, too few answers. *Lancet Neurology* 4, 160–170.
Thwaites, G.E., Simmons, C.P., Than Ha Quyen, N., Thi Hong Chau, T., Phuong Mai, P., Thi Dung, N., Hoan Phu, N., White, N.P., Tinh Hien, T. and Farrar, J.J. (2003) Pathophysiology and prognosis in Vietnamese adults with tuberculous meningitis. *Journal of Infectious Diseases* 188, 1105–1115.
Thwaites, G.E., Macmullen-Price, J., Tran, T.H., Pham, P.M., Nguyen, T.D., Simmons, C.P., White, N.J., Summers, D. and Farrar, J.J. (2007) Serial MRI to determine the effect of dexamethasone on the cerebral pathology of tuberculous meningitis: an observational study. *Lancet Neurology* 6, 230–236.
Tobin, D.M., Vary, J.C., Jr, Ray, J.P., Walsh, G.S., Dunstan, S.J., Bang, N.D., Hagge, D.A., Khadge, S., King, M.C., Hawn, T.R., Moens, C.B. and Ramakrishnan, L. (2010) The *lta4h* locus modulates susceptibility to mycobacterial infection in zebrafish and humans. *Cell* 140, 717–730.
Tobin, D.M., *et al.* (2012) Host genotype-specific therapies can optimize the inflammatory response to mycobacterial infections. *Cell* 148, 434–446.
Tsenova, L., Sokol, K., Freedman, V.H. and Kaplan, G. (1998) A combination of thalidomide plus antibiotics protects rabbits from mycobacterial meningitis-associated death. *Journal of Infectious Diseases* 177, 1563–1572.
Tsenova, L., Bergtold, A., Freedman, V.H., Young, R.A. and Kaplan, G. (1999) Tumor necrosis factor α is a determinant of pathogenesis and disease progression in mycobacterial infection in the central nervous system. *Proceedings of the National Academy of Sciences USA* 96, 5657–5662.
Tsenova, L., Ellison, E., Harbacheuski, R., Moreira, A.L., Kurepina, N., Reed, M.B., Mathema, B., Barry, C.E. 3rd and Kaplan, G. (2005) Virulence of selected *Mycobacterium tuberculosis* clinical isolates in the rabbit model of meningitis is dependent on phenolic glycolipid produced by the bacilli. *Journal of Infectious Diseases* 192, 98–106.
van Kooyk, Y., Appelmelk, B. and Geijtenbeek, T.B. (2003) A fatal attraction: *Mycobacterium tuberculosis* and HIV-1 target DC-SIGN to escape immune surveillance. *Trends in Molecular Medicine* 9, 153–159.
van Well, G.T., Wieland, C.W., Florquin, S., Roord, J.J., van der Poll, T. and van Furth, A.M. (2007) A new murine model to study the pathogenesis of tuberculous meningitis. *Journal of Infectious Diseases* 195, 694–697.
Volkman, H.E., Pozos, T.C., Zheng, J., Davis, J.M., Rawls, J.F. and Ramakrishnan, L. (2010) Tuberculous granuloma induction via interaction of a bacterial secreted protein with host epithelium. *Science* 327, 466–469.
Wolf, A.J., Linas, B., Trevejo-Nunez, G.J., Kincaid, E., Tamura, T., Takatsu, K. and Ernst, J.D. (2007) *Mycobacterium tuberculosis* infects dendritic cells with high frequency and impairs their function in vivo. *Journal of Immunology* 179, 2509–2519.
World Health Organization (2011) *Global tuberculosis control 2011*. Geneva, WHO.

12 Neurosyphilis

Wim Ang*
VU University Medical Center, Amsterdam, The Netherlands

12.1 Introduction

Syphilis is a complex systemic illness that is caused by the spirochaete *Treponema pallidum* and can affect any organ in the body (Radolf *et al.*, 2006). If untreated, a substantial fraction of infected persons will develop neurological signs and symptoms. Syphilis has had a large impact in history. It was a leading cause of neurological disease among middle-aged persons at the turn of the 20th century (Ghanem, 2010). Many famous persons have died from neurosyphilis (Table 12.1). Before the 16th century, there are almost no written reports of disease complexes that we can attribute to neurosyphilis (Rothschild, 2005). In the 17th century, syphilis became widespread and although many explanations have been given for this dramatic expansion, two theories stand out. First, shipmates of Columbus or his successors brought syphilis from the New World back to Europe, where the disease found a new habitat, changed its behaviour slightly and evolved into the disease currently known as syphilis. The second theory states that syphilis has always been present in Europe but that the urbanization of European society facilitated spread of the disease. Large parts of the population in several European cities are believed to have suffered from syphilis but the introduction of antibiotic therapy drastically reduced disease transmission (Rothschild, 2005). Although neurosyphilis still occurs worldwide, the availability of potent antibiotics in developed countries has turned neurosyphilis from a common disease into a rarity, mostly confined to several high-risk groups such as males having sex with males (Ghanem, 2010). There are no population-based studies on the current epidemiology of neurosyphilis and therefore reliable figures on incidence cannot be given.

12.2 Clinical Aspects of Neurosyphilis

The clinical manifestations of syphilis can be divided into several stages (Fig. 12.1). Notably, the central nervous system (CNS) is involved in every stage, although this does not lead to symptomatic illness in all stages. Following exposure to an infectious individual, *T. pallidum* gains access to the body through micro-abrasions in mucosal membranes or skin (LaFond and Lukehart, 2006). Treponemes rapidly disseminate through the body in the bloodstream. During this phase, all organs can become infected.

*w.ang@vumc.nl

Table 12.1. Selected list of famous persons with syphilis.

Composers	Franz Schubert (1797–1828)
	Robert Schumann (1810–1856)
Gangster	Al Capone (1899–1947)
Painters	Paul Gauguin (1848–1903)
	Henri de Toulouse-Lautrec (1864–1901)
	Edouard Manet (1832–1883)
Philosophers	Friedrich Nietzsche (1844–1900)
	Arthur Schopenhauer (1788–1860)
Poets	Charles Baudelaire (1821–1867)
	Heinrich Heine (1797–1856)
Writers	Gustave Flaubert (1821–1880)
	Guy de Maupassant (1850–1893)
	Oscar Wilde (1854–1900)

Within a very short time, invasion of the CNS occurs (LaFond and Lukehart, 2006; Radolf *et al.*, 2006). In rabbits that are exposed to *T. pallidum*, treponemes can be detected in the cerebrospinal fluid (CSF) within hours. Studies at the beginning of the 20th century showed that 15–30% patients with untreated primary syphilis had viable *T. pallidum* in their CSF, which is probably an underestimate. Later studies confirmed the presence of viable *T. pallidum* in the CSF of 30% of patients with primary and secondary syphilis (Lukehart *et al.*, 1988).

12.2.1 Primary syphilis

After an incubation period of a few weeks to a few months, a chancre develops at the site of inoculation. This is called primary syphilis. The chancre consists of a local inflammatory response characterized by spirochaetes and cytokine-producing immunological cells (macrophages, plasma cells, $CD4^+$, $CD8^+$ T-cells) (Radolf *et al.*, 2006). In most cases, this is a painless papule. The chancre heals within 3–6 weeks, irrespective of antibiotic therapy.

12.2.2 Secondary syphilis

Secondary syphilis develops within 3 months of the initial infection and results from multiplication of disseminated spirochaetes. Due to the involvement of many organs, the clinical symptoms of secondary syphilis can be myriad. Most patients have some form of rash, mostly maculopapular, and have

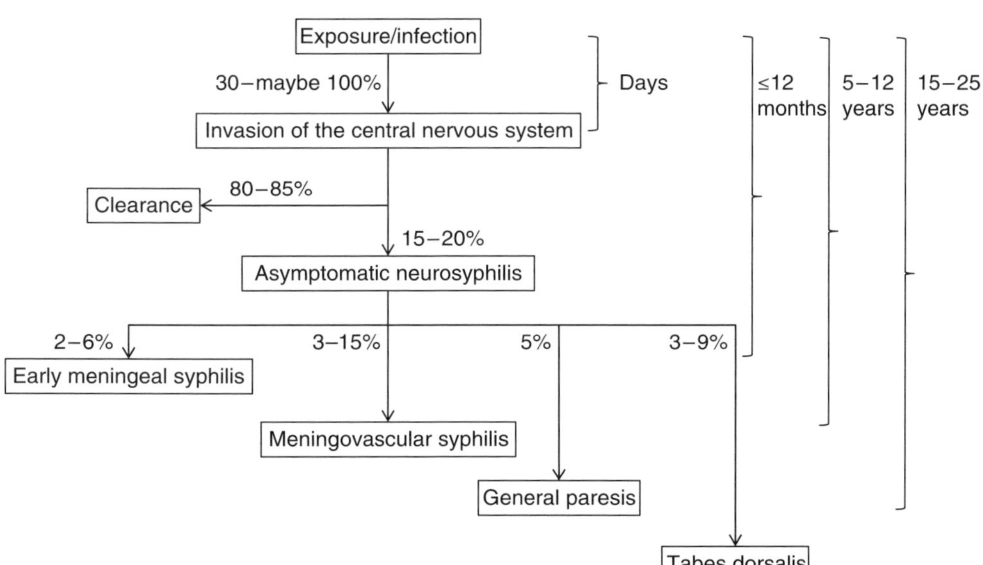

Fig. 12.1. Natural history of untreated syphilis with special emphasis on neurosyphilis. (Adapted from Ghanem, 2010.)

general constitutional symptoms such as fever, malaise, anorexia, weight loss and generalized lymphadenopathy. The CNS is involved in up to 40% of patients with secondary syphilis. The most prominent clinical manifestations are headache and signs of meningeal inflammation, often accompanied by nausea and vomiting. Often one or more cranial nerves are affected, leading to visual disturbances (photophobia), hearing loss, tinnitus and facial paralysis. Occasionally, patients present with seizures (Ghanem, 2010).

Treponemes can be detected by the rabbit infectivity test and by polymerase chain reaction (PCR) in CSF of 20–30% of patients with secondary syphilis (Lukehart *et al.*, 1988; LaFond and Lukehart, 2006). Importantly, patients without CSF abnormalities can harbour viable *T. pallidum* in the CSF. Asymptomatic neurosyphilis is defined by the presence of CSF abnormalities in patients with serological evidence of syphilis but without neurological symptoms. The exact proportion of patients with evidence of CNS inflammation without symptoms is hard to determine because many different study definitions have been used. About 20% of patients with secondary syphilis have abnormalities in the CSF and can be defined as having asymptomatic neurosyphilis. Viable *T. pallidum* can be isolated from the CSF of these patients (Lukehart *et al.*, 1988).

After the phase with florid symptoms, patients enter a subclinical stage, termed 'latent syphilis'. This phase is sometimes subdivided into an 'early latent phase' (the first 1 or 2 years) and a 'late latent phase' (Ghanem, 2010). During this latent phase, patients can relapse and become infectious. The majority of relapses occur in the first year following infection.

12.2.3 Tertiary syphilis

Tertiary syphilis or late syphilis produces clinical illness up to 40–50 years after infection. Any organ can be affected as a result of dissemination. Neurosyphilis and cardiovascular syphilis are the most frequently encountered manifestations of tertiary syphilis. Within the disease entity of tertiary neurosyphilis, different histopathological patterns can be discerned. When patients present between 5 and 10 years after infection, the nervous system pathology consists of a vasculitis (*endarteritis obliterans*) of the small blood vessels of the meninges, brain parenchyma and spinal cord leading to thrombosis and infarction. This is also termed 'meningovascular syphilis'. If untreated, the pathological process eventually leads to destruction of neurons, predominantly in the cerebral cortex. This is called 'parenchymatous neurosyphilis'. A mixture of the two forms is present in most patients that have been investigated, indicating that both inflammation and degeneration are involved in the pathological process (Peeling and Hook, 2006; Ghanem, 2010).

Parenchymatous neurosyphilis includes general paresis ('dementia paralytica', 'paretic neurosyphilis'), as a result of cortical involvement, and tabes dorsalis ('tabetic neurosyphilis'), resulting from spinal cord involvement. General paresis occurs between 15 and 20 years and tabes dorsalis 20–30 years after the initial infection, extending to periods as long as 50 years (Ghanem, 2010). The symptoms and signs are the result of widespread damage and include both psychiatric and neurological findings. Early findings can be very mild, such as irritability or other slight changes in personality, or can affect higher cognitive functions. In later stages, all patients have signs of dementia including impaired memory and judgement, disorientation, depression, hallucinations and psychosis. Occasionally, patients present with seizures. Neurological signs include the typical Argyll–Robertson pupil (irregular form of the pupil), dysarthria and tremors. The involvement of the posterior columns of the spinal cord, the dorsal roots and dorsal root ganglia leads to ataxia (wide-based gait) and typical sudden-onset shooting pains ('like lightning'), bladder disturbances, loss of position and vibratory sense. Syphilis can affect all sections of the eye. In addition to the Argyll–Robertson pupil, uveitis, vitreitis, retinitis and optic atrophy occur.

A final manifestation of neurosyphilis is the 'gumma', a granulomatous-like lesion that can vary in size from microscopic to a large mass. Gummas were frequently observed in the pre-antibiotic era but are very rare nowadays (Fargen *et al.*, 2009). In the pre-antibiotic era, up to 85% of patients would develop some form of tertiary syphilis (LaFond and Lukehart, 2006; Ghanem, 2010). The widespread use of penicillin has diminished the number of cases with general paresis although, even in the 21st century, people with general paresis characterized by psychiatric symptoms can be misdiagnosed. Tabes dorsalis is a rarity in the current era.

12.2.4 Asymptomatic neurosyphilis

It is important to note that it is possible to detect *T. pallidum* and an immune response to the organism in the CSF in all stages of syphilis, irrespective of the presence of neurological symptoms at the time of sampling. The extent of the host response to invasion is related to the probability that infection becomes symptomatic (Lukehart *et al.*, 1988; Radolf *et al.*, 2006). Patients with higher leucocyte counts, higher protein levels and a positive Wasserman test in the CSF had a much higher chance of developing late neurological complications. The relevance of detecting asymptomatic neurosyphilis is still under debate. A significant portion of asymptomatic patients with syphilis will have CSF abnormalities when performing CSF examination. However, there are no data available that unambiguously demonstrate a clinical benefit of screening of all patients with syphilis and subsequent appropriate treatment.

12.2.5 Diagnosis and treatment of neurosyphilis

There is no commonly agreed definition for the diagnosis of neurosyphilis. The two cornerstones for diagnosis are serological testing and determination of markers for CNS inflammation in the CSF. Antibodies used in syphilis diagnosis can be divided into treponemal antibodies and non-treponemal antibodies. The treponemal antibodies can be measured with a variety of techniques such as *T. pallidum* particle agglutination (TPPA), *T. pallidum* haemagglutination (TPHA) and the fluorescent treponemal antibody absorbed (FTA-ABS) test. Recently, the determination of treponemal antibodies with enzyme immunoassays (EIA) and immunoblotting, and chemiluminescence assays using recombinant treponemal antigens such as TP0435 (TpN17) and TP0574 (TpN47) has allowed laboratories to automate their screening methods (Ho and Lukehart, 2011). The non-treponemal antibodies are directed against lipoidal antigens and these antibodies can be detected with the rapid plasma reagin (RPR) or Venereal Disease Research Laboratory (VDRL) test. These are classic agglutination tests that are not yet automated. Most current guidelines also recommend lumbar puncture in all patients with serological evidence of syphilis and neurological signs or symptoms, and in asymptomatic patients when the VDRL does not demonstrate a fourfold or greater decline following therapy.

Most experts agree that the presence of a positive VDRL/RPR test in CSF is diagnostic for neurosyphilis and that the absence of treponemal antibodies in CSF excludes the condition (LaFond and Lukehart, 2006). In the CSF, markers for inflammation include polymorphonuclear leucocytes (PMNLs), protein, immunoglobulin indices and other biomarkers for inflammation such as chemokines (Marra *et al.*, 2010b). The cellular inflammatory response in neurosyphilis is mainly lymphocytic, although PMNLs can be present in acute syphilitic meningitis. CSF protein is elevated in the majority of neurosyphilis patients, although a normal protein level cannot be used to exclude neurosyphilis (Lukehart *et al.*, 1988). A substantial fraction of the CSF protein is albumin, followed by immunoglobulins. Intrathecal synthesis of antibodies can be determined by calculating the IgG index and IgM index, which measures the amount of immunoglobulin in CSF relative to the amount of albumin in serum and CSF. The composition of the CSF proteins in neurosyphilis is largely unknown, which is surprising given that the proteomics approach has been used in other diseases of the CNS

(Angel *et al.*, 2012). No published studies on the proteome of the CSF of neurosyphilis patients are available.

Patients with latent syphilis are usually treated with benzathine penicillin G intramuscularly, but this drug does not reliably produce detectable levels of penicillin in the CSF (Ghanem, 2010). It is still not clear whether treponemicidal levels of penicillin are absolutely needed to adequately treat CNS treponemal invasion. Treatment guidelines for neurosyphilis currently consist of 18–24 million units of intravenous aqueous penicillin G for 10–14 days. An extra layer of difficulty is associated with human immunodefiency virus (HIV) infection. HIV-infected patients often have an increased risk of acquiring syphilis and many of the patients diagnosed nowadays with neurosyphilis are indeed HIV positive. These patients can have slightly different presentation and, due to immune-mediated phenomena, their diagnosis can be more difficult (Marra *et al.*, 2004a). In addition, the risk of developing neurosyphilis in HIV patients may be increased, and the response to therapy may be less than in immunocompetent individuals. The response to therapy depends on the stage of the infection. Non-HIV-infected patients with secondary syphilis with meningeal involvement respond quickly. In HIV-infected patients, signs and symptoms may take much longer to resolve, sometimes more than 1 year (Marra *et al.*, 2004a). In tertiary syphilis, the response to antibiotic therapy may be absent or very difficult to substantiate. Regardless, most treatment protocols advise follow-up lumbar puncture until resolution of the abnormalities.

12.3 Pathogenesis of Neurosyphilis

Despite the well-known clinical manifestations of syphilis, studies on the pathogenesis of non-neurological manifestations of syphilis and neurosyphilis are hampered by the nature of the causative agent. Numerous attempts have been made to culture *T. pallidum in vitro* but it can only be cultured transiently in rabbit epithelial cells (LaFond and Lukehart, 2006). For normal propagation of viable *T. pallidum*, live rabbits have to be used. As a consequence, genetic manipulation of *T. pallidum* is not possible and a great deal of knowledge on *T. pallidum* proteins is inferred from model systems that use heterologous expression of *T. pallidum* genes in other strongly related *Treponema* spp. that can be cultured, such as *Treponema phagedensis* (Cameron, 2006). Another drawback in syphilis research is that the best animal model for neurosyphilis is a rabbit infectivity model, where animals are injected intracisternally or intravenously with treponemes (Marra *et al.*, 1991; Tantalo *et al.*, 2005). Due to the limited availability of reagents for rabbit immunological investigations, many processes have not been studied to the same extent as for other diseases, where mouse models are common. The publication of the complete genetic sequence of the Nichols strain of *T. pallidum* and other treponemes has enhanced syphilis research significantly (Fraser *et al.*, 1998). The lack of *in vitro* experimental methods has led to extensive bioinformatic analyses performed on the *T. pallidum* genome, with promising results (Giacani *et al.*, 2012; Smajs *et al.*, 2012).

12.3.1 Invasion of the CNS

Very shortly after infection, treponemes enter the CNS and this is demonstrated by animal models and the detection of *T. pallidum* in the CSF of early syphilis patients (LaFond and Lukehart, 2006). *T. pallidum* enters the host through mucosal barriers, and the blood–brain barrier (BBB) and blood–CSF barrier (BCSFB) has to be crossed for entry into the CNS. The necessary virulence attributes of *T. pallidum* required for CNS entry and survival for prolonged periods in the host include motility, attachment and persistence.

Motility

T. pallidum displays a corkscrew-like motility, a common feature of other spirochaetes and curved bacteria. This motility allows these bacteria to move in a highly viscous environment such as connective tissue. The cell wall of spirochaetes differs from other

Gram-negative bacteria in the location of the flagella and the lack of lipopolysaccharides (LPSs) (Cameron, 2006; Radolf *et al.*, 2006). Recent studies with cryo-electron microscopy (CEM) tomography have provided detailed knowledge about the structures that are involved in this motility (Izard *et al.*, 2009; Liu *et al.*, 2010a). Spirochaetes have flagella located within the periplasmic space between the cytoplasmic membrane (CM) and the outer membrane (OM) (Fig. 12.2). Bundles of flagella originate at specific structures at both ends of the organism. In contrast to most externally flagellated bacteria, the flagella of *T. pallidum* consist of multiple proteins, FlaB1, FlaB2, FlaB3 and FlaA. The flagella are able to make a rotatory movement and are called flagellar motors (Liu *et al.*, 2010a). The flagella are draped around the cylindrical bacterial cell, and rotation of the flagellar motors results in a conformational change of the flagellar bundle and deformation of the bacterial cell. The thin peptidoglycan layer in the periplasmic space prevents disruption of the fragile treponemal cell (Izard *et al.*, 2009). The combination of forces on the bacterial protoplasmic cell, exerted by the flagellar bundle and the periplasmic peptidoglycan layer, results in the corkscrew-like motion of the bacterium.

Several genes encoding components of treponemal chemotactic sensory systems suggest a possible role for chemotaxis in treponemal pathogenesis. *T. pallidum* contains a chemotaxis operon with four genes with

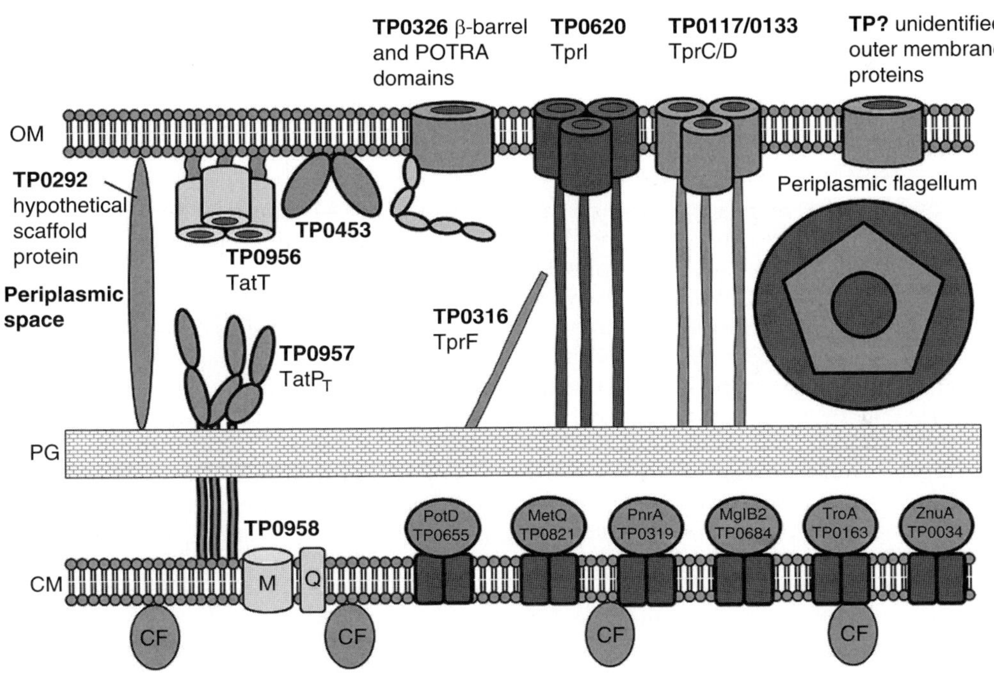

Fig. 12.2. *T. pallidum* cell-wall architecture. The cell wall (CW) consists of an inner cytoplasmic membrane (CM) and an outer membrane (OM), with a thin peptidoglycan (PG) layer and multiple periplasmic flagella inbetween. Between two and five flagella wrap like a ribbon around the CM. Underneath the CM, cytoplasmic filaments are located parallel to the periplasmic flagella. The integrity of the CW is augmented by scaffold proteins (TP0262). Rare OM proteins with β-barrel domains are exposed on the OM. The putative pore-forming lipoprotein TP0453 is anchored to the inner leaflet of the OM. Hydrophobic ligands can be chaperoned through the periplasmic space and over the CM by the TRAP-T complex (TP0956, TP0957 and TP0958). Within the periplasmic space below the PG, ATP-binding cassette transporter substrate-binding proteins for transport of amino acids, metal ions, nucleotides and sugars are located (TP0034, TP0163, TP0319, TP0655, TP0684 and TP0821). POTRA, polypeptide transport-associated.

methyl-accepting chemotaxis transmembrane proteins, TP0040 (Mcp1), TP0488 (Mcp2-1, PrtB), TP0639 (Mcp2-2) and TP0640 (Mcp4) (Fraser *et al.*, 1998). In addition, TP0684 (MglB2, Tp38) has been postulated to be involved in the chemotactic response to glucose. *T. pallidum* also has a set of regulatory genes, CheA (TP0363), CheB (TP0631), CheW1 (TP0364), CheW2 (TP0439), CheR (TP0630), CheX (TP0365) and CheY (TP0366), that are arranged in an operon, but the exact regulation of the chemotactic proteins has not been investigated extensively. High-resolution CEM tomography allowed the visualization of putative chemoreceptor arrays on the surface of *T. pallidum* (Liu *et al.*, 2010a). They show a variable location, 500–1000 nm from the cell end, and have a relatively consistent length of about 27 nm.

Attachment and crossing of epithelial and endothelial barriers

Most identified virulence factors of *T. pallidum* are associated with crossing of epithelial barriers, but many of these factors have not been studied in the context of the BBB. However, the architecture of epithelial barriers and endothelial barriers share many aspects and it seems reasonable to translate most findings of crossing epithelial barriers in the context of the BBB. In experimental animals, treponemes have crossed the epithelial barrier and have entered the bloodstream within hours of infection (Ho and Lukehart, 2011). *In vitro* studies demonstrate that *T. pallidum* is able to penetrate intact endothelial cell monolayers (Thomas *et al.*, 1988) and to upregulate the expression of adhesion molecules on the endothelium. One shared factor in invasive pathogens is the capacity to interact with extracellular matrix (ECM) components, and multiple treponemal proteins have been identified that can bind to ECM components. TP0751 binds to laminin and to fibrinogen: it can also degrade laminin and fibrinogen due to the presence of a protease domain (Houston *et al.*, 2011). TP0136, TP0155 and TP0483 bind to fibronectin (Ho and Lukehart, 2011). TP0155 has a preference for matrix fibronectin, and TP0483 can bind to both soluble and matrix forms of fibronectin (Cameron *et al.*, 2004). Other ECM components such as collagen and hyaluronic acid are able to bind to *T. pallidum*. The organisms attach to cells with their tips, with either one or both ends. The tip structure of *T. pallidum* displays great structural complexity and also high diversity. Multiple tip types can be discriminated with CEM tomography.

For *T. pallidum*, crossing of the BBB is believed to occur in a paracellular fashion. Treponemes traverse between endothelial cells without altering tight junctions, as measured by electrical resistance (Thomas *et al.*, 1988). Heat-killed *T. pallidum* or non-invasive *T. phagedensis* failed to penetrate endothelial cell monolayers. In secondary syphilis, electron microscopy investigations indicated that transcytosis occurs in the skin, but for crossing the BBB this has not been documented (Juanpere-Rodero *et al.*, 2013).

Breaching of the basal membrane and basal lamina by *T. pallidum* has not been elucidated, although for *Treponema denticola*, the protease 'dentisilin' has been described (LaFond and Lukehart, 2006). Proteases are secreted by invading bacteria to destroy structures that are encountered on their way to the brain. Host matrix metalloproteinases (MMPs) degrade various constituents of the ECM (LaFond and Lukehart, 2006), and CNS invasion is associated with an imbalance between MMPs and endogenous tissue inhibitors of MMP (TIMPs) (Tsai *et al.*, 2011). Expression of MMPs is often induced as an inflammatory response by the host, but some pathogens can manipulate this mechanism by suppressing the expression of selective MMPs or TIMPs. In a study in 15 HIV-positive neurosyphilis patients who did not receive anti-retroviral therapy, elevated levels of MMP-9 and higher activity of MMP-9 were found (Tsai *et al.*, 2011). There was also an increased level of TIMP-1 in these patients, and the authors suggested that TIMP-1 is bound to MMP-9. TIMP-4 was found in lower levels, but the authors acknowledged that it is very difficult to dissect the dysregulation caused by the HIV infection from an effect caused by *T. pallidum*.

Direct invasion of neurons by *T. pallidum* has been described in cutaneous nerves in a rabbit chancre model (Sell and Salman, 1992). Although many bacteria were observed in the perineurium, the number of invading bacteria was very low. *In vitro* experiments with cultured neurons demonstrated the capability of treponemes to attach to both neuronal bodies and cell processes (Repesh *et al.*, 1982). Co-incubation of rat dorsal root ganglion cells leads to electrophysiological dysfunction and cellular disruption (Oakes *et al.*, 1982). The relative role of these processes in the development of neurological symptoms is currently unknown.

Persistence

The ability of *T. pallidum* to persist in a host for decades indicates that this organism has developed a set of sophisticated survival tools. One of the most obvious characteristics of *T. pallidum* is its limited metabolic capacity. Analysis of the *T. pallidum* genome indicates that genes encoding glycolysis are present but genes that allow the tricarboxylic acid cycle and electron transport system are lacking. Other metabolic pathways that are absent in the *T. pallidum* genome are those responsible for synthesis of nucleotides, amino acids and lipids. This is probably the result of adaptation to its host and can be viewed as reductive evolution. The oral spirochaete *T. denticola* has almost 2000 genes that are not found in the *T. pallidum* genome (Radolf *et al.*, 2006).

T. pallidum has developed an intricate system for uptake of macromolecules from the host environment, with a minimum of exposure of bacterial molecules on the surface of the bacterium in order to limit antigenicity. This is referred to as a 'stealth-like' strategy. The OM of *T. pallidum* has a few characteristics that provide protection from the host immune system. The number of OM proteins (OMPs) on the surface of *T. pallidum* is only a fraction of that expressed by other Gram-negative bacteria (Cox *et al.*, 2010). Based on freeze fracture electron microscopy, it was estimated that *T. pallidum* has only about 1% of the number of OMPS found in *Escherichia coli*. CEM studies and scanning probe microscopy have revealed the scarcity of OMPS and their location in occasional protrusions of the OM that are often present on the bulge created by the underlying periplasmic flagella (Izard *et al.*, 2009; Liu *et al.*, 2010a).

Sera from syphilis-infected patients bind intact *T. pallidum* and promote opsonization and phagocytosis by macrophages (LaFond and Lukehart, 2006). These results encouraged many researchers to identify the bacterial targets for this effect and to search for possible vaccine candidates. The lack of cultivation and consequent lack of genetic manipulation of *T. pallidum* is compounded by the fact that OMPs are so rare, the sequence relatedness of *T. pallidum* to other organisms may be low and the *T. pallidum* OM is fragile. Despite these hurdles, a combination of bioinformatics and highly sophisticated serological analyses has permitted the delineation of a group of potential OMPs. OM-spanning proteins generally have a β-barrel structure, and Cox *et al.* (2010) identified genes that contained β-barrel structures and subsequently filtered the genes for characteristics such as sub-cellular localization, homology with non-OMPs and signal sequences. This resulted in a set of 19 'candidate OMPs' of which TP0326 and TprC were subsequently demonstrated to be genuine OMPs (Cox *et al.*, 2010). TP0326 has a predicted protein structure that is related to BamA (β-barrel assembly machinery protein A) (Desrosiers *et al.*, 2011). *Borrelia burgdorferi* protein BB0795 is related to TP0326 and is essential for the assembly of OMPs. TP0326 and TprC were shown to be surface expressed, amphiphilic, present in low abundance and to have polypeptide transport-associated (POTRA) domains that comprise the N terminus. Although TP0326 is surface expressed, the exposed parts of the proteins do not elicit an antibody response in infected humans, only in rabbits. Humans do mount an antibody response against the POTRA domains of TP0326, but the periplasmic parts of TprC are not antigenic during human infection (Desrosiers *et al.*, 2011). This indicates that parts of the bacterium can be shielded from the immune system, adding to the survival chances of *T. pallidum*.

TprC is a member of the *T. pallidum* repeat (Tpr) family of proteins. Analysis of the *T. pallidum* genome identified that the Tpr family consists of 12 members (A–L). The set of encoding genes comprise 2% of the total *T. pallidum* genome. There is homology between the Tpr proteins and the major sheath protein (Msp) of *T. denticola*. Msp has been implicated in pathogen binding to the ECM and as having porin capabilities (LaFond and Lukehart, 2006). Another candidate OMP of the Tpr family is TprK (TP0897). Initial observations indicated that TprK was a target for opsonic antibodies, but more recent studies could not confirm these results (Cox *et al.*, 2010). Immuno-labelling with a rat anti-TprK serum failed to stain intact *T. pallidum*, but detergent-treated treponemes and treponemes with a disrupted OM were immune reactive. Furthermore, in contrast to TP0326, TprK lacks amphiphilicity, and therefore doubt has arisen about the localization of TprK within the OM. The investigation of other members of the 'candidate OMP' list is ongoing, and in the coming years much more information on these molecules will become available (Cox *et al.*, 2010).

The lack of metabolic enzymes of *T. pallidum* has forced the organism to a lifestyle in which many nutrients are derived from the host environment, yet the lack of OMPs precludes the active uptake of molecules. The lack of LPS in the *T. pallidum* OM may render the organism more permeable to lipophilic compounds than *E. coli*, and it has been speculated that this may be a general feature of the *T. pallidum* OM (Radolf *et al.*, 2006). Recent investigation of TP0453, the only lipoprotein in *T. pallidum* that is associated with the OM, showed that it consists of an α-β-α fold and amphipathic helices, which make membrane integration possible (Luthra *et al.*, 2011). TP0453 is able to transform from a closed to an open conformation by lateral movement of part of the molecule. The insertion of TP0453 increases membrane permeability at acidic pH and indicates that the polypeptide could be acting as a porin. However, recent studies have shown that increased membrane permeability was not observed at physiological pH. The *Mycobacterium tuberculosis* genes LppX and LprG share structural similarity with TP0453 (Luthra *et al.*, 2011). These mycobacterial genes are involved in translocating complex lipids to the OM. This new information leaves *T. pallidum* again without any porin-like structures, and currently one has to assume that transport of molecules occurs either passively through a relatively permeable OM, or by as yet unidentified transporters.

The transport of nutrients from the periplasmic space to the cytosol is less impervious. Analysis of the *T. pallidum* genome identified 18 putative transporter systems including transporters for amino acids, carbohydrates and cations, and a few of these have already been characterized (Fraser *et al.*, 1998; Ho and Lukehart, 2011). The remainder of these predicted transporters awaits experimental validation. Most of the transporters are lipoproteins and belong to the ATP-binding cassette (ABC) superfamily. They can be viewed as periplasmic receptors located on the CM, inserted by their lipid tails (Cox *et al.*, 2010). For amino acid uptake, TP0655 (PotD) has been shown to be a polyamine receptor, and TP0821 (Tp32, MetQ) was shown to bind methionine. Multiple transporters for metal ions have been identified to date: TP0163 (TroA, formerly TROMP-1) can bind zinc, manganese and iron ions, TP0034 (ZnuA) is able to bind zinc, and TP0971 has been shown to interact with multiple cations and with human lactoferrin. Whether there is lactoferrin present in the periplasmic space and the mechanism by which it collects there through the OM have not been elucidated.

Multiple putative carbohydrate transporters are present in the *T. pallidum* genome and they are predicted transporters for glucose, galactose and ribose. The only ABC transporter that has been investigated extensively to date is TP0684 (LaFond and Lukehart, 2006). TP0684 (MglB2, Tp38) and perhaps also TP0545 (MglB1) can bind glucose and galactose. Although *T. pallidum* has been shown to take up mannose and maltose, the predominant energy source used is probably glucose, leaving the possibility that many other transporters have different specificity, which are only used under special conditions or are non-functional. Recently, a purine transporter (TP0319, PnrA), which is part of the *pnrABCDE* operon, has been found in *T. pallidum*.

Another class of transporter that is present in *T. pallidum* is a subfamily of the tripartite ATP-independent periplasmic transporters (TRAP-T), the so-called TPAT (TPR-protein-associated TRAP-Ts). This molecular complex consists of a TRAP-T plus a T-component (TatT) (Brautigam *et al.*, 2012). TatT forms a trimer that is anchored in the OM. Hydrophobic ligands, which still have to be identified, can be accepted by TatT, chaperoned through the periplasmic space and delivered to TatPt, which is located in the cytosolic membrane and subsequently delivered to the cytosol through TatM.

Transcriptional regulation in *T. pallidum* is only poorly understood. It is apparent that the presence of seven σ factors in *T. pallidum*, which has only one host, compared with *B. burgdorferi*, which has two hosts, indicates that gene regulation may occur at many levels. The *tpr* genes *E*, G and *J* are partially regulated by TP0262 (Giacani *et al.*, 2009), which has homology with the *E. coli* cAMP receptor protein, but the expression of the *tpr* genes is also influenced by an upstream poly(G) tract and possibly other transcription factors. The presence of genes with homology to adenylate cyclase (TP0485) (Matejkova *et al.*, 2008) and carbon catabolite repression proteins (TP0589, TP0591, HprK/Hpr homologues) indicates that intricate regulatory networks exist that allow *T. pallidum* to fine tune its gene expression in a changing environment.

12.3.2 Evasion of, and induction of, the immune response

T. pallidum interacts with components of the immune system in all the different stages of syphilis (LaFond and Lukehart, 2006). The localization of the immune response, such as site of primary infection, the blood or end organs such as the brain, and the stage of the infection (primary, secondary or tertiary) govern the characteristics of the immune response. The natural course of syphilis with a self-limiting primary stage and a secondary stage with relapses followed by the asymptomatic latency indicates that, over the years, a balance between persistence and host clearance is reached. Patients in the latent phase therefore have some degree of protection against progression of disease.

Patients with syphilis can be reinfected, although they have some degree of immunity. Observations in 19th century Dublin showed that mothers from infants with congenital syphilis did not develop chancres of the nipple, whereas wet nurses often did. Immunization of rabbits with γ-irradiated *T. pallidum* induces protection from challenge with intradermally injected homologous bacteria, despite the absence of opsonizing antibodies (LaFond and Lukehart, 2006).

Cellular immune response

During early infection, *T. pallidum* elicits an inflammatory response characterized by a transient influx of PMNLs, quickly followed by infiltrating T-cells, plasma cells and macrophages, which produce interleukin (IL)-2 and interferon (IFN)-γ. The innate immune response is further augmented by recognition of TP0574 (Tp47) by Toll-like receptor (TLR) 2, and stimulation of dendritic cells (DCs) with purified TP0574 leads to production of IL-1β, IL-6, IL-12 and tumour necrosis factor (TNF)-α (Bouis *et al.*, 2001).

The adaptive immune response is characterized by Th1 predominance, with induction of regulatory T-cells and transforming growth factor (TGF)-β production by TP1038 (miniferritin TpF1) (Babolin *et al.*, 2011), resulting in local clearance of the majority of treponemes and resolution of the primary lesions. *T. pallidum* lipoproteins that stimulate DCs are not localized in the OM but are periplasmic. The initiation of an adaptive immune response against these antigens will therefore not begin until the organisms have been degraded, presumably in the draining lymph nodes, and the antigens have been exposed to TLRs or other pattern-recognition receptors. DCs are able to engulf *T. pallidum* by coiling and conventional phagocytosis (Babolin *et al.*, 2011). Subsequently, the bacterium is transferred to membrane-bound vacuoles. The exact mechanisms by which the ingested treponemes are processed and degraded are unknown, but activation of immature DCs takes place during the phagocytic process (Bouis *et al.*, 2001; Shin *et al.*, 2004). *T. pallidum* stimulation of DCs has slower kinetics than for other bacteria. A delay in DC maturation and a consequently slower adaptive immune response could be responsible for a 'head start' for the bacterium and allow more time for haematogeneous dissemination.

There are few data on intracellular signal transduction pathways following infection with *T. pallidum*. Rat Kupffer cells produce reactive oxygen species after incubation with spirochaetes within 30 min of infection (Marangoni *et al.*, 2003). Lipoproteins such as TP0435 (Tp47), TP0574 (Tp47) and TP0751 induce the production of TNF-α, IL-1β and IL-6 in human monocytic cells. Stimulation of monocytes strongly activated nuclear factor (NF)-κB (Norgard *et al.*, 1996; Liu *et al.*, 2010b). Cytokine production could not be inhibited by inhibitors of the stress-activated protein kinase/c-Jun NH_2 terminal kinase (SAPK/JNK) pathway or the extracellular-signal-regulated kinase (ERK). However, blocking of TLR2, p38 and NF-κB signalling strongly reduced cytokine production by *T. pallidum*-infected cells, implicating an important function for these pathways. Other treponemes such as *T. denticola* were shown to induce actin rearrangement in fibroblasts, but for *T. pallidum* such studies are lacking.

In secondary syphilis, the skin lesions contain $CD4^+$ and $CD8^+$ T-cells (Salazar *et al.*, 2007; Cruz *et al.*, 2012), and both perforin and granzyme are expressed, suggesting that cytolytic processes are involved in bacterial clearance, and cross-presentation of treponemal antigens via MHC class I probably takes place. Further evidence for phagosomal processing is the upregulation of TLR7, -8 and -9 (Cruz *et al.*, 2012), which have been implicated in the recognition of bacterial components that are degraded within endosomes. The calculated ratio of spirochaetes to immune cells in the blood of secondary syphilis patients is about 1:1. Elegant experiments by Cruz *et al.* (2012) indicate that treponemes at this ratio do not mount a significant cytokine response and probably do not evoke an immune response when present in the blood. A surprising finding in these studies was the difference in immunophenotypic markers of immune cells and the decrease in natural killer (NK) cells, accompanied by the emergence of a specific subset of NK cells in secondary syphilis patients. The authors hypothesized that *T. pallidum* gained access to the bone marrow and interacted with macrophage–DC progenitors.

Recent studies in secondary syphilis patients have only been done in the skin, and due to ethical and practical reasons not in the brain. The main sources of information on the cellular immune response in neurosyphilis come from animal models or studies in the pre-penicillin era, when people could become severely ill from neurosyphilis and also died from the disease. The cellular reaction in the CSF of intrathecally infected macaques moved from mixed PMNLs/lymphocytic in week 1 to almost exclusively lymphocytic in week 4 after experimental infection (Marra *et al.*, 1998). These CSF lymphocytes were phenotyped in one animal. After 2 weeks, approximately 75% of lymphocytes were B-cells and 25% were T-cells. Two weeks later, the distribution was almost the reverse. The B-cells amounted to only about 20% of total lymphocytes in the CSF. Interestingly, $CD4^+$ and $CD8^+$ T-cells were present in almost equal numbers. PMNLs are present in acute syphilitic meningitis but the percentage is almost never above 25% (Ghanem, 2010). A study on the use of the fraction of B-lymphocytes as an adjunct in the diagnosis of neurosyphilis showed that, in HIV-infected patients, the percentage of B-cells was 0–24% of the total lymphocyte fraction. Unfortunately, the fraction of $CD4^+$ and $CD8^+$ T-cells was not reported (Marra *et al.*, 2004b). Collectively, these data indicate that, in secondary syphilis, the same cell types that are involved in skin lesions probably also govern the immune responses in the CNS.

Cerebral gummata are the manifestations of tertiary syphilis. A gumma consists of a dense inflammatory infiltrate with large numbers of lymphocytes, plasma cells and multinucleated giant cells (Fargen *et al.*, 2009). Sometimes they have a central necrotic core. Vascular proliferation, endarteritis and perivascular inflammation are invariably present. Despite its expected presence, *T. pallidum* is only rarely found in cerebral gummata.

Antibody response

Antibodies against *T. pallidum* lipoproteins can be readily identified in the blood of patients. These IgM and IgG antibodies have the capacity to opsonize bacteria and fix complement. Macrophages clear *T. pallidum* by phagocytosis of opsonized organisms (LaFond and Lukehart, 2006). The targets of the antibody response are widely divergent. Studies using protein arrays of *T. pallidum* identified at least 38 proteins that elicited a significant antibody response in syphilis patients in various stages of the disease (McGill *et al.*, 2010). Immunoreactivity against most of these antigens was present in all stages of the disease, but for selected antigens such as TP0133 (hypothetical protein), TP0136 (hypothetical protein), TP0326 (OMP), TP0398 (flagellar hook–basal body complex protein) and TP0663 (putative OMP), and the hypothetical proteins TP0584, TP0608 and TP0767, the antibody response was only detected in early syphilis patients, making these antigens attractive candidates for early seroscreening (McGill *et al.*, 2010). Other antigens include lipoproteins such as TP0171 (Tp15), TP0435 (Tp17) and TP0574 (Tp47). From the array data, TP0163 (TroA), TP0216 (Hsp70), TP0768 (TmpA) and TP1038 (TpF1) were already known to be targets of the antibody response. The array experiments and immunoblotting of 2D gels also identified new targets such as TP0684 (MglB2, Tp38) a periplasmic glucose/galactose transporter, TP0748 (cytoplasmic filament protein A, CfpA) and TP0965 (putative membrane fusion protein) (Brinkman *et al.*, 2006; McGill *et al.*, 2010).

In secondary syphilis, high titres of circulating antibodies are present in the blood of patients but they cannot prevent spirochaete dissemination. Passive transfer studies in rabbits have shown that immune rabbit serum partially protects against intradermal challenge (LaFond and Lukehart, 2006). Immunohistochemical staining of treponemes in microgel droplets has shown that only 5–10% of treponemes actually bind antibodies from both human syphilis patients and syphilis-infected rabbits (Cox *et al.*, 2010). There were individual differences of staining even within the same treponeme, indicating that treponemes exhibit different expression of antigenic surface molecules and that most *T. pallidum* cells truly earn their 'stealth' status. Other *in vitro* studies have demonstrated that human macrophages destroy a small fraction of opsonized *T. pallidum*, and most of the bacteria can be recovered from the culture medium (LaFond and Lukehart, 2006). These results are in line with earlier observations that a substantial fraction of treponemes evade opsonization and macrophage uptake in syphilis lesions.

VDRL antibodies are directed against cardiolipin, which is present in *T. pallidum* (Cameron, 2006). These antibodies promote opsonization and phagocytosis by macrophages, but VDRL antibodies are not bound to the surface of *T. pallidum*. Although syphilis serum contains antibodies against a number of surface molecules, these molecules are obviously not accessible by circulating antibodies. Disrupted and detergent-treated *T. pallidum* were all readily stained by specific antisera and syphilis serum, confirming the reactivity of the sera (Cox *et al.*, 2010).

Collectively, the results confirm that the immune response against *T. pallidum* antigens is mainly directed against antigens that are shielded in intact treponemes, either because they are located in the periplasm or CM or by as yet undefined mechanisms that take place in the OM. During infection, only a fraction of the bacteria are removed by macrophages and significant amounts of bacteria can make their way to the bloodstream and CNS, without recognition by circulating antibodies.

12.3.3 Genomic variation

T. pallidum can escape detection by the immune system through antigenic variation. Sequence variation has been observed in the TprC, -D, -J and -K regions. The TprK (TP0897) protein is the best studied. During experimental infection, a strong antibody and T-cell immune response is elicited against TprK, and immunization with recombinant TprK provides partial immunity against infectious challenge (Ho and Lukehart, 2011). However, there is debate over whether TprK is surface exposed or a target for opsonizing antibodies (Cox *et al.*, 2010). In the rabbit model, TprK accumulates sequence variation following the development of acquired immunity. Molecular studies of TprK show that new variants are formed during infection by acquiring genetic information from donor sites elsewhere on the chromosome (Giacani *et al.*, 2012). These new variants are not recognized by antibodies that were formed against the TprK variant that infected the individual. Individual *T. pallidum* strains differ in their ability to generate TprK variants in the V6 variable region. Treponemes that have escaped the first line of defence presumably have time to mutate and rearrange their genes. This is a very attractive hypothesis, although the lack of labelling of intact spirochaetes remains puzzling. Detailed examination of the *T. pallidum* SS14 genome indicates that intra-strain variation can also occur in other loci. In addition to *tpr*-related sequences, other genes such as TP0402 (flagellum-specific ATP synthase), TP0971 (membrane antigen) and TP1029 (hypothetical protein) display intra-strain variation (Smajs *et al.*, 2012).

A long-standing question is whether specific strains of *T. pallidum* are more neuroinvasive than others. Until now, only relatively crude typing methods such as restriction fragment length polymorphism of three *tpr* genes (*tprE* (TP0313), *tprG* (TP0317), *tprJ* (TP0621)) combined with determining the number of 60 base pair repeats in the acidic repeat protein (Arp, TP0433) have been used. A study by Marra *et al.* (2010a) demonstrated that 50% of patients with strain type 14d/f had neurosyphilis, compared with only 23% in other types. Other evidence for strain-related factors in the development of neurosyphilis comes from a rabbit study in which six different *T. pallidum* strains showed different patterns of induction of CSF pleiocytosis when infected intravenously (Tantalo *et al.*, 2005). However, the strain that showed the highest level of CSF pleiocytosis, but the lowest level of skin lesions, was the Sea 81-4 strain, type 14 e/b. In South Africa, 14a was the most frequently identified type in neurosyphilis patients (Molepo *et al.*, 2007). In human studies, all types found in patients with neurosyphilis were also found in patients without neurological disease (Marra *et al.*, 2010a). A recent development in *T. pallidum* typing has been the adoption of sequencing-based methods. Initially the sequence of TP0548 was added to the typing scheme and the inclusion of TP0136 and 23S rDNA has also been proposed.

The observations on increased frequency of certain subtypes must be interpreted with caution because these studies are readily subject to inclusion bias, the numbers of patients/strains is low and some of the typing methods do not have high resolution. The results of different typing studies indicate that neuroinvasion is not restricted to specific subtypes, interspecies variation occurs, and genetic diversity within *T. pallidum* strains is geographically specific. Studies that compare the genomes of different *Treponema pallidum* strains and related organisms such as *Treponema pertenue* and *T. paraluiscuniculi* have revealed that these uncultivable treponemes share more than 99% sequence homology and that the *T. pallidum* strains are genetically monomorphic (Smajs *et al.*, 2012). The number of nucleotide changes between the strains examined so far is only a few hundred, which comes close to the number that has been documented within a single strain. Therefore, it is conceivable that, under the influence of the immune system and during the years or decades that *T. pallidum* live in a host, minimal genetic variations arise that influence the biological behaviour of a strain.

12.4 Conclusions

Syphilis is characterized by a continuing quest for the balance between bacterial virulence and host clearance mechanisms. During the initial infection, spirochaetes escape the first line of defence and gain access to many organs through the blood. The special characteristics of the OM allow treponemes to travel through the body in an undisturbed fashion. Once they have penetrated the end organs such as the brain, the immune system keeps the infection localized. With advancing age and immuno-senescence the balance shifts towards the bacterium, leading to an upsurge of inflammatory reactions and consequently a recurrence of symptoms.

References

Angel, T.E., Jacobs, J.M., Smith, R.P., Pasternack, M.S., Elias, S., Gritsenko, M.A., Shukla, A., Gilmore, E.C., McCarthy, C., Camp, D.G., 2nd, Smith, R.D. and Warren, H.S. (2012) Cerebrospinal fluid proteome of patients with acute lyme disease. *Journal of Proteome Research* 11, 4814–4822.

Babolin, C., Amedei, A., Ozolins, D., Zilevica, A., D'Elios, M.M. and de Bernard, M. (2011) TpF1 from *Treponema pallidum* activates inflammasome and promotes the development of regulatory T cells. *Journal of Immunology* 187, 1377–1384.

Bouis, D.A., Popova, T.G., Takashima, A. and Norgard, M.V. (2001) Dendritic cells phagocytose and are activated by *Treponema pallidum*. *Infection and Immunity* 69, 518–528.

Brautigam, C.A., Deka, R.K., Schuck, P., Tomchick, D.R. and Norgard, M.V. (2012) Structural and thermodynamic characterization of the interaction between two periplasmic *Treponema pallidum* lipoproteins that are components of a TPR-protein-associated TRAP transporter (TPAT). *Journal of Molecular Biology* 420, 70–86.

Brinkman, M.B., McKevitt, M., McLoughlin, M., Perez, C., Howell, J., Weinstock, G.M., Norris, S.J. and Palzkill, T. (2006) Reactivity of antibodies from syphilis patients to a protein array representing the *Treponema pallidum* proteome. *Journal of Clinical Microbiology* 44, 888–891.

Cameron, C.E. (2006) The *T. pallidum* outer membrane and outer membrane proteins. In: Radolf, J.D. and Lukehart, S.A. (eds) *Pathogenic Treponema: Molecular and Cellular Biology*. Caister Academic Press, Wymondham, pp. 237–266.

Cameron, C.E., Brown, E.L., Kuroiwa, J.M., Schnapp, L.M. and Brouwer, N.L. (2004) *Treponema pallidum* fibronectin-binding proteins. *Journal of Bacteriology* 186, 7019–7022.

Cox, D.L., Luthra, A., Dunham-Ems, S., Desrosiers, D.C., Salazar, J.C., Caimano, M.J. and Radolf, J.D. (2010) Surface immunolabeling and consensus computational framework to identify candidate rare outer membrane proteins of *Treponema pallidum*. *Infection and Immunity* 78, 5178–5194.

Cruz, A.R., *et al.* (2012) Immune evasion and recognition of the syphilis spirochete in blood and skin of secondary syphilis patients: two immunologically distinct compartments. *PLoS Neglected Tropical Diseases* 6, e1717.

Desrosiers, D.C., Anand, A., Luthra, A., Dunham-Ems, S.M., LeDoyt, M., Cummings, M.A., Eshghi, A., Cameron, C.E., Cruz, A.R., Salazar, J.C., Caimano, M.J. and Radolf, J.D. (2011) TP0326, a *Treponema pallidum* β-barrel assembly machinery A (BamA) orthologue and rare outer membrane protein. *Molecular Microbiology* 80, 1496–1515.

Fargen, K.M., Alvernia, J.E., Lin, C.S. and Melgar, M. (2009) Cerebral syphilitic gummata: a case presentation and analysis of 156 reported cases. *Neurosurgery* 64, 568–575.

Fraser, C.M., *et al.* (1998) Complete genome sequence of *Treponema pallidum*, the syphilis spirochete. *Science* 281, 375–388.

Ghanem, K.G. (2010) Neurosyphilis: a historical perspective and review. *CNS Neuroscience and Therapeutics* 16, e157–168.

Giacani, L., Godornes, C., Puray-Chavez, M., Guerra-Giraldez, C., Tompa, M., Lukehart, S.A. and Centurion-Lara, A. (2009) TP0262 is a modulator of promoter activity of *tpr* subfamily II genes of *Treponema pallidum* ssp. *pallidum*. *Molecular Microbiology* 72, 1087–1099.

Giacani, L., Brandt, S.L., Puray-Chavez, M., Reid, T.B., Godornes, C., Molini, B.J., Benzler, M., Hartig, J.S., Lukehart, S.A. and Centurion-Lara, A. (2012) Comparative investigation of the genomic regions involved in antigenic variation of the TprK antigen among treponemal species, subspecies, and strains. *Journal of Bacteriology* 194, 4208–4225.

Ho, E.L. and Lukehart, S.A. (2011) Syphilis: using modern approaches to understand an old disease. *Journal of Clinical Investigation* 121, 4584–4592.

Houston, S., Hof, R., Francescutti, T., Hawkes, A., Boulanger, M.J. and Cameron, C.E. (2011) Bifunctional role of the *Treponema pallidum* extracellular matrix binding adhesin Tp0751. *Infection and Immunity* 79, 1386–1398.

Izard, J., Renken, C., Hsieh, C.E., Desrosiers, D.C., Dunham-Ems, S., La Vake, C., Gebhardt, L.L., Limberger, R.J., Cox, D.L., Marko, M. and Radolf, J.D. (2009) Cryo-electron tomography elucidates the molecular architecture of *Treponema pallidum*, the syphilis spirochete. *Journal of Bacteriology* 191, 7566–7580.

Juanpere-Rodero, N., Martin-Ezquerra, G., Fernandez-Casado, A., Magan-Perea, L., Garcia-Alguacil, M.A., Barranco-Sanz, C., Serrano-Figueras, S., Pujol-Vallverdu, R.M. and

Lloreta-Trull, J. (2013) Cell and tissue interactions of *Treponema pallidum* in primary and secondary syphilitic skin lesions: an ultrastructural study of serial sections. *Ultrastructural Pathology* 37, 36–42.

LaFond, R.E. and Lukehart, S.A. (2006) Biological basis for syphilis. *Clinical Microbiology Reviews* 19, 29–49.

Liu, J., Howell, J.K., Bradley, S.D., Zheng, Y., Zhou, Z.H. and Norris, S.J. (2010a) Cellular architecture of *Treponema pallidum*: novel flagellum, periplasmic cone, and cell envelope as revealed by cryo electron tomography. *Journal of Molecular Biology* 403, 546–561.

Liu, S., Wang, S., Wu, Y., Zhao, F., Zeng, T., Zhang, Y., Zhang, Q. and Gao, D. (2010b) Production of proinflammatory cytokines in the human THP-1 monocyte cell line following induction by Tp0751, a recombinant protein of *Treponema pallidum*. *Science China Life Sciences* 53, 229–233.

Lukehart, S.A., Hook, E.W., 3rd, Baker-Zander, S.A., Collier, A.C., Critchlow, C.W. and Handsfield, H.H. (1988) Invasion of the central nervous system by *Treponema pallidum*: implications for diagnosis and treatment. *Annals of Internal Medicine* 109, 855–862.

Luthra, A., Zhu, G., Desrosiers, D.C., Eggers, C.H., Mulay, V., Anand, A., McArthur, F.A., Romano, F.B., Caimano, M.J., Heuck, A.P., Malkowski, M.G. and Radolf, J.D. (2011) The transition from closed to open conformation of *Treponema pallidum* outer membrane-associated lipoprotein TP0453 involves membrane sensing and integration by two amphipathic helices. *Journal of Biological Chemistry* 286, 1656–1668.

Marangoni, A., Aldini, R., Guardigli, M., Sambri, V., Giacani, L., Montagnani, M., Roda, A. and Cevenini, R. (2003) Phagocytosis of *Treponema pallidum* and reactive oxygen species production by isolated rat Kupffer cells. *Medical Microbiology and Immunology* 192, 183–188.

Marra, C., Baker-Zander, S.A., Hook, E.W., 3rd and Lukehart, S.A. (1991) An experimental model of early central nervous system syphilis. *Journal of Infectious Diseases* 163, 825–829.

Marra, C.M., Castro, C.D., Kuller, L., Dukes, A.C., Centurion-Lara, A., Morton, W.R. and Lukehart, S.A. (1998) Mechanisms of clearance of *Treponema pallidum* from the CSF in a nonhuman primate model. *Neurology* 51, 957–961.

Marra, C.M., *et al.* (2004a) Cerebrospinal fluid abnormalities in patients with syphilis: association with clinical and laboratory features. *Journal of Infectious Diseases* 189, 369–376.

Marra, C.M., Tantalo, L.C., Maxwell, C.L., Dougherty, K. and Wood, B. (2004b) Alternative cerebrospinal fluid tests to diagnose neurosyphilis in HIV-infected individuals. *Neurology* 63, 85–88.

Marra, C., *et al.* (2010a) Enhanced molecular typing of *Treponema pallidum*: geographical distribution of strain types and association with neurosyphilis. *Journal of Infectious Diseases* 202, 1380–1388.

Marra, C.M., Tantalo, L.C., Sahi, S.K., Maxwell, C.L. and Lukehart, S.A. (2010b) CXCL13 as a cerebrospinal fluid marker for neurosyphilis in HIV-infected patients with syphilis. *Sexually Transmitted Diseases* 37, 283–287.

Matejkova, P., *et al.* (2008) Complete genome sequence of *Treponema pallidum* ssp. *pallidum* strain SS14 determined with oligonucleotide arrays. *BMC Microbiology* 8, 76.

McGill, M.A., Edmondson, D.G., Carroll, J.A., Cook, R.G., Orkiszewski, R.S. and Norris, S.J. (2010) Characterization and serologic analysis of the *Treponema pallidum* proteome. *Infection and Immunity* 78, 2631–2643.

Molepo, J., Pillay, A., Weber, B., Morse, S.A. and Hoosen, A.A. (2007) Molecular typing of *Treponema pallidum* strains from patients with neurosyphilis in Pretoria, South Africa. *Sexually Transmitted Infections* 83, 189–192.

Norgard, M.V., Arndt, L.L., Akins, D.R., Curetty, L.L., Harrich, D.A. and Radolf, J.D. (1996) Activation of human monocytic cells by *Treponema pallidum* and *Borrelia burgdorferi* lipoproteins and synthetic lipopeptides proceeds via a pathway distinct from that of lipopolysaccharide but involves the transcriptional activator NF-κ B. *Infection and Immunity* 64, 3845–3852.

Oakes, S.G., Repesh, L.A., Pozos, R.S. and Fitzgerald, T.J. (1982) Electrophysiological dysfunction and cellular disruption of sensory neurones during incubation with *Treponema pallidum*. *British Journal of Venereal Diseases* 58, 220–227.

Peeling, R.W. and Hook, E.W., 3rd (2006) The pathogenesis of syphilis: the Great Mimicker, revisited. *Journal of Pathology* 208, 224–232.

Radolf, J.D., Hazlett, K.R. and Lukehart, S.A. (2006) Pathogenesis of syphilis. In: Radolf, J.D. and Lukehart, S.A. (eds) *Pathogenic Treponema: Molecular and Cellular Biology*. Caister Academic Press, Wymondham, pp. 197–236.

Repesh, L.A., Fitzgerald, T.J., Oakes, S.G. and Pozos, R.S. (1982) Scanning electron microscopy of the attachment of *Treponema pallidum* to nerve cells in vitro. *British Journal of Venereal Diseases* 58, 211–219.

Rothschild, B.M. (2005) History of syphilis. *Clinical Infectious Diseases* 40, 1454–1463.

Salazar, J.C., Cruz, A.R., Pope, C.D., Valderrama, L., Trujillo, R., Saravia, N.G. and Radolf, J.D. (2007) *Treponema pallidum* elicits innate and adaptive cellular immune responses in skin and blood during secondary syphilis: a flow-cytometric analysis. *Journal of Infectious Diseases* 195, 879–887.

Sell, S. and Salman, J. (1992) Demonstration of *Treponema pallidum* in axons of cutaneous nerves in experimental chancres of rabbits. *Sexually Transmitted Diseases* 19, 1–6.

Shin, J.L., Chung, K.Y., Kang, J.M., Lee, T.H. and Lee, M.G. (2004) The effects of *Treponema pallidum* on human dendritic cells. *Yonsei Medical Journal* 45, 515–522.

Smajs, D., Norris, S.J. and Weinstock, G.M. (2012) Genetic diversity in *Treponema pallidum*: implications for pathogenesis, evolution and molecular diagnostics of syphilis and yaws. *Infection, Genetics and Evolution* 12, 191–202.

Tantalo, L.C., Lukehart, S.A. and Marra, C.M. (2005) *Treponema pallidum* strain-specific differences in neuroinvasion and clinical phenotype in a rabbit model. *Journal of Infectious Diseases* 191, 75–80.

Thomas, D.D., Navab, M., Haake, D.A., Fogelman, A.M., Miller, J.N. and Lovett, M.A. (1988) *Treponema pallidum* invades intercellular junctions of endothelial cell monolayers. *Proceedings of the National Academy of Sciences USA* 85, 3608–3612.

Tsai, H.C., Ye, S.Y., Kunin, C.M., Lee, S.S., Wann, S.R., Tai, M.H., Shi, M.H., Liu, Y.C. and Chen, Y.S. (2011) Expression of matrix metalloproteinases and their tissue inhibitors in the serum and cerebrospinal fluid of patients with HIV-1 infection and syphilis or neurosyphilis. *Cytokine* 54, 106–116.

13 *Streptococcus suis* Meningitis

Marcelo Gottschalk,[1]* Nahuel Fittipaldi[2] and Mariela Segura[1]
[1] *University of Montreal, Québec, Canada;* [2] *The Methodist Hospital Research Institute, Houston, USA*

13.1 Introduction

Streptococcus suis is a major swine pathogen responsible for important economic losses to the porcine industry worldwide. The natural habitat of *S. suis* (not necessarily virulent strains) is the upper respiratory tract of pigs, particularly the tonsils and nasal cavities, and also the genital and alimentary tracts (Gottschalk, 2012). Although pig carrier rates are near 100%, the incidence of disease in swine in a specific farm varies over time and is generally less than 5%, mainly due to the use of preventative or therapeutic antimicrobials (Gottschalk, 2012). However, in the absence of antibiotics, mortality rates can reach 20% (Cloutier *et al.*, 2003). In peracute cases, pigs may be found dead with no premonitory signs. Meningitis is the most striking feature and is often the basis of a presumptive diagnosis, although other kinds of infections also occur such as arthritis, endocarditis, pneumonia and polyserositis (Gottschalk, 2012).

S. suis is an important emerging zoonotic agent, and human cases of *S. suis* infections have been documented in several European and Asian countries as well as in North and South America, Australia and New Zealand (Gottschalk *et al.*, 2010). Infections in humans have been considered for a long time to be sporadic, have low prevalence and only affect people working with pigs or pork-derived products (Gottschalk *et al.*, 2010). However, two important outbreaks that occurred recently in China, which affected more than 200 people with a mortality rate of nearly 20%, changed the perspective and/or the perception of the threat posed by this pathogen to human health (Ye *et al.*, 2006).

From the pathogenesis point of view, highly virulent serotypes of *S. suis*, like Group B *Streptococcus* (GBS), possess a capsule rich in sialic acid. Both pathogens can cause meningitis, but the interactions of *S. suis* with host cells and especially the immune system are quite unique and highly different from those of GBS (Segura, 2012). In this chapter, we will present the current knowledge on the cellular and molecular mechanisms used by *S. suis* to cause meningitis.

13.2 Aetiological Agent and Epidemiology of the Infection

S. suis (originally and wrongly designated as 'Lancefield groups R, S, RS and T') (Gottschalk *et al.*, 2007) is an α-haemolytic encapsulated Gram-positive coccus that possesses cell-wall

*marcelo.gottschalk@umontreal.ca

antigenic determinants somewhat related to Lancefield group D. There are 35 serotypes described to date, and the composition of the capsular polysaccharides (CPS) defines the serotype (Gottschalk, 2012). Most *S. suis* organisms isolated from diseased pigs belong to a limited number of serotypes, often between 1 and 9. However, *S. suis* serotype 2 and, to a lesser extent, serotype 14 strains are considered serious and high-risk zoonotic agents (Gottschalk *et al.*, 2010). Serotypes 1, 4, 5, 16 and 24 have occasionally been isolated from diseased humans (Nghia *et al.*, 2008; Gottschalk *et al.*, 2010; Kerdsin *et al.*, 2011). Available information regarding epidemiology in humans, virulence factors and pathogenesis of the infection are almost exclusively related to serotype 2 strains.

In Western countries, *S. suis* disease has been considered a rare event in humans. Most cases are related to employment in the swine industry: pig farmers, abattoir workers, persons transporting pork, meat inspectors, butchers and veterinarians (Gottschalk *et al.*, 2010). *S. suis* infections are a main cause of piglet deaths in North America (Gottschalk, 2012), but the prevalence of *S. suis* serotype 2 strains isolated from diseased pigs and humans is much lower on this continent than in Europe and Asia, and other non-zoonotic serotypes are also prevalent in swine (Fittipaldi *et al.*, 2009b). The large majority of reported cases in Western countries of *S. suis* infection in humans are from Europe, and only three cases of human infection (two cases of serotype 2 and one of serotype 14) have been reported in Canada (Gottschalk *et al.*, 2010) and only one case (serotype 2) has been confirmed so far in mainland USA (Willenburg *et al.*, 2006). However, a serological survey in the USA indicated that swine-exposed persons had higher titres of antibodies to *S. suis* than non-swine-exposed persons (Smith *et al.*, 2008). A relatively lower virulence of strains has been suggested to be, at least in part, responsible for the low number of *S. suis* human cases in North America (Fittipaldi *et al.*, 2011, 2012).

The situation in South-east Asian countries differs greatly from Western countries. Human disease in these countries is very common and for a long time it has been underdiagnosed. Many characteristics differentiate South-east Asian from developed Western countries: lifestyle, the common use of backyard systems of production and the close contact of humans with pigs (Fig. 13.1), as well as contact among different animal species (Fig. 13.2), which would greatly increase exchange of pathogens. Hogs are sometimes either home slaughtered or handled in improvised open abattoirs. In addition, open markets are very common, increasing the risk of contact with contaminated raw pork or pork products (Wertheim *et al.*, 2009a; Gottschalk *et al.*, 2010). Recent studies have shown that the most important risk factors associated with *S. suis* bacterial meningitis are eating 'high-risk' dishes popular in some countries of Asia, occupational exposure to pigs and pig products, and preparation of pork in the presence of skin lesions (Gottschalk *et al.*, 2010). *S. suis* is the first cause of adult meningitis in Vietnam, the second in Thailand and the third most common cause of community-acquired bacterial meningitis in Hong Kong (Suankratay *et al.*, 2004; Mai *et al.*, 2008; Gottschalk *et al.*, 2010). Although consumption of raw meat is not necessarily common in other parts of Asia, e.g. China, family ingestion of meat from diseased animals may occur, increasing the risk of handling highly contaminated meat. Most strains isolated in Asia possess similar characteristics and virulence to strains isolated in Europe; the exception would be a highly virulent clonal strain isolated in China and responsible not only for meningitis but mainly for streptococcal toxic shock-like syndrome (STSLS) (Ye *et al.*, 2006).

In humans, adults are by far the targeted population affected by this pathogen (Wertheim *et al.*, 2009b). There are several potential routes of entry of the organism: (i) a small cut in the skin, although in some cases no wound was detected; (ii) the nasopharynx, as observed in swine; and (iii) the gastrointestinal tract, as suggested by diarrhoea as a prodromal symptom, as well as the oral route of contamination in some Asian countries, e.g. Vietnam and Cambodia, where consumption of fresh and/or raw pork is a common practice, accounting for most

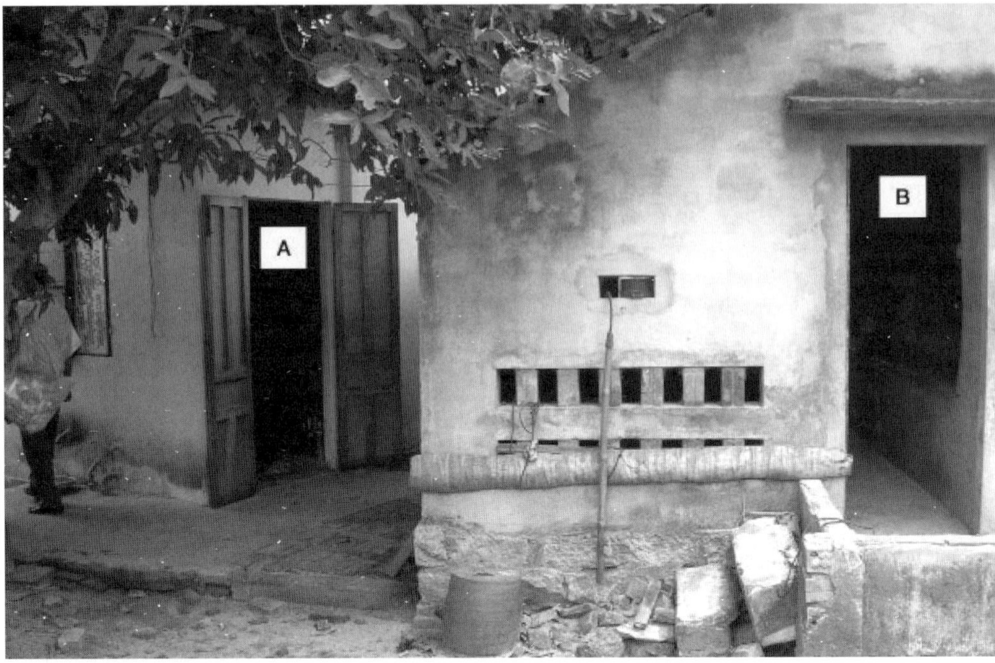

Fig. 13.1. A representative backyard production system in Asian countries: (A) owner's home; (B) pig production site.

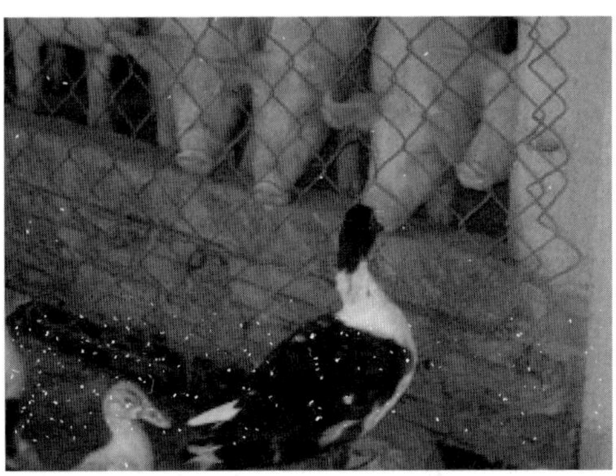

Fig. 13.2. Intimate contact among different animal species in an Asian backyard production system.

infection cases of people who are not normally in contact with the swine industry. The incubation period ranges from a few hours to 2 days. Affected patients have generally been healthy prior to infection with *S. suis,* although predisposing factors such as splenectomy, diabetes mellitus, alcoholism, malignancy and structural heart diseases have been suggested to increase the risk (Wertheim *et al.,* 2009b). Although *S. suis* disease in humans generally occurs sporadically without obvious seasonal change, a certain tendency for infections to occur during the rainy and hottest months of the year has been suggested (Gottschalk *et al.,* 2010). These conditions might favour the persistence of biological aerosols in the environment. Mortality rates vary from less than 3% (mostly developed Western countries) to more than 26% (some Asian countries) (Gottschalk *et al.,* 2010).

13.3 Clinical Pathology of *Streptococcus suis* Meningitis

Usually, patients with acute *S. suis* meningitis will present turbid cerebrospinal fluid (CSF), with more than 10^3 leucocytes/µl (>80% of polymorphonuclear cells), high protein and low glucose concentrations (Fittipaldi *et al.,* 2009a; Huh *et al.,* 2011). Although magnetic resonance imaging sometimes shows abnormal enhancement of the leptomeninges, diffuse cortical oedema and/or vascular congestion/inflammation of the sulci (Fittipaldi *et al.*, 2009a; Huh *et al.*, 2011), in many cases there are no significant changes in images (Camporese *et al.*, 2007). Gram staining of the CSF would usually lead to a misidentification, as *Listeria monocytogenes, Streptococcus pneumoniae* or other pathogens are usually suspected as the causative agent (Huang *et al.*, 2005; Gottschalk *et al.*, 2007). Real-time polymerase chain reaction (PCR) specific for *S. suis* serotype 2 is used in some Asian countries (Mai *et al.*, 2008), but this test will not detect other serotypes causing meningitis, e.g. serotype 14 (Kerdsin *et al.*, 2009; Gottschalk *et al.*, 2010).

A high percentage of *S. suis* meningitis patients will develop significant temporary or long-term hearing loss, with or without vestibular dysfunction. Hearing loss in *S. suis* meningitis is sensineural, is in the high-frequency range and can be profound (Wertheim *et al.*, 2009b). This incidence can reach 50% and 73% in Europe and Asia, respectively (Gottschalk *et al.*, 2010); these figures are consistently higher than those reported for other meningitis-causing bacteria that cause auditory dysfunction, e.g. *S. pneumoniae, Neisseria meningitidis* and *Haemophilus influenzae*. The prognosis for hearing is guarded; some patients improve over time, and others do not. Animal experiments and human electrophysiological studies suggest the cochlea as the site of the lesion and not direct infection of the auditory nerves or brainstem encephalitis. *S. suis* is believed to enter the perilymph via the cochlear aqueduct (Tan *et al.*, 2010). Bilateral labyrinthine haemorrhage, probably secondary to the underlying infective and inflammatory processes, has been described in humans and animal models (Tan *et al.*, 2010; Dominguez-Punaro *et al.*, 2012).

Details available on the pathological lesions caused by *S. suis* in the central nervous system (CNS) concern almost exclusively pigs. In human cases of STSLS, although no clear signs of clinical meningitis were present, mild cerebral, some neuron degeneration, neuronophagia and satellite phenomena could be observed (Yang *et al.*, 2009). An autopsy carried out on a fatal case of human meningitis showed leptomeningitis with moderate arachnoid fibrosis (Hantson *et al.*, 1991). In swine, the dura mater is thickened and congested (Zheng *et al.*, 2009). The surfaces of the gyri are flattened as a result of compression of the swollen brain by the dura mater and inner surface of the skull. The cerebellar sulci are shallow, and the volume of flavescent CSF is increased. Microscopically, haemorrhage and profuse exudates of neutrophils with fewer macrophages are observed in cerebral dura mater and large numbers of neutrophils fill the subarachnoid (SAS) and subpial spaces. The meningeal vessels are turgescent, containing intraluminal neutrophils and macrophages. Encephalitis is sometimes observed, associated with marked cerebral oedema, characterized by broadening of perivascular and pericelluar spaces, massive infiltration of neutrophils and considerable acute necrosis of neurons. Virchow–Robin spaces are distended, and endothelial cells in capillaries are swollen. Choroid plexitis, ventriculitis and optic perineuritis are usually suppurative (Zheng *et al.*, 2009).

13.4 Pathogenesis of Meningitis

13.4.1 Bacteraemia: an essential prerequisite for meningitis

Bacteraemia is a key factor for *S. suis* meningitis. Mechanisms that enable *S. suis* to disseminate throughout the host are not completely understood. The bacterium is able to spread systemically mainly from the nasopharynx (pigs) or through wounds and abrasions in the skin or through the gastrointestinal tract (humans), resulting in bacteraemia and, sometimes, septicaemia (Gottschalk and Segura, 2000). It is not known how *S. suis*, despite its small quantities on mucosal surfaces, is able to traverse this first line of host defence to disseminate and initiate disease (Gottschalk and Segura, 2000). Bacteria must be able to breach respiratory (pigs) and/or intestinal (humans) mucosal epithelia; however, very few studies have investigated the interactions between *S. suis* and epithelial cells, and many of these have produced contradictory results (Gottschalk and Segura, 2000). Cell-wall adhesins of *S. suis* appear to be hindered by the CPS, as suggested by the fact that *S. suis* CPS-deficient mutants adhered better than the encapsulated parental strain to porcine (LLC-PK1 and PK15), canine (MDCK) and human (A549 and HeLa) cell lines (Fittipaldi *et al.*, 2011). In addition, pretreatment of tracheal cells with the 39 kDa glyceraldehyde-3-phosphate dehydrogenase protein of *S. suis* significantly reduced pathogen adherence to porcine tracheal rings and the HEp-2 epithelial cell line, suggesting its involvement in the first steps of bacterial colonization (Fittipaldi *et al.*, 2012). Many other putative virulence factor proteins have been shown to interfere with the adhesion of *S. suis* to HEp-2 cells, but the mechanisms for such reduced adherence have not yet been deduced (Fittipaldi *et al.*, 2012).

To achieve high levels of bacteraemia, *S. suis* must avoid phagocytosis and killing. An early theory suggested uptake of bacteria by monocytes (in the absence of specific antibodies), intracellular survival and invasion of the CNS by the 'Trojan horse theory' (Williams and Blakemore, 1990a). Early studies carried out with flow cytometry also indicated high uptake of *S. suis* by swine and human phagocytes (Busque *et al.*, 1998). However, positive results obtained by flow cytometry studies were the result of high numbers of bacteria associated with (but not inside) phagocytes and the lack of appropriate quenching. In fact, high levels of adhesion (without phagocytosis) of *S. suis* to macrophages has been described (Segura and Gottschalk, 2002), which led to a 'modified Trojan horse theory', where bacteria can be largely bound but not ingested by phagocytes, thus being responsible for persistent bacteraemia and disseminated infection (Gottschalk and Segura, 2000). The fact that *S. suis* should be considered as a real extracellular pathogen has been well documented during the last 15 years, with studies showing that CPS protects *S. suis* from neutrophil-monocyte/macrophage- and dendritic cell-mediated phagocytosis and killing, in models using murine, swine and human cells (Gottschalk and Segura, 2000; Fittipaldi *et al.*, 2012; Meijerink *et al.*, 2012). Mechanisms used by *S. suis* to avoid phagocytosis have recently been suggested: upon contact with macrophages, encapsulated *S. suis*, as well as purified CPS, were shown to destabilize lipid microdomains at the cell surface, to block nitric oxide (NO) production, and to prevent lactosylceramide accumulation at the phagocytic cup (Houde *et al.*, 2012). Several different *in vitro* and *in vivo* experiments using isogenic unencapsulated mutant strains have conclusively shown that the absence of CPS correlates with highly increased phagocytosis and/or killing of these strains by phagocytic cells, and a rapid clearance of the bacteria from circulation (Gottschalk and Segura, 2000; Fittipaldi *et al.*, 2012). The structure of the *S. suis* serotype 2 CPS shows the presence of galactose (Gal), 6-linked Gal, 3,4-linked Gal, 4-linked *N*-acetyl-glucosamine (GlcNAc) and 3,4-linked rhamnose. In addition, *S. suis* CPS, similar to GBS, also contains *N*-acetyl-neuraminic acid (sialic acid) residues that are terminally linked (different linkage in both pathogens) to the CPS chain (Van Calsteren *et al.*, 2010). Capsular sialic acid is important for preventing deposition of the complement protein C3 on the surface of GBS, therefore blocking activation of the alternative pathway and allowing GBS resistance to opsonin-dependent intracellular killing (Marques *et al.*, 1992). Such a role has not yet been demonstrated for *S. suis* sialic acid. It is worth noting that the capsules of *S. suis* serotypes 2 and 14, which cause most disease in humans, possess sialic acid (Van Calsteren *et al.*, 2010).

Despite the critical role played by CPS in *S. suis* virulence, the fact that a strain is encapsulated does not imply that the strain is virulent. Some avirulent serotype 2 field strains are well encapsulated (Gottschalk and Segura, 2000; Fittipaldi *et al.*, 2012), indicating that *S. suis* survival in blood does not rely solely on encapsulation. For instance, it has been shown that well-encapsulated avirulent strains are eliminated from blood within 48 h, whereas a virulent strain persists in circulation at relatively high titres for several days (Dominguez-Punaro *et al.*, 2007). Resistance to phagocytosis is multifactorial and seems to also require modification of the cell-wall peptidoglycan and lipoteichoic acid (LTA) (Fittipaldi *et al.*, 2008a,b; Lecours *et al.*, 2011). Although not considered a critical virulence factor, a haemolysin (called suilysin) (Jacobs *et al.*, 1994), which is closely related to the pneumolysin of *S. pneumoniae*, has been suggested to play a role in *S. suis* survival, being toxic for different cells (Fittipaldi *et al.*, 2012). Suilysin was also shown to modulate complement-mediated opsonophagocytosis (Lecours *et al.*, 2011). Unlike the strains isolated in Europe and Asia, more than 95% of serotype 2 *S. suis* strains recovered in North America do not produce this toxin (Gottschalk and Segura, 2000; Fittipaldi *et al.*, 2009b). Other factors, such as nutrients, may also be important for survival in blood (Fittipaldi *et al.*, 2012).

13.4.2 How does *S. suis* reach the CNS?

Interactions with brain microvascular endothelial cells: blood–brain barrier (BBB)

Presence of *S. suis* in the bloodstream may be followed by septicaemia, septic shock and/or STSLS (Gottschalk *et al.*, 2010). However, in many cases, septic disease is not present, and bacteria can remain in the blood for many days without any clinical signs, as shown in mouse models. High levels of bacteraemia will usually lead to CNS invasion and meningitis (Dominguez-Punaro *et al.*, 2007). As with other blood-borne pathogens, *S. suis* must cross the BBB and/or the blood–CSF barrier (BCSFB) in order to cause CNS infections. The main cellular type of the BBB is the brain microvascular endothelial cell (BMEC). It has been reported that *S. suis* could reach the CNS by either adhesion and invasion of these cells (transcytosis) or by a toxic effect, which would increase the permeability of the barrier, allowing the access of free bacteria and/or monocyte-attached bacteria (modified Trojan horse) using a paracellular pathway (Fig. 13.3a). Adhesion to but not invasion of human BMECs has been shown for *S. suis* (Charland *et al.*, 2000). Conversely, *S. suis* not only attached to immortalized porcine BMECs, but also invaded these cells, as demonstrated by antibiotic protection assays and electron microscopy (Vanier *et al.*, 2004). *S. suis* survived up to 7 h within porcine BMECs, which is an interesting finding because a crucial element for the development of meningitis is the ability of pathogens to cross the BBB as live bacteria (Vanier *et al.*, 2004). These results suggest transcytosis, but they remain to be confirmed with a Transwell model of infection. It is difficult to assess whether or not differences between human and porcine BMECs are due to the model, the type of cells (methodology used to immortalize cells) or the species (human versus porcine). Interpretation of the results may also vary among different laboratories. In fact, using the same porcine cell line and a highly similar methodology, Benga *et al.* (2005) also showed internalization of *S. suis*. However, these authors did not consider the number of internalized bacteria to be significant and reported inability of *S. suis* to invade porcine BMECs. There are no general criteria to designate bacterial strains as invasive or not on the basis of the number of internalized bacteria, which may lead to different conclusions. In fact, most researchers arbitrarily decide a threshold to define the event as bacterial invasion. Immortalization per se was not responsible for the observed invasion, because Vanier *et al.* (2007) obtained similar results (invasion) with primary porcine BMECs. More studies from independent laboratories using primary human BMECs are necessary to assess the ability of *S. suis* to adhere to and, especially, invade human BMECs.

The bacterial factors involved in endothelial cell adhesion/invasion have not been fully elucidated. The CPS partially, but significantly, interferes with bacterial adhesion to (human) and adhesion/invasion (porcine) of BMECs, because it may hinder the display of putative adhesins (Charland *et al.*, 2000; Vanier *et al.*, 2004). A possible downregulation of CPS expression that would allow bacteria to increase adhesion to the BBB has been suggested but remains to be demonstrated (Fittipaldi *et al.*, 2012). Further characterization of *S. suis* invasion of porcine BMECs also suggested the involvement of cell-wall-associated proteins (Vanier *et al.*, 2007). An

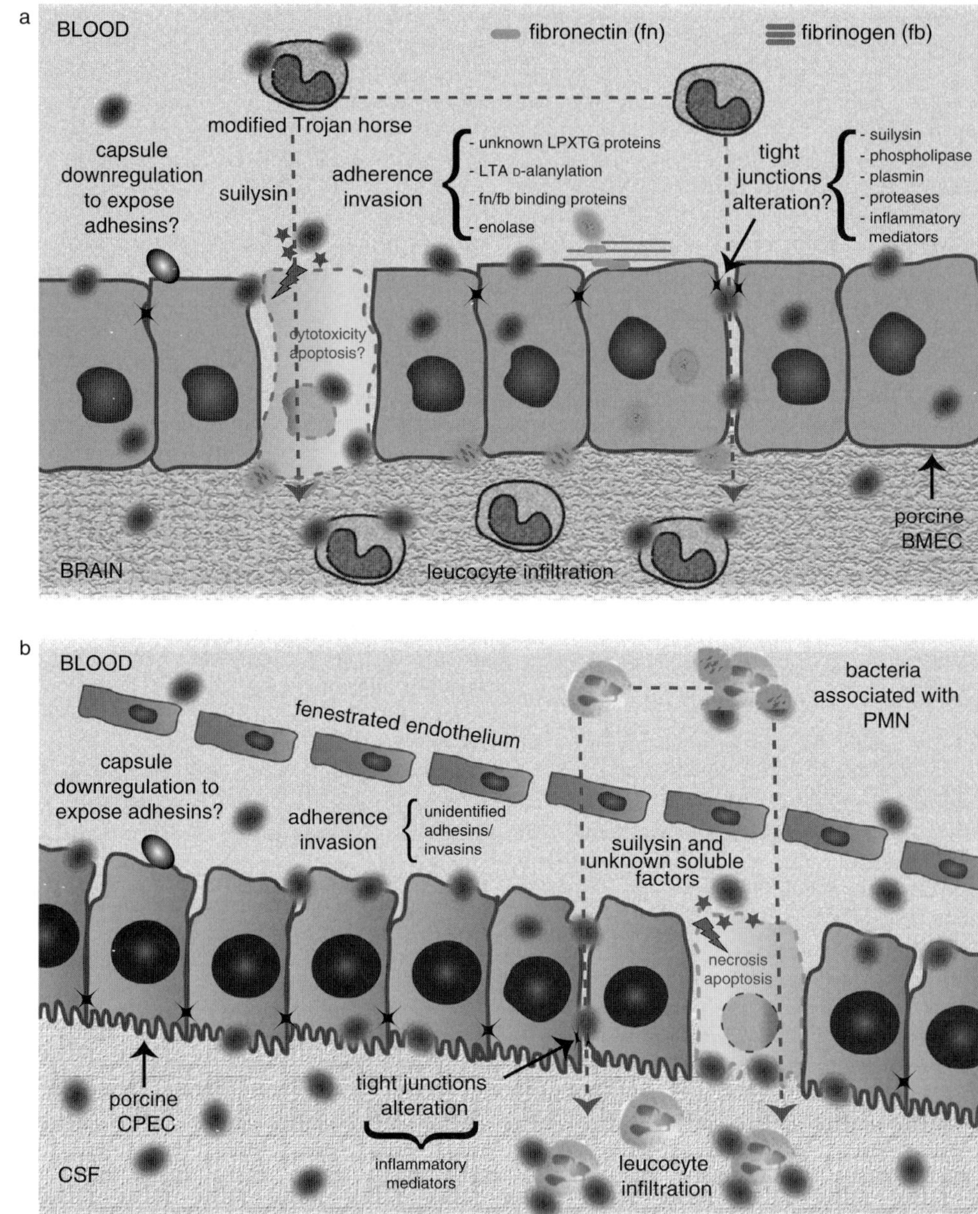

Fig. 13.3. A porcine model of *S. suis* invasion of the CNS is presented. (a) Invasion through the BBB: interactions with BMECs. BMEC adhesion but not invasion has been described so far for human cells. (b) Invasion through the BCSFB: interactions with CPECs.

S. suis mutant defective in the production of a sortase (SrtA$^-$) showed reduced adherence and invasion of porcine BMECs, suggesting that LPXTG-motif cell-wall-anchored proteins may serve as adhesins/invasins (Vanier *et al.*, 2008). A poorly characterized LPXTG protein and a transmembrane protein (a component from an ATP-binding cassette transporter) were more specifically identified as being involved in invasion of porcine endothelial cells and in *S. suis* virulence in mouse and pig models of infection (Vanier *et al.*, 2009a). A non-LPXTG protein, α-enolase, was also shown to be involved in adhesion/invasion of porcine BMECs (Esgleas *et al.*, 2005, 2008). In addition, mutants impaired in LTA D-alanylation adhered to and invaded porcine BMECs to a significantly lesser extent than the wild-type parent strain (Fittipaldi *et al.*, 2008b). Serum components may also participate in the interactions between *S. suis* and porcine BMECs (Vanier *et al.*, 2007). For example, *S. suis* possess different fibronectin-binding proteins, such as α-enolase, an autolysin and a fibronectin/fibrinogen-binding protein that may be involved in such a role (de Greeff *et al.*, 2002; Esgleas *et al.*, 2008; Ju *et al.*, 2012). Interactions of *S. suis* with BMECs probably involve multiple adhesins as well as serum components that may act as a bridge between the bacterium and the cell (Vanier *et al.*, 2007).

Paracellular invasion of the BBB by *S. suis* may rely on the secretion of toxic factors that would affect endothelial cells. Such factors could increase BBB permeability, which could lead to the development of cerebral oedema, increased intracranial pressure and cerebral blood flow blockage characteristic of bacterial meningitis. They may also increase CNS invasion by either free or phagocyte-associated bacteria. Indeed, histopathological findings indicating necrosis of vessel walls in association with inflammatory cellular aggregates have been reported (Sanford, 1987). Suilysin has been suggested to contribute to BBB dysfunction, because it is highly toxic for both human and porcine BMECs (Charland *et al.*, 2000; Vanier *et al.*, 2004). In addition, *S. suis* can bind porcine and human plasminogens on its surface, which can then be activated into plasmin by an endogenous plasminogen activator (Jobin *et al.*, 2005). Acquisition of plasmin activity enables invasive bacteria to enhance their capabilities to destroy cell integrity and penetrate more deeply into tissues. A subtilisin-like protease produced by *S. suis* was also shown to be toxic for human BMECs (Bonifait *et al.*, 2010). *S. suis* can also induce the production of metalloproteinase (MMP)-9 in a monocyte/BMEC co-culture model. MMP-9 is active against extracellular matrix (ECM) proteins such as fibronectin, laminin and type IV collagen, and it has been suggested to enable monocytes to migrate through the BBB. Increased BBB permeability mediated by MMP-9 may also contribute to the migration of pathogens, including *S. suis*, to the CNS, thus causing further damage (Tanabe and Grenier, 2009).

S. suis could also modify the permeability of the BBB by increasing inflammation (see below). This pathogen can stimulate the production of interleukin (IL)-6, IL-8/CXCL8 and monocyte chemotactic protein-1 (MCP-1/CCL2) by human BMECs (Vadeboncoeur *et al.*, 2003). Finally, it has been reported that human BMECs activated by *S. suis* supernatant (containing suilysin and a phospholipase C) release membrane-associated arachidonic acid. Host-derived lipids and prostaglandins are important inflammatory mediators that can promote tissue destruction and cell migration and modulate BBB permeability (Jobin *et al.*, 2005).

Interaction with choroid plexus epithelial cells: blood–cerebrospinal fluid barrier (BCSFB)

Another suggested CNS entry portal for *S. suis* is the BCSFB, maintained by choroid plexus epithelial cells (CPECs) (Fig. 13.3b). In fact, disruption of the plexus brush border, with fibrin and inflammatory cell exudate present in the ventricles, has been described during natural or experimentally induced *S. suis* meningitis in mice and pigs (Williams and Blakemore, 1990b). Although the BCSFB has a smaller surface area than the BBB, it may play an important role in bacterial translocation as well as in leucocyte transmigration (Wewer *et al.*, 2011). First studies carried out with different *S. suis* isolates and primary porcine CPECs showed that bacterial apical application significantly decreased transepithelial resistance and significantly increased paracellular [^{3}H]-mannitol flux. *S. suis* induces CPEC necrosis, although apoptosis, through caspase-3 and caspase-9 activity, is also important (Tenenbaum *et al.*, 2006). Interestingly, some isolates were able to disrupt the BCSFB whether they were applied to the apical or to the basolateral compartment, signifying that soluble virulence factors, in addition to direct bacteria-cell contact, may alter the tightness of the porcine CPEC barrier. It seems that suilysin plays an important role as a toxin affecting BCSFB function; however, other non-identified soluble factors would also be involved (Tenenbaum *et al.*, 2005, 2006). *S. suis* is able to cause disorganization of the tight junction proteins occludin, ZO-1 and claudin-1 in porcine CPECs, loss of actin at the apical cell pole and basolateral stress fibre formation (Tenenbaum *et al.*, 2008). Inflammatory mediators have also been suggested to induce porcine CPEC necrosis with increased permeability (Tenenbaum *et al.*, 2009).

Recently, *in vitro* studies with a human choroid plexus papilloma cell line showed invasion and translocation of *S. suis* across the BCSFB using an inverted transwell model (Schwerk *et al.*, 2012). This invasion was suggested to involve three potential steps: (i) invasion of CPECs from the basolateral side; (ii) transport within membrane-bound endocytic vacuoles to the apical side; and (iii) exocytosis onto the apical membrane of the BCSFB. *S. suis* adhered to and invaded cells better when applied to basolateral membranes of CPECs, suggesting that direct access to the ECM was required. CPS expression compromised *S. suis* CPEC invasion, as compared with unencapsulated mutants, indicating that as yet unidentified bacterial cell-wall components and/or surface proteins are needed (Schwerk *et al.*, 2012). A fibronectin-binding protein, the enolase and a dipeptidylpeptidase (DppIV) of *S. suis* were involved in mediating bacterial adherence to different ECM proteins (Fittipaldi *et al.*, 2012). Downregulation of CPS expression during *S. suis*–epithelial cell interactions remains to be demonstrated (Fittipaldi *et al.*, 2012).

13.4.3 Inflammation: hallmark of *S. suis* meningitis

Meningitis-associated brain injury and neuronal death is mainly associated with a host reaction to bacterial components (Gerber and Nau, 2010). An interesting *S. suis* mouse model has been developed, consistently reproducing the clinical signs of affected nervous system and CNS damage in adult animals by means of a haematogenous infection, with bacteraemia leading to late meningitis and encephalitis (Dominguez-Punaro *et al.*, 2007). Most *S. suis*-infected mice that survived septicaemia later developed CNS clinical signs such as locomotor problems, episthotonus, opisthotonus, bending of the head laterally and walking in circles, which could all be considered characteristic of brain inflammation (Dominguez-Punaro *et al.*, 2007). *In situ* hybridization of sampled brains showed strong activation of Toll-like receptor (TLR) 2 in regions of the brain where *S. suis* was present. TLR2 activation by suilysin coincided with upregulated expression of CD14 receptor and activation of IκBα (index of NF-κB activation) in similar anatomical regions among mice with CNS symptoms. Unlike the related pneumolysin, suilysin does not appear to activate TLR4 (Dominguez-Punaro *et al.*, 2007). Transcriptional activation of IL-1β, tumour necrosis factor (TNF)-α and MCP-1 in the CNS at a time coincident with the presence of clinical signs may also indicate an important role for pro-inflammatory cytokines in the development of *S. suis*-related meningitis (Dominguez-Punaro *et al.*, 2007).

S. suis could reach the CNS by interacting with CPECs and/or BMECs, but only one report indicates that, after infection with *S. suis*, epithelial cells from the choroid plexus contribute to inflammation by producing cytokines and chemokines (Schwerk *et al.*, 2011). By contrast, many studies demonstrate the involvement of BMECs in *S. suis*-induced inflammation. Shortly after infection of a mouse model, upregulation of TLR2 and pro-inflammatory cytokine mRNAs in cells lining the brain microvasculature was observed (Dominguez-Punaro *et al.*, 2007). *In vitro* studies showed that *S. suis* infection of human and porcine BMECs induced the release of pro-inflammatory cytokines and chemokines (Vadeboncoeur *et al.*, 2003; Vanier *et al.*, 2009b). The fact that human BMECs were highly activated demonstrates that induction of such cytokines was not related to bacterial invasion. Interestingly, a certain threshold of bacterial concentration was shown to be critical, which correlates with the need, *in vivo*, for high levels of bacteraemia to reproduce clinical signs of meningitis in mouse and pig models (Pallares *et al.*, 2003; Berthelot-Herault *et al.*, 2005; Dominguez-Punaro *et al.*, 2008).

Using porcine BMECs, *S. suis* was also shown to induce, at first, the production of high levels of IL-6 and IL-8; however, at later incubation times, degradation of IL-8 was observed, probably due to the presence of a serine protease (Vanier *et al.*, 2009b). A first burst of IL-8 probably causes the recruitment of leucocytes and subsequent BBB breakdown, facilitating the pathogenesis of *S. suis*-induced meningitis. Subsequently, *S. suis* modulates this response by degrading IL-8, thereby delaying the recruitment of neutrophils to the site of inflammation and allowing the pathogen to survive and to cause more damage (Vanier *et al.*, 2009b).

Leucocyte influx into the SAS and increased BBB and/or BCSFB permeability are considered hallmarks of bacterial meningitis. Leucocyte recruitment to sites of inflammation is mediated by several families of adhesion molecules present on the surface of leucocytes and endothelial cells. These molecules work together, as shown by a synergistic activation of both cells by *S. suis* in an endothelial cell/macrophage co-culture model, with an increased production of pro-inflammatory mediators (Tanabe and Grenier, 2009). *S. suis* is able to induce an upregulation of intercellular adhesion molecule-1 (ICAM-1), CD11c/CD18 and CD11a/CD18 on human monocytes as well as inducing the shedding of ICAM-1 from human BMECs in a dose-dependent manner (Al-Numani *et al.*, 2003; Grenier and Bodet, 2008). This leads to increased adhesion of monocytes to endothelial cells, thus providing a mechanism for some of the inflammatory features of meningitis caused by this pathogen. Using an inverted Transwell culture model of the BCSFB, it has been shown that neutrophils migrate across porcine CPECs previously activated with *S. suis* using a transcellular route via funnel-like structures developing from the apical membrane (Wewer *et al.*, 2011). Flow cytometric and transmigration inhibition studies with integrin-specific antibodies showed that neutrophil traversal is dependent on CD11b/CD18, ICAM-1 and vascular cell adhesion protein 1 (VCAM-1) expression after *S. suis* stimulation (Schwerk *et al.*, 2012). Interestingly, the role of infiltrating leucocytes has not been studied *in vivo*. Moreover, the contribution of resident meningeal macrophages and leptomeningeal cells to inflammation is not known. Infiltrated monocytes may contribute not only to *in situ* inflammation but also to *S. suis* invasion into the CNS by the modified Trojan horse theory.

Although BMECs and CPECs may significantly contribute to inflammation in the CNS, *in vivo* studies strongly indicate an active role of microglial cells and, to a lesser extent, astrocytes. In fact, microglia play an ambiguous role, because they may protect neurons by preventing the entry of pathogens into the brain, but they can also be toxic to surrounding neurons by releasing NO, glutamate and pro-inflammatory cytokines. Studies carried out with mouse cells showed that, similarly to other phagocytes, microglial cells hardly ingest well-encapsulated *S. suis*, but they are highly activated by this pathogen (Dominguez-Punaro *et al.*, 2010). Indeed, high levels of TNF-α and MCP-1 as well as NO synthase expression and further NO production were induced after *S. suis* activation, mainly through a TLR2 pathway (Dominguez-Punaro *et al.*, 2010). After *S. suis* contact with microglial cells, a pattern of low and biphasic phosphorylation of protein kinase C (PKC) substrates and tyrosyl residues was observed. Higher levels of phosphorylation were obtained when using a non-encapsulated mutant. It was concluded that encapsulated *S. suis*, once in contact with microglia, is able to modulate intracellular signalling events, probably to avoid phagocytosis and delay activation of the inflammatory response. These findings support previous research on *S. suis* modulation of murine macrophage functions, in which it was observed that the capsule was responsible for weak activation of the PI3K/Akt/PKCα signalling pathway, as well as several protein tyrosine events, which correlated with low levels of phagocytosis (Segura *et al.*, 2004).

The fact that poorly identified cell-wall components were mostly involved in activation of microglia was confirmed by the high levels of phosphorylation of mitogen-activated protein kinases (MAPKs), in particular those of p-ERK (extracellular signal-regulated kinase) 1/2, p38 and p-JNK (c-Jun NH_2-terminal kinase), induced by non-encapsulated *S. suis*. In fact, recent studies revealed that a capsule-deficient mutant of *S. suis* was able to induce higher levels of transcriptional expression of different putative genes from the MAPK pathway than the capsulated parental strain (de Greeff *et al.*, 2010), and purified cell-wall preparations from *S. suis* were shown to trigger the phosphorylation of the MAPK signal transduction pathway (Tanabe *et al.*, 2008). Finally, the involvement of murine astrocytes in local CNS inflammation has been reported, confirming data obtained after *in vivo* infection of mice (Zheng *et al.*, 2011).

In most studies, *S. suis* cell-wall components have been mainly involved in cell activation (Segura *et al.*, 2006). Although these components have not been clearly identified, a putative prolipoprotein, diacylglyceryl transferase present in the *S. suis* cell wall, is required for innate immune activation (Wichgers Schreur *et al.*, 2010, 2011). Similar to other streptococci, soluble peptidoglycan/cell-wall fragments (including LTA) may be released into the SAS by exponentially growing bacteria as well as by antibiotic treatment (especially β-lactams), thereby causing a burst of meningeal inflammation. Although not directly implicated in inflammation, suilysin may indirectly play a role by releasing haemoglobin, which has been shown to significantly potentiate the induction of pro-inflammatory mediators by acting in synergy with *S. suis* cell-wall components (Tanabe *et al.*, 2008).

13.5 Conclusions

S. suis is an important swine pathogen and an emerging zoonotic agent. Our understanding of the pathogenesis of meningitis in swine and humans has improved tremendously in recent years. However, it is still difficult to associate most described bacterial virulence factors with different stages of CNS infection (Fittipaldi *et al.*, 2012). In addition, nothing is known about the human/swine cell receptors that interact with these bacterial ligands as well as the cellular rearrangements that follow such interactions.

In any case, results obtained during the last decade clearly indicate that strains from different geographical areas possess different virulence potentials. Further studies are necessary to compare swine and human strains from different continents and evaluate their capacity to induce meningitis. In addition, more *in vitro* studies are needed with human primary cells from the CNS and to elucidate the role of BMECs and CPECs in the pathogenesis of *S. suis* meningitis. In fact, most available data are either from swine or mice, and very few studies have been performed with human cells.

Finally, the immune response against this pathogen is a relatively neglected area that needs to be addressed. There are no effective vaccines available for swine, and no vaccine has ever been developed for humans. Indeed, the adaptive humoral immune response against *S. suis* is usually low (in mice and pigs) and no data are available regarding cellular immune responses. Surprisingly, different single antigens included in many subunit vaccination trials during the last few years appear to be highly protective (Fittipaldi *et al.*, 2012). The methodology to measure protection against *S. suis* infection is not standardized, and conflicting results can be obtained with the same vaccine candidate. This area will require intensive research in the years to come.

Health agencies and physicians in Asian countries should increase awareness among the population regarding the risks associated with eating raw pork products from uncontrolled sources and/or meat from clinically diseased pigs. Increased collaboration between laboratories in veterinary and human medicine with diverse but complementary expertise, in different parts of the world, is necessary in order to significantly increase our understanding of the pathogenesis of meningitis caused by this challenging zoonotic pathogen.

References

Al-Numani, D., Segura, M., Dore, M. and Gottschalk, M. (2003) Up-regulation of ICAM-1, CD11a/CD18 and CD11c/CD18 on human THP-1 monocytes stimulated by *Streptococcus suis* serotype 2. *Clinical and Experimental Immunology* 133, 67–77.

Benga, L., Friedl, P. and Valentin-Weigand, P. (2005) Adherence of *Streptococcus suis* to porcine endothelial cells. *Journal of Veterinary Medicine B. Infectious Diseases and Veterinary and Public Health* 52, 392–395.

Berthelot-Herault, F., Gottschalk, M., Morvan, H. and Kobisch, M. (2005) Dilemma of virulence of *Streptococcus suis*: Canadian isolate 89-1591 characterized as a virulent strain using a standardized experimental model in pigs. *Canadian Journal of Veterinary Research* 69, 236–240.

Bonifait, L., de la Cruz Dominguez-Punaro, M., Vaillancourt, K., Bart, C., Slater, J., Frenette, M., Gottschalk, M. and Grenier, D. (2010) The cell envelope subtilisin-like proteinase is a virulence determinant for *Streptococcus suis*. *BMC Microbiology* 10, 42.

Busque, P., Higgins, R., Senechal, S., Marchand, R. and Quessy, S. (1998) Simultaneous flow cytometric measurement of *Streptococcus suis* phagocytosis by polymorphonuclear and mononuclear blood leukocytes. *Veterinary Microbiology* 63, 229–238.

Camporese, A., Tizianel, G., Bruschetta, G., Cruciatti, B. and Pomes, A. (2007) Human meningitis caused by *Streptococcus suis*: the first case report from north-eastern Italy. *Infezioni in Medicina* 15, 111–114.

Charland, N., Nizet, V., Rubens, C.E., Kim, K.S., Lacouture, S. and Gottschalk, M. (2000) *Streptococcus suis* serotype 2 interactions with human brain microvascular endothelial cells. *Infection and Immununity* 68, 637–643.

Cloutier, G., D'Allaire, S., Martinez, G., Surprenant, C., Lacouture, S. and Gottschalk, M. (2003) Epidemiology of *Streptococcus suis* serotype 5 infection in a pig herd with and without clinical disease. *Veterinary Microbiology* 97, 135–151.

de Greeff, A., Buys, H., Verhaar, R., Dijkstra, J., van Alphen, L. and Smith, H.E. (2002) Contribution of fibronectin-binding protein to pathogenesis of *Streptococcus suis* serotype 2. *Infection and Immunity* 70, 1319–1325.

de Greeff, A., Benga, L., Wichgers Schreur, P.J., Valentin-Weigand, P., Rebel, J. and Smith, H.E. (2010) Involvement of NF-κB and MAP-kinases in the transcriptional response of alveolar macrophages to *Streptococcus suis*. *Veterinary Microbiology* 141, 59–67.

Dominguez-Punaro, M.C., Segura, M., Plante, M.M., Lacouture, S., Rivest, S. and Gottschalk, M. (2007) *Streptococcus suis* serotype 2, an important swine and human pathogen, induces strong systemic and cerebral inflammatory responses in a mouse model of infection. *Journal of Immunology* 179, 1842–1854.

Dominguez-Punaro, M.C., Segura, M., Radzioch, D., Rivest, S. and Gottschalk, M. (2008) Comparison of the susceptibilities of C57BL/6 and A/J mouse strains to *Streptococcus suis* serotype 2 infection. *Infection and Immunity* 76, 3901–3910.

Dominguez-Punaro, M.C., Segura, M., Contreras, I., Lachance, C., Houde, M., Lecours, M.P., Olivier, M. and Gottschalk, M. (2010) In vitro characterization of the microglial inflammatory response to *Streptococcus suis*, an important emerging zoonotic agent of meningitis. *Infection and Immunity* 78, 5074–5085.

Dominguez-Punaro, M.C., Koedel, U., Hoegen, T., Demel, C., Klein, M. and Gottschalk, M. (2012) Severe cochlear inflammation and vestibular syndrome in an experimental model of *Streptococcus suis* infection in mice. *European Journal of Clinical Microbiology and Infectious Diseases* 31, 2391–2400.

Esgleas, M., Lacouture, S. and Gottschalk, M. (2005) *Streptococcus suis* serotype 2 binding to extracellular matrix proteins. *FEMS Microbiology Letters* 244, 33–40.

Esgleas, M., Li, Y., Hancock, M.A., Harel, J., Dubreuil, J.D. and Gottschalk, M. (2008) Isolation and characterization of α-enolase, a novel fibronectin-binding protein from *Streptococcus suis*. *Microbiology* 154, 2668–2679.

Fittipaldi, N., Sekizaki, T., Takamatsu, D., Dominguez-Punaro Mde, L., Harel, J., Bui, N.K., Vollmer, W. and Gottschalk, M. (2008a) Significant contribution of the *pgdA* gene to the virulence of *Streptococcus suis*. *Molecular Microbiology* 70, 1120-35.

Fittipaldi, N., Sekizaki, T., Takamatsu, D., Harel, J., Dominguez-Punaro Mde, L., Von Aulock, S., Draing, C., Marois, C., Kobisch, M. and Gottschalk, M. (2008b) D-Alanylation of lipoteichoic acid contributes to the virulence of *Streptococcus suis*. *Infection and Immunity* 76, 3587–3594.

Fittipaldi, N., Collis, T., Prothero, B. and Gottschalk, M. (2009a) *Streptococcus suis* meningitis, Hawaii. *Emerging Infectious Diseases* 15, 2067–2069.

Fittipaldi, N., Fuller, T.E., Teel, J.F., Wilson, T.L., Wolfram, T.J., Lowery, D.E. and Gottschalk, M. (2009b) Serotype distribution and production of muramidase-released protein, extracellular factor and suilysin by field strains of *Streptococcus suis* isolated in the United States. *Veterinary Microbiology* 139, 310–317.

Fittipaldi, N., Xu, J., Lacouture, S., Tharavichitkul, P., Osaki, M., Sekizaki, T., Takamatsu, D. and Gottschalk, M. (2011) Lineage and virulence of *Streptococcus suis* serotype 2 isolates from North America. *Emerging Infectious Diseases* 17, 2239–2244.

Fittipaldi, N., Segura, M., Grenier, D. and Gottschalk, M. (2012) Virulence factors involved in the pathogenesis of the infection caused by the swine pathogen and zoonotic agent *Streptococcus suis. Future Microbiology* 7, 259–279.

Gerber, J. and Nau, R. (2010) Mechanisms of injury in bacterial meningitis. *Current Opinion in Neurology* 23, 312–318.

Gottschalk, M. (2012) Streptococcocis. In: Straw, B.E., Zimmerman, J.J., D'Allaire, S. and Taylor, D.J. (eds) *Diseases of Swine*, 10th edn. Blackwell Publishing, Ames, IA, pp. 841–855.

Gottschalk, M. and Segura, M. (2000) The pathogenesis of the meningitis caused by *Streptococcus suis*: the unresolved questions. *Veterinary Microbiology* 76, 259–272.

Gottschalk, M., Segura, M. and Xu, J. (2007) *Streptococcus suis* infections in humans: the Chinese experience and the situation in North America. *Animal Health Research Reviews* 8, 29–45.

Gottschalk, M., Xu, J., Calzas, C. and Segura, M. (2010) *Streptococcus suis*: a new emerging or an old neglected zoonotic pathogen? *Future Microbiology* 5, 371–391.

Grenier, D. and Bodet, C. (2008) *Streptococcus suis* stimulates ICAM-1 shedding from microvascular endothelial cells. *FEMS Immunology and Medical Microbiology* 54, 271–276.

Hantson, P., Vekemans, M.C., Gautier, P., Mahieu, P., Sindic, C.J., Guerit, J.M., Wauters, G. and Nannan, M. (1991) Fatal *Streptococcus suis* meningitis in man. *Acta Neurologica Belgica* 91, 165–168.

Houde, M., Gottschalk, M., Gagnon, F., Van Calsteren, M.R. and Segura, M. (2012) *Streptococcus suis* capsular polysaccharide inhibits phagocytosis through destabilization of lipid microdomains and prevents lactosylceramide-dependent recognition. *Infection and Immunity* 80, 506–517.

Huang, Y.T., Teng, L.J., Ho, S.W. and Hsueh, P.R. (2005) *Streptococcus suis* infection. *Journal of Microbiology and Immunology and Infection* 38, 306–313.

Huh, H.J., Park, K.J., Jang, J.H., Lee, M., Lee, J.H., Ahn, Y.H., Kang, C.I., Ki, C.S. and Lee, N.Y. (2011) *Streptococcus suis* meningitis with bilateral sensorineural hearing loss. *Korean Journal of Laboratory Medicine* 31, 205–210.

Jacobs, A.A., Loeffen, P.L., van den Berg, A.J. and Storm, P.K. (1994) Identification, purification, and characterization of a thiol-activated hemolysin (suilysin) of *Streptococcus suis. Infection and Immunity* 62, 1742–1748.

Jobin, M.C., Fortin, J., Willson, P.J., Gottschalk, M. and Grenier, D. (2005) Acquisition of plasmin activity and induction of arachidonic acid release by *Streptococcus suis* in contact with human brain microvascular endothelial cells. *FEMS Microbiology Letters* 252, 105–111.

Ju, C.X., Gu, H.W. and Lu, C.P. (2012) Characterization and functional analysis of atl, a novel gene encoding autolysin in *Streptococcus suis. Journal of Bacteriology* 194, 1464–1473.

Kerdsin, A., Oishi, K., Sripakdee, S., Boonkerd, N., Polwichai, P., Nakamura, S., Uchida, R., Sawanpanyalert, P. and Dejsirilert, S. (2009) Clonal dissemination of human isolates of *Streptococcus suis* serotype 14 in Thailand. *Journal of Medical Microbiology* 58, 1508–1513.

Kerdsin, A., Dejsirilert, S., Sawanpanyalert, P., Boonnark, A., Noithachang, W., Sriyakum, D., Simkum, S., Chokngam, S., Gottschalk, M., Akeda, Y. and Oishi, K. (2011) Sepsis and spontaneous bacterial peritonitis in Thailand. *Lancet* 378, 960.

Lecours, M.P., Gottschalk, M., Houde, M., Lemire, P., Fittipaldi, N. and Segura, M. (2011) Critical role for *Streptococcus suis* cell wall modifications and suilysin in resistance to complement-dependent killing by dendritic cells. *Journal of Infectious Diseases* 204, 919–929.

Mai, N.T., *et al.* (2008) *Streptococcus suis* meningitis in adults in Vietnam. *Clinical Infectious Diseases* 46, 659–667.

Marques, M.B., Kasper, D.L., Pangburn, M.K. and Wessels, M.R. (1992) Prevention of C3 deposition by capsular polysaccharide is a virulence mechanism of type III group B streptococci. *Infection and Immunity* 60, 3986–3993.

Meijerink, M., Ferrando, M.L., Lammers, G., Taverne, N., Smith, H.E. and Wells, J.M. (2012) Immunomodulatory effects of *Streptococcus suis* capsule type on human dendritic cell responses, phagocytosis and intracellular survival. *PLoS One* 7, e35849.

Nghia, H.D., Hoa, N.T., le Linh, D., Campbell, J., Diep, T.S., Chau, N.V., Mai, N.T., Hien, T.T.,

Spratt, B., Farrar, J. and Schultsz, C. (2008) Human case of *Streptococcus suis* serotype 16 infection. *Emerging Infectious Diseases* 14, 155–157.

Pallares, F.J., Halbur, P.G., Schmitt, C.S., Roth, J.A., Opriessnig, T., Thomas, P.J., Kinyon, J.M., Murphy, D., Frank, D.E. and Hoffman, L.J. (2003) Comparison of experimental models for *Streptococcus suis* infection of conventional pigs. *Canadian Journal of Veterinary Research* 67, 225–228.

Sanford, S.E. (1987) Gross and histopathological findings in unusual lesions caused by *Streptococcus suis* in pigs. II. Central nervous system lesions. *Canadian Journal of Veterinary Research* 51, 486–489.

Schwerk, C., *et al.* (2011) In vitro transcriptome analysis of porcine choroid plexus epithelial cells in response to *Streptococcus suis*: release of pro-inflammatory cytokines and chemokines. *Microbes and Infections* 13, 953–962.

Schwerk, C., *et al.* (2012) Polar invasion and translocation of *Neisseria meningitidis* and *Streptococcus suis* in a novel human model of the blood–cerebrospinal fluid barrier. *PLoS One* 7, e30069.

Segura, M. (2012) Fisher scientific award lecture – the capsular polysaccharides of Group B *Streptococcus* and *Streptococcus suis* differently modulate bacterial interactions with dendritic cells. *Canadian Journal of Microbiology* 58, 249–260.

Segura, M. and Gottschalk, M. (2002) *Streptococcus suis* interactions with the murine macrophage cell line J774: adhesion and cytotoxicity. *Infection and Immunity* 70, 4312–4322.

Segura M, Gottschalk, M. and Olivier, M. (2004) Encapsulated *Streptococcus suis* inhibits activation of signaling pathways involved in phagocytosis. *Infection and Immunity* 72, 5322–5330.

Segura, M., Vanier, G., Al-Numani, D., Lacouture, S., Olivier, M. and Gottschalk, M. (2006) Proinflammatory cytokine and chemokine modulation by *Streptococcus suis* in a whole-blood culture system. *FEMS Immunology and Medical Microbiology* 47, 92–106.

Smith, T.C., Capuano, A.W., Boese, B., Myers, K.P. and Gray, G.C. (2008) Exposure to *Streptococcus suis* among US swine workers. *Emerging Infectious Diseases* 14, 1925–1927.

Suankratay, C., Intalapaporn, P., Nunthapisud, P., Arunyingmongkol, K. and Wilde, H. (2004) *Streptococcus suis* meningitis in Thailand. *Southeast Asian Journal of Tropical Medicine and Public Health* 35, 868–876.

Tan, J.H., Yeh, B.I. and Seet, C.S. (2010) Deafness due to haemorrhagic labyrinthitis and a review of relapses in *Streptococcus suis* meningitis. *Singapore Medical Journal* 51, e30–33.

Tanabe, S. and Grenier, D. (2009) Endothelial cell/macrophage cocultures as a model to study *Streptococcus suis*-induced inflammatory responses. *FEMS Immunology and Medical Microbiology* 55, 100–106.

Tanabe, S., Gottschalk, M. and Grenier, D. (2008) Hemoglobin and *Streptococcus suis* cell wall act in synergy to potentiate the inflammatory response of monocyte-derived macrophages. *Innate Immunity* 14, 357–363.

Tenenbaum, T., Adam, R., Eggelnpohler, I., Matalon, D., Seibt, A., K Novotny, G.E., Galla, H.J. and Schroten, H. (2005) Strain-dependent disruption of blood-cerebrospinal fluid barrier by *Streptoccocus suis* in vitro. *FEMS Immunology and Medical Microbiology* 44, 25–34.

Tenenbaum, T., Essmann, F., Adam, R., Seibt, A., Janicke, R.U., Novotny, G.E., Galla, H.J. and Schroten, H. (2006) Cell death, caspase activation, and HMGB1 release of porcine choroid plexus epithelial cells during *Streptococcus suis* infection in vitro. *Brain Research* 1100, 1–12.

Tenenbaum, T., Matalon, D., Adam, R., Seibt, A., Wewer, C., Schwerk, C., Galla, H.J. and Schroten, H. (2008) Dexamethasone prevents alteration of tight junction-associated proteins and barrier function in porcine choroid plexus epithelial cells after infection with *Streptococcus suis* in vitro. *Brain Research* 1229, 1–17.

Tenenbaum, T., Papandreou, T., Gellrich, D., Friedrichs, U., Seibt, A., Adam, R., Wewer, C., Galla, H.J., Schwerk, C. and Schroten, H. (2009) Polar bacterial invasion and translocation of *Streptococcus suis* across the blood–cerebrospinal fluid barrier in vitro. *Cell Microbiology* 11, 323–336.

Vadeboncoeur, N., Segura, M., Al-Numani, D., Vanier, G. and Gottschalk, M. (2003) Pro-inflammatory cytokine and chemokine release by human brain microvascular endothelial cells stimulated by *Streptococcus suis* serotype 2. *FEMS Immunology and Medical Microbiology* 35, 49–58.

Van Calsteren, M.R., Gagnon, F., Lacouture, S., Fittipaldi, N. and Gottschalk, M. (2010) Structure determination of *Streptococcus suis* serotype 2 capsular polysaccharide. *Biochemical and Cellular Biology* 88, 513–525.

Vanier, G., Segura, M., Friedl, P., Lacouture, S. and Gottschalk, M. (2004) Invasion of porcine brain microvascular endothelial cells by

Streptococcus suis serotype 2. *Infection and Immunity* 72, 1441–1449.

Vanier, G., Segura, M. and Gottschalk, M. (2007) Characterization of the invasion of porcine endothelial cells by *Streptococcus suis* serotype 2. *Canadian Journal of Veterinary Research* 71, 81–89.

Vanier, G., Sekizaki, T., Dominguez-Punaro, M.C., Esgleas, M., Osaki, M., Takamatsu, D., Segura, M. and Gottschalk, M. (2008) Disruption of *srtA* gene in *Streptococcus suis* results in decreased interactions with endothelial cells and extracellular matrix proteins. *Veterinary Microbiology* 127, 417–424.

Vanier, G., Fittipaldi, N., Slater, J.D., de la Cruz Dominguez-Punaro, M., Rycroft, A.N., Segura, M., Maskell, D.J. and Gottschalk, M. (2009a) New putative virulence factors of *Streptococcus suis* involved in invasion of porcine brain microvascular endothelial cells. *Microbial Pathogenesis* 46, 13–20.

Vanier, G., Segura, M., Lecours, M.P., Grenier, D. and Gottschalk, M. (2009b) Porcine brain microvascular endothelial cell-derived interleukin-8 is first induced and then degraded by *Streptococcus suis*. *Microbial Pathogenesis* 46, 135–143.

Wertheim, H.F., Nghia, H.D., Taylor, W. and Schultsz, C. (2009a) *Streptococcus suis*: an emerging human pathogen. *Clinical and Infectious Diseases* 48, 617–625.

Wertheim, H.F., *et al.* (2009b) *Streptococcus suis*, an important cause of adult bacterial meningitis in northern Vietnam. *PLoS One* 4, e5973.

Wewer, C., Seibt, A., Wolburg, H., Greune, L., Schmidt, M.A., Berger, J., Galla, H.J., Quitsch, U., Schwerk, C., Schroten, H. and Tenenbaum, T. (2011) Transcellular migration of neutrophil granulocytes through the blood–cerebrospinal fluid barrier after infection with *Streptococcus suis*. *Journal of Neuroinflammation* 8, 51.

Wichgers Schreur, P.J., Rebel, J.M., Smits, M.A., van Putten, J.P. and Smith, H.E. (2010) Differential activation of the Toll-like receptor 2/6 complex by lipoproteins of *Streptococcus suis* serotypes 2 and 9. *Veterinary Microbiology* 143, 363–370.

Wichgers Schreur, P.J., Rebel, J.M., Smits, M.A., van Putten, J.P. and Smith, H.E. (2011) Lgt processing is an essential step in *Streptococcus suis* lipoprotein mediated innate immune activation. *PLoS One* 6, e22299.

Willenburg, K.S., Sentochnik, D.E. and Zadoks, R.N. (2006) Human *Streptococcus suis* meningitis in the United States. *New England Journal of Medicine* 354, 1325.

Williams, A.E. and Blakemore, W.F. (1990a) Pathogenesis of meningitis caused by *Streptococcus suis* type 2. *Journal of Infectious Diseases* 162, 474–481.

Williams, A.E. and Blakemore, W.F. (1990b) Pathology of Streptococcal meningitis following intravenous intracisternal and natural routes of infection. *Neuropathology and Applied Neurobiology* 16, 345–356.

Yang, Q.P., Liu, W.P., Guo, L.X., Jiang, Y., Li, G.D., Bai, Y.Q., Li, S.H., Wu, T. and Jing, H.Q. (2009) Autopsy report of four cases who died from *Streptococcus suis* infection, with a review of the literature. *European Journal of Clinical Microbiology and Infectious Diseases* 28, 447–453.

Ye, C., *et al.* (2006) *Streptococcus suis* sequence type 7 outbreak, Sichuan, China. *Emerging Infectious Diseases* 12, 1203–1208.

Zheng, H., Punaro, M.C., Segura, M., Lachance, C., Rivest, S., Xu, J., Houde, M. and Gottschalk, M. (2011) Toll-like receptor 2 is partially involved in the activation of murine astrocytes by *Streptococcus suis*, an important zoonotic agent of meningitis. *Journal of Neuroimmunology* 234, 71–83.

Zheng, P., Zhao, Y.X., Zhang, A.D., Kang, C., Chen, H.C. and Jin, M.L. (2009) Pathologic analysis of the brain from *Streptococcus suis* type 2 experimentally infected pigs. *Veterinary Pathology* 46, 531–535.

14 *Listeria monocytogenes:* An Intracellular Pathogen of Monocytes and the Central Nervous System

Nancy E. Freitag,[1] Michael S. Bronze[2] and Douglas A. Drevets[2,3*]

[1]*University of Illinois at Chicago, Chicago, USA;* [2]*University of Oklahoma Health Sciences Center, Oklahoma City, USA;* [3]*Department of Veterans Affairs Medical Center, Oklahoma City, USA*

14.1 Introduction

Listeria monocytogenes is a facultative intracellular bacterium that is an important cause of zoonosis in animals and has emerged as an important cause of food-borne illness and central nervous system (CNS) infection in humans. The relevance of *L. monocytogenes* as a human pathogen was recently underscored by a cantaloupe-associated outbreak in the USA that sickened 146 people and caused 30 deaths and one miscarriage (http://www.cdc.gov/Listeria/outbreaks/cantaloupes-jensen-farms/index.html). Although it is not the most common of the neuroinvasive bacteria, *L. monocytogenes* is one of the most efficient organisms at causing meningitis once invasive infection of a host has been established. For example, in a study of invasive bacterial diseases, meningitis was present in 36% of invasive *L. monocytogenes* infection compared with 4% each for *Streptococcus pneumoniae* and Group B *Streptococcus* (Schuchat *et al.*, 1997). *L. monocytogenes* is unique among neuroinvasive bacteria in that *in vitro* and *in vivo* data suggest it can invade the CNS by at least three different mechanisms (Drevets *et al.*, 2004b). These are: (i) transport across the blood–brain barrier (BBB) or blood–cerebrospinal fluid barrier (BCSFB) within parasitized leucocytes, i.e. the 'Trojan horse model'; (ii) direct invasion of endothelial cells by extracellular blood-borne bacteria; and (iii) a neural route in which there is retrograde (centripetal) migration of bacteria into the brain within the axons of cranial nerves.

14.2 Basic Microbiology

L. monocytogenes is a Gram-positive, non-spore-forming facultative anaerobic bacterium that is widely distributed in the outside environment and found in soil, silage, groundwater, sewage and decaying vegetation and as part of the faecal flora of mammals, including humans (Freitag *et al.*, 2009). The organism is able to resist many forms of stress and endure large fluctuations in temperature (−1.5 to 45°C), and high salt concentrations (10–14%, w/v) and pH

*douglas-drevets@ouhsc.edu

(Chaturongakul *et al.*, 2008). Moreover, it can adapt to long periods of starvation without any detectable loss in bacterial virulence (Bruno and Freitag, 2011).

14.3 Epidemiology and Transmission

The incidence of invasive listeriosis varies by country, ranging from 0.1 to 11.3 cases per million of the population (Swaminathan and Gerner-Smidt, 2007). Estimates suggest there are 1591 cases/year (range 557–3161) of invasive listeriosis in the USA with a 15.9% case fatality rate (Scallan *et al.*, 2011). Highest rates of infection are seen in those at extremes of age, pregnant women and their neonates, transplant patients, those immunosuppressed by either disease or medications, and those with chronic illnesses such as diabetes, chronic liver disease or malignancy, especially haematologic malignancy (Drevets and Bronze, 2008). Examples of conditions that increase risk for listeriosis include alcoholism (relative risk (RR) 12.3, 95% confidence interval (CI) 9.4, 16.1), diabetes mellitus (RR 11.4, 95% CI 9.0, 14.5), liver disease (RR 22.4, 95% CI 17.7, 28.4) and lymphoid and haematopoietic malignancies (RR 17.6, 95% CI 15.1, 20.6) (Mook *et al.*, 2011).

Human *L. monocytogenes* infections are largely transmitted by consumption of contaminated food, in particular unpasteurized dairy products, soft cheeses, ready-to-eat meats and delicatessen products, and produce items. Its ubiquity in the food supply is demonstrated by the fact that *L. monocytogenes* contamination prompted 32% of US Department of Agriculture food recalls between 2002 and 2006 (Drevets and Bronze, 2008). Uncommon routes include transplacental or transvaginal transmission from mother to child, direct contact with infected animals or as nosocomial infections.

14.4 Clinical Features: One Pathogen, Multiple Syndromes

Human *L. monocytogenes* infections are typically divided into non-invasive and invasive infections (Vazquez-Boland *et al.*, 2001). Non-invasive infections manifest as a self-limited febrile gastroenteritis, whereas invasive infections produce bacteraemia, CNS infections or sundry focal infections derived from haematogenous spread. CNS infection may take the form of meningitis, meningoencephalitis, brain abscess or, less commonly, rhombencephalitis (Vazquez-Boland *et al.*, 2001; Drevets and Bronze, 2008). Recent data show that *L. monocytogenes* causes nearly 4% of all cases of bacterial meningitis in the USA (Thigpen *et al.*, 2011). However, it accounts for a much higher percentage of meningitis cases in neonates and in adults older than 60 years. The classic triad of fever, stiff neck and altered mental status is seen in approximately 50% of patients while focal neurological findings and seizures are observed in 32% and 9% of patients, respectively (Amaya-Villar *et al.*, 2010). Most patients have underlying risk factors for *L. monocytogenes* infection, and the mortality rate is high. Two less common presentations are those of encephalitis (cerebritis) and rhombencephalitis. *Listeria* encephalitis probably represents a localized cortical infection predating progression to true brain abscess. Ampicillin and penicillin, without the addition of aminoglycosides, are usually considered the drugs of choice as *L. monocytogenes* is innately resistant to cephalosporins and earlier-generation fluoroquinolones. The case fatality rate of *L. monocytogenes* meningitis ranges from 20% to 30% (Swaminathan and Gerner-Smidt, 2007).

Clinical features include altered consciousness and cognitive dysfunction. Rhombencephalitis (brainstem encephalitis) is a biphasic illness usually seen in healthy individuals. The classical syndrome begins with headache, fever and nausea/vomiting followed by sudden onset of asymmetrical cranial nerve deficits (especially cranial nerves 5, 6, 7, 9 and 10), cerebellar signs and hemiparesis. A CSF Gram stain is usually negative, but CSF and blood cultures are positive in 33% and 60% of cases, respectively (Armstrong and Fung, 1993). Neuropathological examination in humans and affected animals reveals brain oedema and extensive inflammation, necrosis and vasculitis in the medulla and pons, and micro-abscesses in the cerebral white matter (Krueger *et al.*, 1995; Vazquez-Boland *et al.*, 2001; Drevets *et al.*, 2004b; Antal *et al.*, 2005). In those with meningitis, there is pyogenic suppuration of the leptomeninges with necrosis, micro-abscesses and vasculitis. In an ovine model, cellular infiltrates include neutrophils and mononuclear phagocytes, but few T- and B-lymphocytes (Krueger *et al.*, 1995).

14.5 Molecular and Cellular Pathogenicity

14.5.1 Extracellular survival

Survival within the gastrointestinal tract is a critical component of *L. monocytogenes* pathogenicity. Pre-adaptation of *L. monocytogenes* to acidic pH increases bacterial survival following macrophage infection and following intragastric inoculation of mice (Saklani-Jusforgues *et al.*, 2000; Gahan and Hill, 2005). The alternative sigma factor σ^B induces genes required for acid resistance in the stomach (*gadD2*, *gadT2*) and for osmotic stress and bile resistance within the duodenum (*opuC*, *bilE*, *bsh*, *pva*) (Gray *et al.*, 2006; O'Byrne and Karatzas, 2008). The GadD2 glutamate decarboxylase contributes to acid resistance by consuming hydrogen ions to produce γ-aminobutyric acid, which is then removed from the bacterial cell by the GadT2 antiporter in exchange for extracellular glutamate (Karatzas *et al.*, 2010). BilE and Bsh function as a bile exclusion system and a bile salt hydrolase, respectively, while OpuC functions as part of an osmolyte transporter and Pva contributes to bile resistance in an as yet undefined manner. Alternative sigma factor σ^B also induces expression of gene products required for host cell invasion (InlA and InlB), thus priming *L. monocytogenes* for invasion of the small intestine. *L. monocytogenes* also replicates extracellularly within the gall bladder (Hardy *et al.*, 2004; Gahan and Hill, 2005) and requires expression of *bsh*, *bilE* and *pva* as well as *brtA*, which encodes a bile-sensing regulatory protein that contributes to bile resistance (O'Byrne and Karatzas, 2008; Quillin *et al.*, 2011).

14.5.2 Cellular invasion

Invasion of non-professional phagocytes

Bacterial translocation across the intestinal epithelium is prerequisite for development of systemic listeriosis (Lecuit, 2007). Internalin (InlA) is a surface protein that mediates *L. monocytogenes* invasion of intestinal epithelial cells *in vitro* and *in vivo*. InlA binds to E-cadherin, an epithelial cell transmembrane protein associated with tight junction formation, exposed at the apical surface of enterocytes (Pentecost *et al.*, 2006). This interaction stimulates bacterial engulfment through clatherin-dependent endocytosis, which coordinates actin remodelling (Bonazzi *et al.*, 2009). A second surface protein, InlB, recognizes and binds the growth factor receptor tyrosine kinase Met, which is expressed on many cell types (Ireton, 2007). This interaction stimulates cytoskeletal rearrangements required for bacterial engulfment through Gab1-mediated recruitment of CrkII and activation of phosphoinositide 3-kinase (Gavicherla *et al.*, 2010; Jiwani *et al.*, 2012). InlB mediates *L. monocytogenes* invasion of a wide variety of cell types, including cultured brain microvascular endothelial cells (Greiffenberg *et al.*, 1998).

Entry into phagocytes

L. monocytogenes binding of C3 and C1q increases bacterial binding to macrophage CR3 and C1q receptors, respectively (Drevets and Campbell, 1991; Alvarez-Dominguez *et al.*, 1993). The macrophage non-selective cation channel TRPV2 is involved in the early steps of phagocytosis via its role in membrane depolarization, which subsequently triggers clustering of macrophage Fcγ receptors, substrate binding and phagocytosis. Transgenic mice lacking the TRPV2 channel are significantly more susceptible to *L. monocytogenes* infection (Link *et al.*, 2010).

14.5.3 Intracellular survival

LIPI-1 and secreted virulence factors

Having gained entry into the host cell, *L. monocytogenes* secretes a variety of factors that promote phagosome rupture, replication within the cytosol, and spread to adjacent cells. Several of these virulence factors are encoded on a 9 kb chromosomal element known as the *Listeria* pathogenicity island 1 (LIPI-1), while others are dispersed within other regions of the *L. monocytogenes* chromosome (Vazquez-Boland *et al.*, 2001).

Phagosome escape

L. monocytogenes disrupts phagosomal membranes via the secretion of a pore-forming cholesterol-dependent cytotoxin (CDC) known as listeriolysin O, or LLO (encoded by *hly*) (Hamon *et al.*, 2012). LLO is unique in its relationship to other CDC family members in that it has a low pH optimum that contributes to efficient vacuole lysis while reducing plasma membrane damage. LLO acts in concert with phosphatidylinositol-specific phospholipase C (PI-PLC), encoded by *plcA*, and phosphatidylcholine-specific phospholipase C (PC-PLC), encoded by *plcB*, to mediate bacterial escape into the cytosol. In addition, two host factors have been identified for their roles in promoting LLO-dependent pore formation. GILT (gamma-interferon (IFN-γ)-inducible lysosomal thiol reductase) is a lysosomal thiol reductase reported to activate LLO by maintaining the unique cysteine residue in a reduced state (Singh *et al.*, 2008). CFTR (cystic fibrosis transmembrane conductance regulator) is a host cell chloride channel that can facilitate *Listeria* escape by increasing phagosomal chloride concentration and potentiating LLO pore formation (Radtke *et al.*, 2011). LLO has also been associated with a variety of host cell-related activities that include enhancing *L. monocytogenes* invasion, inhibition of phagosomal NADPH oxidase (NOX2) activity, and evasion of autophagy (Hamon *et al.*, 2012).

Intracellular replication, actin motility and escape from autophagy

Within the cytosol, *L. monocytogenes* scavenges nutrients including hexose phosphate sugars, glycerol and other three-carbon sugars, lipoic acid, branched-chain amino acids and peptides (Marquis *et al.*, 1993; O'Riordan *et al.*, 2003; Eylert *et al.*, 2008; Sun and O'Riordan, 2010). Polar expression of the *L. monocytogenes* surface protein ActA provides a scaffold for the recruitment of actin and actin-binding proteins, a process that enables bacterial movement via actin polymerization and escape of autophagic recognition (Yoshikawa *et al.*, 2009). ActA binds actin monomers and also binds and activates the Arp2/3 complex, which catalyses nucleation of actin filament growth (Pizarro-Cerdá and Cossart, 2006). Another secreted protein, InlK, also contributes to bacterial evasion of autophagy through the recruitment of host cell major vault protein (MVP) to the bacterial surface (Dortet *et al.*, 2012). Secreted InlC has a dual role in promoting *L. monocytogenes* intracellular survival and cell-to-cell spread. InlC binds IKKα, a catalytic subunit of the IκB kinase complex (IKK), and inhibits IKKα-dependent activation of nuclear factor (NF)-κB, thereby dampening the host cell innate immune response (Gouin *et al.*, 2010). InlC also functions to relieve membrane cortical tension to facilitate the formation of *L. monocytogenes*-driven membrane protrusions and bacterial spread to adjacent cells (Rajabian *et al.*, 2009). Following entry into adjacent cells, *L. monocytogenes* lyses the double membrane-bound vacuole using LLO, PI-PLC and PC-PLC to return to the cytosol.

Regulation of virulence gene expression and virulence factor secretion

The majority of secreted virulence factors identified in *L. monocytogenes* are regulated at the level of gene expression by a transcriptional activator known as PrfA (Xayarath and Freitag, 2012). Following *L. monocytogenes* contact with host cells, PrfA induces the expression of several gene products directly associated with virulence, including *hly*, *plcA*, *actA*, *plcB*, *inlA*, *inlB* and *inlC* (de las Heras *et al.*, 2011). Bacteria containing deletions or loss-of-function mutations within the *prfA* gene fail to replicate in host cells and are > 100,000-fold less virulent in murine models (Freitag *et al.*, 1993). PrfA also regulates expression of genes that contribute to bile resistance (Dussurget *et al.*, 2002; Sleator *et al.*, 2005; Quillin *et al.*,

2011). An additional regulator, VirR, also contributes to *L. monocytogenes* virulence through bacterial surface modifications (Mandin *et al.*, 2005).

The dramatic increase in numbers of secreted virulence gene products that occurs following *L. monocytogenes* invasion of host cells indicates additional factors are needed to facilitate folding and activity of proteins during transit across the bacterial cell membrane. Induced by the virulence regulator PrfA, the post-translocation secretion chaperone known as PrsA2 (Forster *et al.*, 2012) appears specifically adapted to regulate the folding and activity of virulence factors at the membrane–cell wall interface (Alonzo *et al.*, 2011). *L. monocytogenes* mutants lacking PrsA2 exhibit normal growth characteristics in broth culture but exhibit reduced viability when PrfA becomes activated (Alonzo and Freitag, 2010), presumably due to the accumulation of misfolded proteins at the membrane–cell wall interface. PrsA2 works in concert with a second secreted chaperone, HtrA, which also possesses protease activity. Together, PrsA2 and HtrA promote the folding of secreted virulence factors at the membrane–cell wall interface, thereby maintaining *L. monocytogenes* cytosolic viability under conditions of increased protein secretion.

Virulence factors and inflammatory mediators within the brain

Experimental intracerebral inoculation of mice with *L. monocytogenes* shows that replicating bacteria infect choroid plexus epithelial cells, ependymal cells, macrophages, microglia and neurons (Schluter *et al.*, 1996). These animals exhibited signs of meningitis, ventriculitis and encephalitis, and finally succumbed to necrotizing brainstem encephalitis. Several studies suggest that, along with a requirement for LLO-mediated phagosomal escape, ActA and PC-PLC are key virulence factors for haemolytic *L. monocytogenes*. For example, mice infected intracerebrally with *L. monocytogenes* Δ*actA* mutants survived and cleared bacteria from the brain within 14 days (Virna *et al.*, 2006). This study also showed that Δ*actA* bacteria migrated from the site of inoculation, presumably as a result of macrophage infection. Additionally, although mice infected with Δ*plcB* mutants ultimately succumbed, they survived significantly longer than did mice infected with wild-type bacteria (Schluter *et al.*, 1998). Other reports noted an association of particular alleles of *actA* with isolates from CNS infections (particularly rhombencephalitis), further supporting a functional role for ActA in *L. monocytogenes* neurovirulence (Balandyté *et al.*, 2011).

Intracerebral inoculation of bacteria into mice elicits a rapid influx of neutrophils within 12 h that shifts to an infiltrate in which monocytes predominate by 72 h (Seebach *et al.*, 1995). Infection triggers immediate and large increases in pro-inflammatory cytokines including tumour necrosis factor (TNF)-α, interleukin (IL)-6, IL-1α and -β, and later also IFN-γ and inducible nitric oxide synthase (iNOS) (Frei *et al.*, 1993; Deckert *et al.*, 2007). TNF-α and IL-1 trigger intrathecal production of the chemoattractants macrophage inflammatory protein (MIP)-1α (CCL3) and MIP-2 (CXCL2) and the anaphlyatoxin C5a, which mediate recruitment of neutrophils and other leucocytes bearing the cognate receptors CCR1, CXCR2 and C5aR, respectively (Seebach *et al.*, 1995; Stahel *et al.*, 1997). LLO also triggers NF-κB-dependent upregulation of adhesion molecules E-selectin, ICAM-1 and VCAM-1, which mediate adhesion of monocytes and neutrophils to endothelial cells (Drevets, 1997; Kayal *et al.*, 1999).

The inflammatory response in this context is a downstream manifestation of innate immune pathways triggered by intracellular infection with *L. monocytogenes* (Witte *et al.*, 2012). Bacteria within phagosomes elicit a MyD88-dependent pathway that triggers expression of pro-inflammatory cytokines, whereas LLO-expressing bacteria exiting from phagosomes trigger the cytosolic surveillance pathway, thereby activating a stimulator of IFN genes (STING)/IFN regulatory factor 3 (IRF3)-dependent pathway, leading to expression of IFN-β and IFN-β-related genes (O'Riordan *et al.*, 2002; Sauer *et al.*, 2011). LLO-mediated phagosomal rupture and cathepsin B release is also critical for triggering a caspase-1-dependent, inflammasome pathway requiring the adaptor molecule ASC and NOD-like receptor family, pyrin domain containing 3 (NLRP3) that results in proteolytic activation of pro-IL-1β and secretion of IL-1β and IL-18 (Hara *et al.*, 2008; Meixenberger *et al.*, 2010). Interestingly, innate immune responses to intracellular infection in systemic organs also can remotely activate key systems in the CNS including upregulation of ICAM-1, P-selectin and E-selectin, as well as expression of chemokines and recruitment of leucocytes apart from infection of the CNS (Lopez *et al.*, 1999). This is most likely due to non-specific stimulation of cerebral endothelial cells by elevated levels of systemic cytokines, in particular IFN-γ along with TNF-α or IL-1α/β.

14.6 Mechanisms of CNS Invasion

14.6.1 Trojan horse model

Background

The Trojan horse mechanism of CNS invasion is transportation of a microbe across the BBB/BCSFB within a parasitized leucocyte. This mechanism is used by a wide variety of neuroinvasive bacteria that share an intracellular lifestyle and a proclivity to infect monocytes (Drevets *et al.*, 2004b). A long history of experimental data in the mouse model shows that mononuclear phagocytes are targets for *L. monocytogenes* parasitism (Mackaness, 1962). This fundamental observation, coupled with the absence of vascular infection as a common feature of CNS listeriosis, and the appearance of *L. monocytogenes*-infected mononuclear phagocytes in the brains of experimentally infected mice lead to the notion that monocytes transport *L. monocytogenes* into the brain (Prats *et al.*, 1992). The mouse model of experimental *L. monocytogenes* infection has been invaluable for elucidating the mechanisms of CNS invasion *in vivo*. In this model system, bacteria injected intravenously are cleared rapidly from the bloodstream by the liver and spleen in less than 60 min (Gregory *et al.*, 1996). Bacteria replicate in lymphoid tissues, predominantly the liver and spleen, but also in bone marrow and lymph nodes. Secondary bacteraemia appears 12–48 h later, depending on the inoculum, and precedes brain invasion (Berche, 1995; Drevets *et al.*, 2004a).

Monocyte biology

Classical and non-classical monocytes form the largest subsets of monocytes numerically, whereas monocyte cells with the intermediate phenotype are typically found at lower frequency. Mouse Ly-6C^{high}CD43^{low} (referred to as Ly-6C^{high} monocytes) and human CD14^{pos}CD16^{neg} monocytes are CCR2^{high} CX3CR1^{pos} whereas mouse Ly-6C^{low}CD43^{high} (referred to as Ly-6C^{low} monocytes) and human CD14^{low}CD16^{high} monocytes are CCR2^{neg}CX3CR1^{high}. Ly-6C^{high} monocytes exit the bone marrow in a CCR2-dependent manner in response to Toll-like receptor (TLR) ligands in the bloodstream (Shi *et al.*, 2011). Systemic infection with LLO-expressing *L. monocytogenes*, but not non-haemolytic *L. monocytogenes* mutants or avirulent *Listeria* spp., skews the steady-state ratio of Ly-6^{neg} to Ly-6C^{high} monocytes to significantly greater representation of Ly-6C^{high} monocytes (Drevets *et al.*, 2004a).

Bone marrow Ly-6C^{high} monocytes that develop during lethal infection acquire a novel CD115$^{neg/low}$CD121b^{high} phenotype (Drevets *et al.*, 2010b). Changes in surface molecules are accompanied by excessive upregulation of intracellular regulators of cytokine signalling (SOCS1 and SOCS3) and TLR signalling (IRAK-M), and by decreased lipopolysaccharide-induced IL-6 production. Monocytes from lethally infected mice also bind and internalize significantly more *L. monocytogenes* than do monocytes from sub-lethally infected animals, yet do not produce more reactive oxygen intermediates. The lack of phagocytic activity by immature myeloid cells is considered a protective feature that prevents pathogens from gaining access to the intracellular environment of phagocytes not capable of bactericidal activity. Collectively, these data show that *L. monocytogenes* infection promotes monopoiesis and that, during lethal infection, monocyte development and function are subverted in favour of the pathogen.

Parasitism of blood monocytes

L. monocytogenes parasitizes bone marrow monocytes, specifically identified as Ly-$6C^{high}CD11b^{pos}Ly\text{-}6G^{low}$ cells, along with other myeloid cells of monocytic and granulocytic lineages in various stages of development (Join-Lambert *et al.*, 2005). Importantly, infected monocytes in blood and bone marrow compartments display the same phenotype, supporting the idea that parasitized blood monocytes originate in the bone marrow (Join-Lambert *et al.*, 2005). A variety of data indicate that parasitized monocytes found in the bloodstream are able to initiate CNS infection (Fig. 14.1) (Drevets, 1999). Injection of *L. monocytogenes*-infected peripheral blood monocytes is more efficient for establishing brain infection than injection of naked bacteria (Drevets, 1999; Join-Lambert *et al.*, 2005). Additionally, CNS infection is not impeded when extracellular bacteria are eliminated from the bloodstream by gentamicin (Drevets *et al.*, 2001). Elegant electron micrographic studies have identified migration of bacteria-laden monocytes from the bloodstream into the CNS (Join-Lambert *et al.*, 2005). Finally, *L. monocytogenes* that have parasitized monocytes are fully capable of invading heterologous cell types, including neurons and endothelial cells, by cell-to-cell spread, suggesting a key means by which bacteria are transmitted from parasitized monocytes to resident cells of the CNS (Drevets *et al.*, 1995; Dramsi *et al.*, 1998; Greiffenberg *et al.*, 1998; Drevets, 1999).

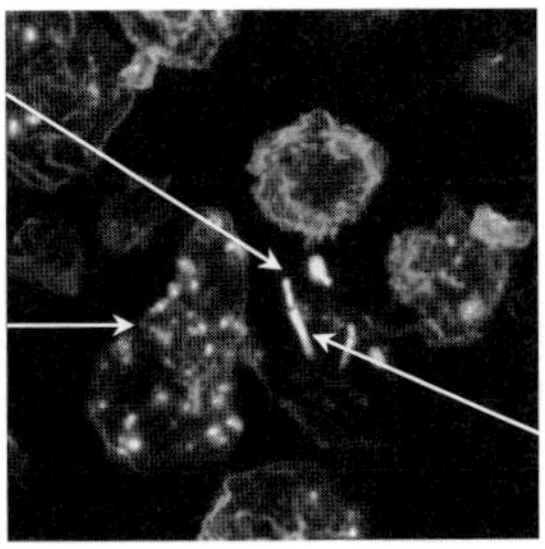

Fig. 14.1. Intracellular parasitism of peripheral blood leucocytes. Gentamicin-treated mice were infected with *L. monocytogenes* NF-L512, which contains an *actA–gfpuv–plcB* transcriptional fusion enabling preferential expression of green fluorescent protein (GFP) during intracellular growth. Cells were stained with Alexa Fluor 568 phalloidin to reveal F-actin. Images were collected on a confocal microscope. GFP-positive bacteria are associated with polarized F-actin tails proving cytoplasmic location and productive intracellular parasitism.

Systemic Listeria monocytogenes *infection triggers monocyte influxes in the brain*

A key concept of the Trojan horse mechanism is that bacterial infection of the brain does not trigger the initial influxes of infected leucocytes into the brain. In systemic *L. monocytogenes* infection, influxes of Ly-$6C^{high}$ monocytes into the brain are triggered by infection of peripheral organs that activates the cytosolic surveillance system and its downstream cytokines (Drevets *et al.*, 2008). This was demonstrated *in vivo* with *L. monocytogenes* highly attenuated Δ*actA* and Δ*hly* mutants, which neither cause bacteraemia nor invade the CNS. Δ*actA* mutants escape from phagosomes and activate the IRF3-dependent cytosolic response and caspase-1, which is a critical step for IL-1, IL-18 and IFN-γ production (Hara *et al.*, 2008; Meixenberger *et al.*, 2010). Systemic infection of mice with Δ*actA* mutants upregulates mRNA expression in the brain for endothelial cell adhesion molecules and monocyte-attracting chemokines, and triggers significant influxes of Ly-$6C^{high}$ monocytes into the brain. In contrast, infection with 100-fold more Δ*hly* mutants, which do not escape phagosomes or activate the cytosolic response, does not trigger brain influxes of Ly-$6C^{high}$ monocytes (Drevets *et al.*, 2008). A critical difference between infection with Δ*actA* and Δ*hly* mutants is that Δ*hly* mutants increase serum IFN-γ, IL-6 and TNF-α concentrations only marginally and much less than infection with Δ*actA* mutants. Interestingly, Δ*actA* infection of IFN-$\gamma^{-/-}$ mice did not elicit measurable influxes of Ly-$6C^{high}$ monocytes into the brain, despite normal monocyte emigration from the bone marrow to bloodstream and trafficking to the spleen. Additionally, mRNA upregulation of most monocyte-attracting chemokines and endothelial cell adhesion molecules in the brain was greatly diminished. Thus, IFN-γ has a critical role linking the cytosolic surveillance system with events in the brain that facilitate monocyte influxes. None the less, it is likely that other pro-inflammatory mediators such as TNF-α and IL-1 act with IFN-γ to promote maximum CNS inflammation (Drevets *et al.*, 2010a).

Mechanisms of monocyte trafficking to brain

CCR2-binding chemokines including CCL2 (MCP-1) and CCL7 (MCP-3) are critical for directing migration of Ly-6C^{high} monocytes to inflamed foci, including into the brain in some models of infection (Jia *et al.*, 2008; Mildner *et al.*, 2008). Systemic *L. monocytogenes* infection increases CCR2-binding chemokines including CCL2, CCL7, CCL8 and CCL12, suggesting that CCR2 could have a key role in mediating monocyte influxes (Drevets *et al.*, 2008, 2010a). However, despite transient retention of Ly-6C^{high} monocytes in the bone marrow of CCR2$^{-/-}$ mice, monocyte influxes to the brain were not decreased in *L. monocytogenes*-infected CCR2$^{-/-}$ and CCL2$^{-/-}$ mice compared with normal controls. Moreover, adoptively transferred Ly-6C^{high} monocytes from infected CCR2$^{+/+}$ and CCR2$^{-/-}$ were equally able to migrate from the bloodstream into the brains of infected mice (Table 14.1). These data suggest that the initial Ly6C^{high} monocyte influxes are CCR2 independent, although CCR2 and chemokines that bind it may have roles in monocyte recruitment to the brain after infection has been established. In addition, neither monocyte trafficking nor CNS infection were reduced in *L. monocytogenes*-infected mice lacking CCR1, CCR5, CX3CR1 or CXCR3 (Drevets *et al.*, 2010a). Recently, Shi and colleagues identified CCR2-independent trafficking of inflammatory monocytes into the liver during experimental *L. monocytogenes* infection and showed that the adhesion molecules CD11b, ICAM-1 and CD44 were important for directing monocyte recruitment (Shi *et al.*, 2010). The extent to which these molecules mediate monocyte recruitment to the brain during *L. monocytogenes* infection is not clear. However, upregulation of CAM-1, JAM-A and VCAM-1 was significantly lower in IFN-γ$^{-/-}$ mice than in normal animals, and ALCAM was upregulated only in normal mice (Drevets *et al.*, 2010a).

Table 14.1. Adoptive transfer shows no role for CCR2 in monocyte migration from blood to brain during *L. monocytogenes* infection.

Monocytes injected	FL1$^+$ cells/brain monocytes (× 100)[a]
CCR2$^{+/+}$[b]	8.8 ± 1.7[c]
CCR2$^{-/-}$[b]	8.3 ± 1.9[c]
None (control)	3.5 ± 0.5

[a]Results presented as mean ± SEM of three to seven mice.
[b]Infected mice received 1 × 10^6 labelled monocytes of the indicated genotype.
[c]p<0.01 compared with background control.

14.6.2 Neural route

L. monocytogenes can invade the CNS via a neural route in which bacteria enter axons in the periphery and then migrate centripetally within them into the brainstem. This mechanism is the likely cause of rhombencephalitis, a brainstem encephalitis that is the most common natural form of CNS listeriosis in ruminants (Oevermann *et al.*, 2010) and is also found less frequently, but in a highly analogous form, in humans (Antal *et al.*, 2005). Several investigators have replicated the natural finding of *L. monocytogenes* in axons of the trigeminal nerve in mice by inoculating bacteria into oral tissues/muscle or the facial nerve (Antal *et al.*, 2001; Jin *et al.*, 2001). Post-mortem analyses of ruminants indicate that bacteria spread in a caudal–rostral direction via nerve fibre tracts, which is consistent with *in vitro* studies showing that *L. monocytogenes* can propagate in anterograde or retrograde directions within axons (Dons *et al.*, 1999; Oevermann *et al.*, 2010). Analysis of virulence genes and alleles associated with CNS infection suggests that the *actA*3 and *inlJ1* alleles are associated with ruminant rhombencephalitis (Balandyté *et al.*, 2011).

In vitro studies show that *L. monocytogenes* can invade a variety of cultured brain parenchymal cells including neurons, microglia, astrocytes and oligodendrocytes

(Peters and Hewicker-Trautwein, 1996; Dramsi *et al.*, 1998). Non-neuronal cells take up bacteria more avidly than do neurons, with microglia and macrophages the most easily infected. In addition, *L. monocytogenes* can spread from infected macrophages to neurons via cell-to-cell spread (Dramsi *et al.*, 1998). This finding is important with respect to *in vivo* mechanisms as *L. monocytogenes* inoculated into oral tissues of macrophage-deficient op$^{-/-}$ (M-CSFR$^{-/-}$) mice were less able to enter neurons than after injection into normal mice (Jin *et al.*, 2002). Binding and invasion of neurons may occur once bacteria have been inoculated into oral tissues and may be internalin-dependent as E-cadherin is expressed by peripheral Schwann cells and oral epithelium, but does not co-localize with foci of brainstem infection in ruminants (Madarame *et al.*, 2011).

14.6.3 Direct invasion of blood vessel endothelial cells of the CNS

L. monocytogenes can invade endothelial cells *in vitro* either by direct bacterium–endothelial cell interactions or via cell-to-cell spread from adherent phagocytes that harbour intracellular bacteria (Drevets *et al.*, 1995; Greiffenberg *et al.*, 1998). Direct invasion *in vitro* is mediated by InlB under serum-free conditions (Greiffenberg *et al.*, 1998), but is independent of InlA and InlB in the presence of serum (Greiffenberg *et al.*, 1997). Autret and colleagues used signature-tagged mutagenesis to identify bacteria with attenuated brain invasion *in vivo* but that also had preserved LLO secretion (Autret *et al.*, 2001). Wang and Lin found that *L. monocytogenes* lacking IscP, a cell wall-anchored autolysin, had reduced virulence *in vivo* including brain invasion (Wang and Lin, 2008). These mutants had decreased *in vitro* binding to sheep choroid plexus cells but not to brain endothelial cells, and were attenuated in cell-to-cell spread and intracellular growth. They also showed greater reductions in the number of colony-forming units per organ in the liver than in the brain, whereas cultures of blood and bone marrow were not performed. Thus, lack of brain invasion by these mutants is probably a by-product of reduced virulence in general, rather than a specific lack of brain tropism. The role of direct endothelial cell invasion for establishing CNS infection in humans is unclear. Normal human serum contains antibodies that strongly inhibit InlB-mediated *L. monocytogenes* invasion of human brain microvascular endothelial cells (Hertzig *et al.*, 2003) and so-called 'natural' antibodies protect mice against CNS invasion by *L. monocytogenes* (Ochsenbein *et al.*, 1999). Additionally, studies in humans comparing expression of full-length internalin transcripts and protein in food and clinical isolates concluded that this invasion protein is not used for CNS invasion from the blood (Jacquet *et al.*, 2004).

14.7 Conclusions

L. monocytogenes came to clinical attention as a human pathogen after World War II but remained an obscure cause of CNS infection until the end of the 20th century. Its emergence as a notable CNS pathogen occurred largely due to increased numbers of people at risk and perhaps also to declines in the incidence of vaccine-preventable causes of CNS infection. *L. monocytogenes* is a remarkably resourceful pathogen, capable of crossing the BBB/BCSFB by at least three distinct mechanisms. This organism is a model pathogen for the next phase of discovery research aimed at elucidating the mechanisms that underlie the neurobiological consequences of host responses to systemic infectious diseases.

References

Alonzo, F., III and Freitag, N.E. (2010) *Listeria monocytogenes* PrsA2 is required for virulence factor secretion and bacterial viability within the host cell cytosol. *Infection and Immunity* 78, 4944–4957.

Alonzo, F., III, Xayarath, B., Whisstock, J.C. and Freitag, N.E. (2011) Functional analysis of the *Listeria monocytogenes* secretion chaperone PrsA2 and its multiple contributions to bacterial virulence. *Molecular Microbiology* 80, 1530–1548.

Alvarez-Dominguez, C., Carrasco-Marin, E. and Leyva-Cobian, F. (1993) Role of complement component C1q in phagocytosis of *Listeria monocytogenes* by murine macrophage-like cell lines. *Infection and Immunity* 61, 3664–3672.

Amaya-Villar, R., Garcia-Cabrera, E., Sulleiro-Igual, E., Fernandez-Viladrich, P., Fontanals-Aymerich, D., Catalan-Alonso, P., Rodrigo-Gonzalo de Liria, C., Coloma-Conde, A., Grill-Diaz, F., Guerrero-Espejo, A., Pachon, J. and Prats-Pastor, G. (2010) Three-year multicenter surveillance of community-acquired *Listeria monocytogenes* meningitis in adults. *BMC Infectious Diseases* 10, 324.

Antal, E.A., Loberg, E.M., Bracht, P., Melby, K.K. and Maehlen, J. (2001) Evidence for intraaxonal spread of *Listeria monocytogenes* from the periphery to the central nervous system. *Brain Pathology* 11, 432–438.

Antal, E.A., Dietrichs, E., Loberg, E.M., Melby, K.K. and Maehlen, J. (2005) Brain stem encephalitis in listeriosis. *Scandinavian Journal of Infectious Diseases* 37, 190–194.

Armstrong, R.W. and Fung, P.C. (1993) Brainstem encephalitis (rhombencephalitis) due to *Listeria monocytogenes*: case report and review. *Clinical Infectious Diseases* 16, 689–702.

Autret, N., Dubail, I., Trieu-Cuot, P., Berche, P. and Charbit, A. (2001) Identification of new genes involved in the virulence of *Listeria monocytogenes* by signature-tagged transposon mutagenesis. *Infection and Immunity* 69, 2054–2065.

Balandyté, L., Brodard, I., Frey, J., Oevermann, A. and Abril, C. (2011) Ruminant rhombencephalitis-associated *Listeria monocytogenes* alleles linked to a multilocus variable-number tandem-repeat analysis complex. *Applied and Environmental Microbiology* 77, 8325–8335.

Berche, P. (1995) Bacteremia is required for invasion of the murine central nervous system by *Listeria monocytogenes*. *Microbial Pathogenesis* 18, 323–336.

Bonazzi, M., Lecuit, M. and Cossart, P. (2009) *Listeria monocytogenes* internalin and E-cadherin: from structure to pathogenesis. *Cellular Microbiology* 11, 693–702.

Bruno, J.C. and Freitag, N.E. (2011) *Listeria monocytogenes* adapts to long term stationary phase survival without compromising bacterial virulence. *FEMS Microbiology Letters* 323, 171–179.

Chaturongakul, S., Raengpradub, S., Wiedmann, M. and Boor, K.J. (2008) Modulation of stress and virulence in *Listeria monocytogenes*. *Trends in Microbiology* 16, 388–396.

de las Heras, A., Cain, R.J., Bielecka, M.K. and Vazquez-Boland, J.A. (2011) Regulation of *Listeria* virulence: PrfA master and commander. *Current Opinion in Microbiology* 14, 118–127.

Deckert, M., Virna, S., Sakowicz-Burkiewicz, M., Lutjen, S., Soltek, S., Bluethmann, H. and Schluter, D. (2007) Interleukin-1 Receptor Type 1 is essential for control of cerebral but not systemic listeriosis. *American Journal of Pathology* 170, 990–1002.

Dons, L., Weclewicz, K., Jin, Y., Bindseil, E., Olsen, J. and Kristenson, K. (1999) Rat dorsal root ganglia neurons as a model for *Listeria monocytogenes* infections in culture. *Medical Microbiology and Immunology* 188, 15–21.

Dortet, L., Mostowy, S. and Cossart, P. (2012) Listeria and autophagy escape: involvement of InlK, an internalin-like protein. *Autophagy* 8, 132–134.

Dramsi, S., Levi, S., Triller, A. and Cossart, P. (1998) Entry of *Listeria monocytogenes* into neurons occurs by cell-to-cell spread: an in vitro study. *Infection and Immunity* 66, 4461–4468.

Drevets, D.A. (1997) *Listeria monocytogenes* infection of cultured endothelial cells stimulates neutrophil adhesion and adhesion molecule expression. *Journal of Immunology* 158, 5305–5313.

Drevets, D.A. (1999) Dissemination of *Listeria monocytogenes* by infected phagocytes. *Infection and Immunity* 67, 3512–3517.

Drevets, D.A. and Bronze, M.S. (2008) *Listeria monocytogenes*: epidemiology, human disease, and mechanisms of brain invasion. *FEMS Immunology and Medical Microbiology* 53, 151–165.

Drevets, D.A. and Campbell, P.A. (1991) Roles of complement and complement receptor type 3 in phagocytosis of *Listeria monocytogenes* by inflammatory mouse peritoneal macrophages. *Infection and Immunity* 59, 2645–2652.

Drevets, D.A., Sawyer, R.T., Potter, T.A. and Campbell, P.A. (1995) *Listeria monocytogenes* infects human endothelial cells by two distinct mechanisms. *Infection and Immunity* 63, 4268–4276.

Drevets, D.A., Jelinek, T.A. and Freitag, N.E. (2001) *Listeria monocytogenes*-infected phagocytes can initiate central nervous system infection in mice. *Infection and Immunity* 69, 1344–1350.

Drevets, D.A., Dillon, M.J., Schawang, J.S., Van Rooijen, N., Ehrchen, J., Sunderkotter, C. and Leenen, P.J. (2004a) The Ly-6C^{high} monocyte subpopulation transports *Listeria monocytogenes* into the brain during systemic infection of mice. *Journal of Immunology* 172, 4418–4424.

Drevets, D.A., Leenen, P.J. and Greenfield, R.A. (2004b) Invasion of the central nervous system by intracellular bacteria. *Clinical Microbiology Reviews* 17, 323–347.

Drevets, D.A., Schawang, J.E., Dillon, M.J., Lerner, M.R., Bronze, M.S. and Brackett, D.J. (2008) Innate responses to systemic infection by intracellular bacteria trigger recruitment of Ly-6C^{high} monocytes to the brain. *Journal of Immunology* 181, 529–536.

Drevets, D.A., Dillon, M.J., Schawang, J.E., Stoner, J.A. and Leenen, P.J. (2010a) IFN-γ triggers CCR2-independent monocyte entry into the brain during systemic infection by virulent *Listeria monocytogenes*. *Brain Behaviour and Immunology* 24, 919–929.

Drevets, D.A., Schawang, J.E., Mandava, V.K., Dillon, M.J. and Leenen, P.J.M. (2010b) Severe *Listeria monocytogenes* infection induces development of monocytes with distinct phenotypic and functional features. *Journal of Immunology* 185, 2432–2441.

Dussurget, O., Cabanes, D., Dehoux, P., Lecuit, M., Buchrieser, C., Glaser, P. and Cossart, P. (2002) *Listeria monocytogenes* bile salt hydrolase is a PrfA-regulated virulence factor involved in the intestinal and hepatic phases of listeriosis. *Molecular Microbiology* 45, 1095–1106.

Eylert, E., Schar, J., Mertins, S., Stoll, R., Bacher, A., Goebel, W. and Eisenreich, W. (2008) Carbon metabolism of *Listeria monocytogenes* growing inside macrophages. *Molecular Microbiology* 69, 1008–1017.

Forster, B.M., Zemansky, J., Portnoy, D.A. and Marquis, H. (2012) Posttranslocation chaperone PrsA2 regulates the maturation and secretion of *Listeria monocytogenes* proprotein virulence factors. *Journal of Bacteriology* 193, 5961–5970.

Frei, K., Nadal, D., Pfister, H.W. and Fontana, A. (1993) *Listeria* meningitis: identification of a cerebrospinal fluid inhibitor of macrophage listericidal function as interleukin 10. *Journal of Experimental Medicine* 178, 1255–1261.

Freitag, N.E., Rong, L. and Portnoy, D.A. (1993) Regulation of the *prfA* transcriptional activator of *Listeria monocytogenes*: multiple promoter elements contribute to intracellular growth and cell-to-cell spread. *Infection and Immunity* 61, 2537–2544.

Freitag, N.E., Port, G.C. and Miner, M.D. (2009) *Listeria monocytogenes* – from saprophyte to intracellular pathogen. *Nature Reviews Microbiology* 7, 623–628.

Gahan, C.G. and Hill, C. (2005) Gastrointestinal phase of *Listeria monocytogenes* infection. *Journal of Applied Microbiology* 98, 1345–1353.

Gavicherla, B., Ritchey, L., Gianfelice, A., Kolokoltsov, A.A., Davey, R.A. and Ireton, K. (2010) Critical role for the host GTPase-activating protein ARAP2 in InlB-mediated entry of *Listeria monocytogenes*. *Infection and Immunity* 78, 4532–4541.

Gouin, E., Adib-Conquy, M., Balestrino, D., Nahori, M.A., Villiers, V., Colland, F., Dramsi, S., Dussurget, O. and Cossart, P. (2010) The *Listeria monocytogenes* InlC protein interferes with innate immune responses by targeting the IkB kinase subunit IKKa. *Proceedings of the National Academy of Sciences USA* 107, 17333–17338.

Gray, M.J., Freitag, N.E. and Boor, K.J. (2006) How the bacterial pathogen *Listeria monocytogenes* mediates the switch from environmental Dr. Jekyll to pathogenic Mr. Hyde. *Infection and Immunity* 74, 2505–2512.

Gregory, S.H., Sagnimeni, A.J. and Wing, E.J. (1996) Bacteria in the bloodstream are trapped in the liver and killed by immigrating neutrophils. *Journal of Immunology* 157, 2514–2520.

Greiffenberg, L., Sokolovic, Z., Schnittler, H.J., Spory, A., Bockmann, R., Goebel, W. and Kuhn, M. (1997) *Listeria monocytogenes*-infected human umbilical vein endothelial cells: internalin-independent invasion, intracellular growth, movement, and host cell responses. *FEMS Microbiology Letters* 157, 163–170.

Greiffenberg, L., Goebel, W., Kim, K.S., Weiglein, I., Bubert, A., Engelbrecht, F., Stins, M. and Kuhn, M. (1998) Interaction of *Listeria monocytogenes* with human brain microvascular endothelial cells: InlB-dependent invasion, long-term intracellular growth, and spread from macrophages to endothelial cells. *Infection and Immunity* 66, 5260–5267.

Hamon, M.A., Ribet, D., Stavru, F. and Cossart, P. (2012) Listeriolysin O: the Swiss army knife of Listeria. *Trends in Microbiology* 20, 360–368.

Hara, H., Tsuchiya, K., Nomura, T., Kawamura, I., Shoma, S. and Mitsuyama, M. (2008) Dependency of caspase-1 activation induced in macrophages by *Listeria monocytogenes* on cytolysin, listeriolysin O, after evasion from phagosome into the cytoplasm. *Journal of Immunology* 180, 7859–7868.

Hardy, J., Francis, K.P., DeBoer, M., Chu, P., Gibbs, K. and Contag, C.H. (2004) Extracellular replication of *Listeria monocytogenes* in the murine gall bladder. *Science* 303, 851–853.

Hertzig, T., Weber, M., Greiffenberg, L., Holthausen, B.S., Goebel, W., Kim, K.S. and Kuhn, M. (2003) Antibodies present in normal human serum inhibit invasion of human brain microvascular endothelial cells by *Listeria monocytogenes*. *Infection and Immunity* 71, 95–100.

Ireton, K. (2007) Entry of the bacterial pathogen *Listeria monocytogenes* into mammalian cells. *Cellular Microbiology* 9, 1365–1375.

Jacquet, C., Doumith, M., Gordon, J.I., Martin, P.M., Cossart, P. and Lecuit, M. (2004) A molecular marker for evaluating the pathogenic potential of foodborne *Listeria monocytogenes*. *Journal of Infectious Diseases* 189, 2094–2100.

Jia, T., Serbina, N.V., Brandl, K., Zhong, M.X., Leiner, I.M., Charo, I.F. and Pamer, E.G. (2008) Additive roles for MCP-1 and MCP-3 in CCR2-mediated recruitment of inflammatory monocytes during *Listeria monocytogenes* infection. *Journal of Immunology* 180, 6846–6853.

Jin, Y., Dons, L., Kristensson, K. and Rottenberg, M.E. (2001) Neural route of cerebral *Listeria monocytogenes* murine infection: role of immune response mechanisms in controlling bacterial neuroinvasion. *Infection and Immunity* 69, 1093–1100.

Jin, Y., Dons, L., Kristensson, K. and Rottenberg, M.E. (2002) Colony-stimulating factor 1-dependent cells protect against systemic infection with *Listeria monocytogenes* but facilitate neuroinvasion. *Infection and Immunity* 70, 4682–4686.

Jiwani, S., Wang, Y., Dowd, G.C., Gianfelice, A., Pichestapong, P., Gavicherla, B., Vanbennekom, N. and Ireton, K. (2012) Identification of components of the host type IA phosphoinositide 3-kinase pathway that promote internalization of *Listeria monocytogenes*. *Infection and Immunity* 80, 1252–1266.

Join-Lambert, O.F., Ezine, S., Le Monnier, A., Jaubert, F., Okabe, M., Berche, P. and Kayal, S. (2005) *Listeria monocytogenes*-infected bone marrow myeloid cells promote bacterial invasion of the central nervous system. *Cellular Microbiology* 7, 167–180.

Karatzas, K.-A.G., Brennan, O., Heavin, S., Morrissey, J. and O'Byrne, C.P. (2010) Intracellular accumulation of high levels of α-aminobutyrate by *Listeria monocytogenes* 10403S in response to low pH: uncoupling of α-aminobutyrate synthesis from efflux in a chemically defined medium. *Applied and Environmental Microbiology* 76, 3529–3537.

Kayal, S., Lilienbaum, A., Poyart, C., Memet, S., Israel, A. and Berche, P. (1999) Listeriolysin O-dependent activation of endothelial cells during infection with *Listeria monocytogenes*: activation of NF-κ B and upregulation of adhesion molecules and chemokines. *Molecular Microbiology* 31, 1709–1722.

Krueger, N., Low, C. and Donachie, W. (1995) Phenotypic characterization of the cells of the inflammatory response in ovine encephalitic listeriosis. *Journal of Comparative Pathology* 113, 263–275.

Lecuit, M. (2007) Human listeriosis and animal models. *Microbes and Infection* 9, 1216–1225.

Link, T.M., Park, U., Vonakis, B.M., Raben, D.M., Soloski, M.J. and Caterina, M.J. (2010) TRPV2 has a pivotal role in macrophage particle binding and phagocytosis. *Nature Immunology* 11, 232–239.

Lopez, S., Prats, N. and Marco, A.J. (1999) Expression of E-selectin, P-selectin, and intercellular adhesion molecule-1 during experimental murine listeriosis. *American Journal of Pathology* 155, 1391–1397.

Mackaness, G.B. (1962) Cellular resistance to infection. *Journal of Experimental Medicine* 116, 407.

Madarame, H., Seuberlich, T., Abril, C., Zurbriggen, A., Vandevelde, M. and Oevermann, A. (2011) The distribution of E-cadherin expression in listeric rhombencephalitis of ruminants indicates its involvement in *Listeria monocytogenes* neuroinvasion. *Neuropathology and Applied Neurobiology* 37, 753–767.

Mandin, P., Fsihi, H., Dussurget, O., Vergassola, M., Milohanic, E., Toledo-Arana, A., Lasa, I., Johansson, J. and Cossart, P. (2005) VirR, a response regulator critical for *Listeria monocytogenes* virulence. *Molecular Microbiology* 57, 1367–1380.

Marquis, H., Bouwer, H.G., Hinrichs, D.J. and Portnoy, D.A. (1993) Intracytoplasmic growth and virulence of *Listeria monocytogenes* auxotrophic mutants. *Infection and Immunity* 61, 3756–3760.

Meixenberger, K., Pache, F., Eitel, J., Schmeck, B., Hippenstiel, S., Slevogt, H., N'Guessan, P., Witzenrath, M., Netea, M.G., Chakraborty, T., Suttorp, N. and Opitz, B. (2010) *Listeria monocytogenes*-infected human peripheral blood mononuclear cells produce IL-1β, depending on listeriolysin O and NLRP3. *Journal of Immunology* 184, 922–930.

Mildner, A., Djukic, M., Garbe, D., Wellmer, A., Kuziel, W.A., Mack, M., Nau, R. and Prinz, M. (2008) Ly-6G^{+}CCR2^{-} myeloid cells rather than Ly-6C^{high}CCR2^{+} monocytes are required for the control of bacterial infection in the central nervous system. *Journal of Immunology* 181, 2713–2722.

Mook, P., O'Brien, S.J. and Gillespie, I.A. (2011) Concurrent conditions and human listeriosis, England, 1999–2009. *Emerging Infectious Diseases* 17, 38–43.

O'Byrne, C.P. and Karatzas, K.A. (2008) The role of sigma B (σ^B) in the stress adaptations of *Listeria monocytogenes*: overlaps between stress adaptation and virulence. *Advances in Applied Microbiology* 65, 115–140.

O'Riordan, M., Yi, C.H., Gonzales, R., Lee, K.D. and Portnoy, D.A. (2002) Innate recognition of bacteria by a macrophage cytosolic surveillance pathway. *Proceedings of the National Academy of Sciences USA* 99, 13861–13866.

O'Riordan, M., Moors, M.A. and Portnoy, D.A. (2003) *Listeria* intracellular growth and virulence require host-derived lipoic acid. *Science* 302, 462–464.

Ochsenbein, A.F., Fehr, T., Lutz, C., Suter, M., Brombacher, F., Hengartner, H. and Zinkernagel, R.M. (1999) Control of early viral and bacterial distribution and disease by natural antibodies. *Science* 286, 2156–2159.

Oevermann, A., Di Palma, S., Doherr, M.G., Abril, C., Zurbriggen, A. and Vandevelde, M. (2010) Neuropathogenesis of naturally occurring encephalitis caused by *Listeria monocytogenes* in ruminants. *Brain Pathology* 20, 378–390.

Pentecost, M., Otto, G., Theriot, J.A. and Amieva, M.R. (2006) *Listeria monocytogenes* invades the epithelial junctions at sites of cell extrusion. *PLoS Pathogens* 2, e3.

Peters, M. and Hewicker-Trautwein, M. (1996) Studies on the cell tropism of *Listeria monocytogenes* in ovine fetal brain cell cultures. *Veterinary Microbiology* 49, 169–179.

Pizarro-Cerdá, J. and Cossart, P. (2006) Subversion of cellular functions by *Listeria monocytogenes*. *Journal of Pathology* 208, 215–223.

Prats, N., Briones, V., Blanco, M.M., Altimira, J., Ramos, J.A., Dominguez, L. and Marco, A. (1992) Choroiditis and meningitis in experimental murine infection with *Listeria monocytogenes*. *European Journal of Clinical Microbiology and Infectious Diseases* 11, 744–747.

Quillin, S.J., Schwartz, K.T. and Leber, J.H. (2011) The novel *Listeria monocytogenes* bile sensor BrtA controls expression of the cholic acid efflux pump MdrT. *Molecular Microbiology* 81, 129–142.

Radtke, A.L., Anderson, K.L., Davis, M.J., DiMagno, M.J., Swanson, J.A. and O'Riordan, M.X. (2011) *Listeria monocytogenes* exploits cystic fibrosis transmembrane conductance regulator (CFTR) to escape the phagosome. *Proceedings of the National Academy of Sciences USA* 108, 1633–1638.

Rajabian, T., Gavicherla, B., Heisig, M., Muller-Altrock, S., Goebel, W., Gray-Owen, S.D. and Ireton, K. (2009) The bacterial virulence factor InlC perturbs apical cell junctions and promotes cell-to-cell spread of *Listeria*. *Nature Cell Biology* 11, 1212–1218.

Saklani-Jusforgues, H., Fontan, E. and Goossens, P.L. (2000) Effect of acid-adaptation on *Listeria monocytogenes* survival and translocation in a murine intragastric infection model. *FEMS Microbiology Letters* 193, 155–159.

Sauer, J.-D., Sotelo-Troha, K., von Moltke, J., Monroe, K.M., Rae, C.S., Brubaker, S.W., Hyodo, M., Hayakawa, Y., Woodward, J.J., Portnoy, D.A. and Vance, R.E. (2011) The *N*-ethyl-*N*-nitrosourea-induced *Goldenticket* mouse mutant reveals an essential function of *Sting* in the *in vivo* interferon response to *Listeria monocytogenes* and cyclic dinucleotides. *Infection and Immunity* 79, 688–694.

Scallan, E., Hoekstra, R.M., Angulo, F.J., Tauxe, R.V., Widdowson, M.A., Roy, S.L., Jones, J.L. and Griffin, P.M. (2011) Foodborne illness acquired in the United States – major pathogens. *Emerging Infectious Diseases* 17, 7–15.

Schluter, D., Chahoud, S., Lassmann, H., Schumann, A., Hof, H. and Deckert-Schluter, M. (1996) Intracerebral targets and immunomodulation of murine *Listeria monocytogenes* meningoencephalitis. *Journal of Neuropathology and Experimental Neurology* 55, 14–24.

Schluter, D., Domann, E., Buck, C., Hain, T., Hof, H., Chakraborty, T. and Deckert-Schluter, M. (1998) Phosphatidylcholine-specific phospholipase C from *Listeria monocytogenes* is an important virulence factor in murine cerebral listeriosis. *Infection and Immunity* 66, 5930–5938.

Schuchat, A., Robinson, K., Wenger, J.D., Harrison, L.H., Farley, M., Reingold, A.L., Lefkowitz, L. and Perkins, B.A. (1997) Bacterial meningitis in the United States in 1995. Active Surveillance Team. *New England Journal of Medicine* 337, 970–976.

Seebach, J., Bartholdi, D., Frei, K., Spanaus, K.S., Ferrero, E., Widmer, U., Isenmann, S., Strieter, R.M., Schwab, M., Pfister, H. and Fontana, A. (1995) Experimental *Listeria* meningoencephalitis. Macrophage inflammatory protein-1α and -2 are produced intrathecally and mediate chemotactic activity in cerebrospinal fluid of infected mice. *Journal of Immunology* 155, 4367–4375.

Shi, C., Velazquez, P., Hohl, T.M., Leiner, I., Dustin, M.L. and Pamer, E.G. (2010) Monocyte trafficking to hepatic sites of bacterial infection is chemokine independent and directed by focal intercellular adhesion molecule-1 expression. *Journal of Immunology* 184, 6266–6274.

Shi, C., Jia, T., Mendez-Ferrer, S., Hohl, T.M., Serbina, N.V., Lipuma, L., Leiner, I., Li, M.O., Frenette, P.S. and Pamer, E.G. (2011) Bone marrow mesenchymal stem and progenitor cells induce monocyte emigration in response to circulating Toll-like receptor ligands. *Immunity* 34, 590–601.

Singh, R., Jamieson, A. and Cresswell, P. (2008) GILT is a critical host factor for *Listeria monocytogenes* infection. *Nature* 455, 1244–1247.

Sleator, R.D., Wemekamp-Kamphuis, H.H., Gahan, C.G., Abee, T. and Hill, C. (2005) A PrfA-regulated bile exclusion system (BilE) is a novel virulence factor in *Listeria monocytogenes*. *Molecular Microbiology* 55, 1183–1195.

Stahel, P.F., Frei, K., Eugster, H.P., Fontana, A., Hummel, K.M., Wetsel, R.A., Ames, R.S. and Barnum, S.R. (1997) TNF-α-mediated expression of the receptor for anaphylatoxin C5a on neurons in experimental *Listeria* meningoencephalitis. *Journal of Immunology* 159, 861–869.

Sun, Y. and O'Riordan, M.X. (2010) Branched-chain fatty acids promote *Listeria monocytogenes* intracellular infection and virulence. *Infection and Immunity* 78, 4667–4673.

Swaminathan, B. and Gerner-Smidt, P. (2007) The epidemiology of human listeriosis. *Microbes and Infection* 9, 1236–1243.

Thigpen, M.C., *et al.* (2011) Bacterial meningitis in the United States, 1998–2007. *New England Journal of Medicine* 364, 2016–2025.

Vazquez-Boland, J.A., Kuhn, M., Berche, P., Chakraborty, T., Dominguez-Bernal, G., Goebel, W., Gonzalez-Zorn, B., Wehland, J. and Kreft, J. (2001) *Listeria* pathogenesis and molecular virulence determinants. *Clinical Microbiology Reviews* 14, 584–640.

Virna, S., Deckert, M., Lutjen, S., Soltek, S., Foulds, K.E., Shen, H., Korner, H., Sedgwick, J.D. and Schluter, D. (2006) TNF is important for pathogen control and limits brain damage in murine cerebral listeriosis. *Journal of Immunology* 177, 3972–3982.

Wang, L. and Lin, M. (2008) A novel cell wall-anchored peptidoglycan hydrolase (autolysin), IspC, essential for *Listeria monocytogenes* virulence: genetic and proteomic analysis. *Microbiology* 154, 1900–1913.

Witte, C.E., Archer, K.A., Rae, C.S., Sauer, J.-D., Woodward, J.J. and Portnoy, D.A. (2012) Innate immune pathways triggered by *Listeria monocytogenes* and their role in the induction of cell-mediated immunity. *Advances in Immunology* 113, 135–156.

Xayarath, B. and Freitag, N.E. (2012) Optimizing the balance between host and environmental survival skills: lessons learned from *Listeria monocytogenes*. *Future Microbiology* 7, 839–852.

Yoshikawa, Y., Ogawa, M., Hain, T., Chakraborty, T. and Sasakawa, C. (2009) *Listeria monocytogenes* ActA is a key player in evading autophagic recognition. *Autophagy* 5, 1220–1221.

15 Meningitis in Neuroborreliosis

Diego Cadavid[1,2*]

[1]*Center for Immunology and Inflammatory Diseases, Massachusetts General Hospital, Boston, USA;* [2]*Neurology Clinical Development, Biogen Idec, Cambridge, USA*

15.1 *Borrelia* Meningitis

15.1.1 Lyme meningitis

Lyme disease, or Lyme borreliosis, is an arthropod-borne infection caused by the pathogenic spirochaete *Borrelia burgdorferi* (Burgdorfer *et al.*, 1982). Since its discovery in 1975, during an epidemic of oligoarthritis in children and adults in Lyme, Connecticut, Lyme disease has become recognized as the most prevalent arthropod-borne infection in the western hemisphere. Meningitis is a known complication of infection with all three pathogenic genospecies of *B. burgdorferi*, *B. burgdorferi* sensu stricto, *B. garinii* and *B. afzelii*. The most common neurological abnormalities in early disseminated Lyme disease are aseptic meningitis, cranial neuritis and radiculitis, and any of these can be the first clinical manifestation of the illness (Pachner and Steere, 1985). The reported frequency of meningeal symptoms in Lyme disease is variable, ranging from 30% to over 90%, depending partly on the method of ascertainment and the endemic area. Children are more likely to be symptomatic than adults (Christen, 1993). Headache is the single most common symptom of Lyme meningitis, affecting 30–90% of patients with cerebrospinal fluid (CSF) inflammation, is usually frontal or occipital, and ranges from mild to severe and can be disabling in intensity. Neck stiffness is less common, affecting less than 20% of those with CSF pleocytosis, and, when present, is found only on extreme flexion. Kernig's and Brudzinski's signs are infrequent. Other meningeal symptoms, such as photophobia, nausea and vomiting, are intermediate in frequency between headache and neck stiffness (20–30%). Papilloedema has been reported, but it is uncommon. Accompanying systemic symptoms are present in up to two-thirds of cases and include malaise and fatigue (40%), myalgias (30%), fever (30%), arthralgias (20%) and weight loss. Fever is usually low grade but can be higher. The symptoms usually begin acutely and can last from a month to a year or more in the absence of treatment, often lasting 1–2 months before resolving gradually over weeks. Untreated patients may experience recurrent attacks of meningeal symptoms lasting weeks. Most patients with symptomatic Lyme meningitis have other manifestations of neuroborreliosis, particularly facial palsy. When Lyme disease presents as isolated meningitis, it has to be differentiated from other causes of aseptic meningitis. Prospective studies have

*cadavid.diego@gmail.com

implicated Lyme disease in 10–40% of cases of isolated aseptic meningitis in Europe (Christen, 1993). Magnetic resonance imaging may show gadolinium-enhancement of the leptomeninges and CSF (Good and Jager, 2000). Lyme meningitis often presents in Europe in combination with poly-radiculoneuritis in a syndrome first described by Bannwarth (1941).

15.1.2 CSF abnormalities in Lyme meningitis

Several abnormalities are found in the CSF in Lyme meningitis (Pachner, 1995). The lumbar pressure is usually normal but may be increased, up to 50 cm H_2O. Expected CSF abnormalities include pleocytosis of usually 100–200 cells/mm^3 (up to 4000), mostly lymphocytic (> 90% lymphocytes in 75% of cases), although plasma cells are not uncommon (~ 10%). CSF cell pellet cytology can show prominent immunoblasts and frequent mitoses, but the cells are polyclonal in origin. The CSF protein is usually increased to 100–300 mg/dl and can be higher than 1 g/dl in cases of longer duration. Increases in CSF IgG (90%), IgM (90%) and IgA (75%) and the presence of oligoclonal bands of IgG (mostly in European cases) and specific anti-*B. burgdorferi* antibodies (75–100%) are characteristic, particularly in cases of at least 3 weeks' duration. CSF levels of the B-cell chemokine CXCL13 are often elevated in Lyme meningitis and have been proposed as both a diagnostic marker and a therapy-response marker in human neuroborreliosis (Tumani and Cadavid, 2011). The CSF glucose is most often normal but can be low in cases of longer duration. The CSF abnormalities eventually subside, even without treatment. Cell counts may not return to normal for 4 months or longer. The CSF protein falls even more slowly: it still may be elevated after 5 or 6 months. Immunoglobulin abnormalities and specific antibody can persist for years without evidence of further disease activity (Kruger *et al.*, 1989). *B. burgdorferi* DNA can be demonstrated by polymerase chain reaction (PCR) in the CSF of patients with Lyme meningitis, but the sensitivity is 40% at best (Nocton *et al.*, 1996). This low sensitivity probably reflects the low number of organisms free in the CSF as opposed to the tissues surrounding the subarachnoid space (SAS), as shown in experimental animals (Cadavid *et al.*, 2000). A proposed advantage of a positive CSF-PCR is the demonstration of active infection, which is possible only rarely by CSF culture.

15.1.3 Meningitis in relapsing fever

Relapsing fever is another disease caused by *Borrelia* spp. and occurs in two major forms: epidemic and endemic (Barbour and Hayes, 1986). The epidemic form, caused by *B. recurrentis*, is transmitted by the human body louse *Pediculus humanus*. Humans are the principal vertebrate hosts for *B. recurrentis*. Louse-borne relapsing fever has been reported on most continents and still occurs in East Africa. By contrast, soft-bodied ticks of the genus *Ornithodoros* transmit endemic relapsing fever, and several different species are responsible for infection across the world (Barbour and Hayes, 1986). The clinical hallmark of relapsing fever is two or more episodes of high fever and constitutional symptoms, such as headache and myalgias, spaced by periods of relative well-being. The recurrent febrile periods and spirochaetaemia are the consequences of antigenic variation of the variable major proteins that confer serotype identity to relapsing fever borreliae (Barbour, 1990). The most common neuro-logical complications of relapsing fever borreliosis are meningitis and facial palsy (Cadavid and Barbour, 1998). The frequency of meningitis in tick-borne relapsing fever can be ≥ 50%, CSF opening pressure is frequently increased and the mean leucocyte count is around 200/μl CSF, but can be as high as 2000/μl CSF. As in Lyme meningitis, the leucocytes are predominantly mononuclear cells. The mean CSF protein is around 300 mg/dl (range 50–1000) and CSF glucose is usually normal but can be low. Borreliae can be found in the CSF. The large number of spirochaetes in the blood during relapsing fever provides the opportunity for the simplest method of laboratory diagnosis: a

Wright stain of a thin blood smear or dark-field or phase-contrast microscopy of a wet mount of plasma obtained during or just before a febrile peak. Between fever peaks, spirochaetes can be demonstrated by inoculations of blood and/or CSF into culture media or into experimental animals.

15.1.4 Treatment of *Borrelia* meningitis

Treatment of *Borrelia* meningitis traditionally has called for the use, for at least 2 weeks, of parenteral antibiotics, such as penicillin G, cefotaxime or ceftriaxone, or oral antibiotics such as amoxycillin or doxycycline. However, very few comparative studies of antibiotic regimens in neuroborreliosis have been reported and all with small numbers of patients.

15.2 Virulence Factors

15.2.1 Pathogen factors

The complete genome of the *B. burgdorferi* type strain B31 was sequenced in 1997 (Fraser *et al.*, 1997). It showed a linear chromosome of 910,725 base pairs and 21 linear and circular extrachromosomal DNA elements with a combined size of 610,694 base pairs, the largest number known for any bacterium; the total genome size is 1,521,419 base pairs. Borreliae are unique as they can cause chronic infection and persist in the infected human, even though a robust host humoral and cellular immune response is produced. Persistent infection by *Borrelia* spp. requires antigenic variation through a complex DNA rearrangement process at the *vlsE* locus for Lyme disease borreliae and at the *vlp*/*vsp* locus for the relapsing fever borreliae (Zhang *et al.*, 1997). All members of the *B. burgdorferi* complex share a number of protein components. These include the 60 kDa heat-shock protein, which is strongly immunogenic and cross-reactive, a 41 kDa flagellar antigen that is similar to the flagellar antigens of other spirochaetes, and the highly conserved and immunogenic 83 kDa protoplasmic antigen and the 39 kDa family of basic membrane proteins. Borreliae proteins localized to the outer membrane (OM) play a key role in pathogen dissemination, virulence, tissue tropism and immune evasion. Many of the *Borrelia* OM proteins are lipoproteins. Lipoproteins are not only differentially expressed during the stages of the borrelial enzootic life cycle, but they also can be shuttled to and from the surface of this organism at different points during infection. Recently, we demonstrated that purified OM lipoproteins can disseminate systemically and enter the brain to cause inflammation (Londono and Cadavid, 2010). Nearly all differentially expressed *Borrelia* lipoproteins identified to date are plasmid encoded. Lipoprotein-encoding plasmids are essential for borrelial virulence, including antigenic variation (Barbour, 1993) and neuro-invasiveness (Cadavid *et al.*, 1994). This notion is further supported by the finding that changes in plasmid content correlate with loss of infectivity (Purser and Norris, 2000). Pathogenic *B. burgdorferi* strains vary in several abundant OM lipoproteins, notably outer surface protein (Osp) A, OspB and OspC (Bergstrom *et al.*, 1989; Wilske *et al.*, 1993). OspA and OspB are essential for colonization of and survival within tick midguts, events crucial for sustaining the natural enzootic life cycle (Yang *et al.*, 2004). By contrast, OspC is essential for mammalian infection (Grimm *et al.*, 2004) and for dissemination to remote tissues (Seemanapalli *et al.*, 2010). OspC has also been shown to bind a tick salivary protein, Salp15, indicating a possible role in transmission and/or survival during host colonization, while it is not required for *Borrelia* persistence.

Several proteins that mediate the interactions of borreliae with host ligands have been identified. These include decorin-binding proteins A and B, which are not essential for mammalian infection but are critical for virulence (Fischer *et al.*, 2003). *B. burgdorferi* BBK32 protein mediates the adhesion of *Borrelia* spp. to vascular endothelium (Moriarty *et al.*, 2012). *B. burgdorferi* also express up to five complement regulator-acquiring surface lipoproteins (CRASPs) that bind to complement regulatory proteins like factor H, factor H like-1 and complement factor H-related protein 1 for protection against complement-mediated killing (Wallich *et al.*, 2005). In fact, the direct deposition of membrane attack complex on microscopically intact spirochaetes observed in tissues from rhesus macaques infected with *B. burgdorferi* is consistent with complement resistance (Cadavid *et al.*, 2000).

15.2.2 Host factors

After transmission by an infected tick or louse, borreliae colonize the mammalian skin and often disseminate systemically to distant sites including the meninges and SAS. As an extracellular pathogen, borreliae outside the central nervous system (CNS) reside during mammalian infection primarily in the extracellular matrix (ECM) and connective tissues and between host cells, while inside the CNS they reside primarily in the leptomeninges (Cadavid *et al.*, 2000, 2001). Colonization is probably promoted by borreliae ligand adherence to multiple host adhesive molecules on target tissues. For example, the proteoglycan decorin and the glycosaminoglycan (GAG) dermatan sulfate bind *Borrelia* membrane proteins such as decorin-binding proteins A and B and Bgp. Decorin is a proteoglycan that consists of a protein core substituted with the GAG chains dermatan sulfate or chondroitin sulfate. Decorin interacts with collagen fibres and can be found in numerous tissues as a component of connective tissue. Both pathogen dissemination and inflammation to distant tissues is reduced in decorin-deficient mice (Brown *et al.*, 2001). *Borrelia* lipoproteins also bind fibronectin (Szczepanski *et al.*, 1990). Heparin and dermatan sulfate and GAGs expressed on the surface of cultured endothelial cells bind to host-adapted *B. burgdorferi* (Parveen *et al.*, 2003). Several host ligands for *B. burgdorferi* lipoproteins have been identified, including bone morphogenic protein 2, collagen I, collagen III, collagen IV, fibronectin, laminin and plasminogen. Several CRASPs are plasminogen-binding proteins (Brissette *et al.*, 2009) and plasminogen on CRASP-1 is converted to plasmin by host urokinase-type plasminogen activator. Activation of host plasminogen facilitates *Borrelia* dissemination during infection (Gebbia *et al.*, 1999; Nordstrand *et al.*, 2001) and there is evidence that host plasminogen can bind to other *Borrelia* proteins like OspA (Fuchs *et al.*, 1994).

15.3 Pathology, Host Response and Brain Tissue Damage in *Borrelia* Meningitis

Little is known about the molecular mechanisms of inflammation and tissue injury in *Borrelia* meningitis. More than 8% of the coding sequence of *B. burgdorferi* corresponds to putative lipoproteins (Fraser *et al.*, 1997). The lipidation corresponds to a tripalmitoyl-*S*-glyceryl-cysteine (Pam3Cys) modification, common to many bacterial species (Erdile and Guy, 1997). Lipoproteins are probably responsible for the inflammatory response in *Borrelia* meningitis, largely via induction of pro-inflammatory cytokines like interleukin (IL)-1β, IL-6, IL-12 and tumour necrosis factor (TNF)-α (Radolf *et al.*, 1995) and chemokines (Cadavid, 2006; Rupprecht *et al.*, 2007). *Borrelia* lipoproteins can directly activate endothelial cells, as shown by induction of nuclear factor (NF)-κB and increased production of IL-6, CXCL-8, E-selectin, VCAM-1 and ICAM-1 (Wooten *et al.*, 1996). The ability of eukaryotic cells to respond to *Borrelia* lipoproteins correlates with expression of Toll-like receptor (TLR) 2 (Hirschfeld *et al.*, 1999), although other TLRs like TLR1 and/or TLR6 are also involved (Bulut *et al.*, 2001). TLR 2-independent pathways are also involved in induction of *Borreliae* inflammation (Behera *et al.*, 2006).

15.3.1 *Borrelia* meningitis in immunocompetent mice

We have studied *Borrelia* meningitis in immunocompetent mice using various strains of inbred and outbred mice for up to 1 month after intraperitoneal inoculation with serotype 1 of the relapsing fever spirochaete *Borrelia turicatae* (Cadavid *et al.*, 2006). TLR2-deficient mice were also studied for comparison. Haematoxylin and eosin (H&E) staining revealed mild meningitis of similar severity in all immunocompetent mouse strains tested and in the TLR2-deficient mice (Cadavid *et al.*, 2006). Immunostaining with an antibody to the membrane glycoprotein F4/80, a marker of microglia/macrophage activation, revealed increased activation/ infiltration in the leptomeninges and to a lesser extent in the brain parenchyma. Cultures of blood and perfused brains revealed that 20% of mice had residual brain infection, meaning persistence of infection in the brain but not the blood (Cadavid *et al.*, 2006). Examination of serotypes causing residual brain infection revealed that in one case it was the same serotype originally inoculated. This indicates that borreliae can avoid immune eradication by hiding in the brain, a phenomenon recognized by earlier investigators a century ago (Cadavid and Barbour, 1998). Interestingly, although none of the inbred or TLR2-deficient mice developed any signs of disease, 25% of the outbred mice developed signs of severe vestibular dysfunction starting about 3 weeks after inoculation. It is likely that vestibular disease was the result of a lack of pathogen clearance from the peripheral vestibular system in the inner ear.

15.3.2 *Borrelia* meningitis in B-cell-deficient mice

We have used B-cell-deficient mice to investigate disease outcome when the host is unable to clear the infection. The first studies were done in CB17-SCID mice, which are both B- and T- cell deficient, and revealed multiple complications of persistent infection at high pathogen loads, including ruffled fur, conjunctival secretion, tibiotarsal arthritis, carditis, meningitis, hepatitis and vestibular dysfunction (Cadavid *et al.*, 1994, 2001). On regular H&E staining, the main finding in the brain of infected SCID mice was mild meningitis. Immunohistochemistry with F4/80 revealed macrophage infiltration/microglial activation in the meninges and brain parenchyma. A comparison of infection in SCID mice of three different genetic backgrounds, CB17, C3H-HeJ and C57BL/6, showed similar meningitis and brain inflammation. One notable finding of these studies was that isogenic serotype 1, defined by expression of the OM lipoprotein Vsp1, caused much more brain infection and inflammation than isogenic serotype 2, defined by expression of Vsp2 (Cadavid *et al.*, 1994, 1997, 2001; Pennington *et al.*, 1999). This was the first observation linking *Borrelia* brain infection to expression of a specific protein. Another notable finding was that in none of these studies was there any evidence of brain injury despite persistence infection at high pathogen loads.

In subsequent studies, we focused on mice deficient only in B-cells using Igh6$^{-/-}$ mice (B6.129S2-Igh-6tm1Cgn). These allowed us to investigate the contribution of T-cells to pathogen control and tissue injury during persistent infection by comparing them with Rag1$^{-/-}$ mice (B6.129S7-Rag1tm1Mom), which are deficient in both B- and T-cells. Igh6$^{-/-}$ mice developed more severe clinical disease than Rag1$^{-/-}$ mice (Gelderblom *et al.*, 2007a,b). However, Rag1$^{-/-}$ had a much higher pathogen load than Igh6$^{-/-}$ mice. Examination of meningitis and brain inflammation by F4/80 immunohistochemistry revealed similar intensity of microgliosis/ brain macrophage infiltration in both and only a paucity of T-cells in the brain of Igh6$^{-/-}$ mice. The reason why Rag1$^{-/-}$ mice had a higher pathogen load but less severe clinical manifestations became clear when we compared the cytokine and chemokine response to infection. Rag1$^{-/-}$ mice had extraordinarily high levels of circulating IL-10, analogous to the observation in a clinical trial of louse-borne relapsing fever in Ethiopia (Cooper *et al.*, 2000). Furthermore, a strong negative correlation between levels of IL-10 and levels of TNF-α, IL-6, IL-12 and granulocyte–macrophage colony-stimulating factor was found. Importantly, high levels of IL-10 were found not only systemically but also in infected tissues including the brain and the heart (Gelderblom *et al.*, 2007a,b). In the brain, there was a significant positive correlation between the pathogen load and production of IL-10. Activated microglia/ infiltrating macrophages were the source of most of the IL-10 in the brain, which was sufficient to completely prevent TNF-α production. Similar to the SCID mice, H&E

staining of persistently infected Igh6$^{-/-}$ and Rag1$^{-/-}$ mice showed mild meningeal inflammation without any evidence of tissue injury. There was no ischaemia, haemorrhage, vasculitis or evidence of demyelination. Immunostaining for markers of astrocyte proliferation (GFAP), neuronal cell loss (NeuN) and synaptic loss (synaptophysin) showed no difference between infected and uninfected control mice of either genotype.

Affymetrix oligoarray analysis revealed that the 110 genes significantly upregulated in the brain of Igh6$^{-/-}$ mice persistently infected with serotype 1 of *B. turicatae* for 1 month were not involved in neural stress responses or brain damage and repair but rather were all involved with the immune response to the pathogen. The highest upregulated gene in infected brains was the B-cell chemokine CXCL13. The first evidence that CXCL13 plays a distinct role in borrelial infection came from a study in tissues from rhesus macaques persistently infected with *B. burgdorferi* (Pachner *et al.*, 2002). Soon after, we documented very high levels of CXCL13 in the blood and tissues of mice infected with relapsing fever borreliae (Cadavid, 2006; Gelderblom *et al.*, 2007a; Londono *et al.*, 2008; Cadavid and Londono, 2009). We concluded that production of large amounts of IL-10 in response to higher pathogen loads was the most likely explanation for the differences in clinical disease observed between Igh6$^{-/-}$ and Rag1$^{-/-}$ mice. The eventual complete suppression of TNF-α in the brain, but not the heart, may be one reason for finding heart injury (Londono *et al.*, 2005) but not brain injury (Cadavid *et al.*, 2001; Sethi *et al.*, 2006) in these mice.

15.3.3 Protective role of IL-10 in *Borrelia* meningitis

The protective role of IL-10 in *Borrelia* infection first became apparent in a double-blind, placebo-controlled trial in Ethiopian men with louse-borne relapsing fever, who were randomized to receive a single intravenous bolus of recombinant human IL-10 or vehicle, 5 min before treatment with intramuscular penicillin to investigate a potential protective role from the Jarish–Herxheimer reaction (Cooper *et al.*, 2000). In this trial, patients already had extraordinarily high levels of circulating IL-10 prior to treatment, 5–60 times greater than those found in humans with septic shock. Because these patients were ambulatory and capable of signing the informed consent at the time, this suggested that IL-10 plays an important protective role in *Borrelia* infection. Furthermore, peripheral blood mononuclear cells from healthy humans exposed *in vitro* to *B. burgdorferi* produced significantly more IL-10 and less TNF-α than if exposed to lipopolysaccharide (Diterich *et al.*, 2003). IL-10 was shown to act on endothelial cells exposed to *B. burgdorferi* to reduce migration of monocytes and T-cells and decrease production of pro-inflammatory cytokines (Lisinski and Furie, 2002). Monocytes *in vitro* also produced abundant IL-10 upon stimulation with *B. burgdorferi* lipoproteins, which in turn downregulated pro-inflammatory cytokines (Giambartolomei *et al.*, 1998). Elevated IL-10 levels were also found in the CSF in humans with Lyme neuroborreliosis (Rupprecht *et al.*, 2005).

To investigate the protective role of IL-10 further, we measured the effects of giving exogenous IL-10 to Igh6$^{-/-}$ mice infected with isogenic serotype 1 or 2 of *B. turicatae*. Daily doses of 50 μg/kg of recombinant IL-10 given from days 0 to 8 after inoculation prevented the development of all the clinical manifestations of infection (Gelderblom *et al.*, 2007b). In addition, treatment with 100 μg/kg/day given daily on days 11–13 after inoculation significantly reduced established clinical manifestations of disease in infected Igh6$^{-/-}$ mice. Furthermore, exogenous IL-10 significantly reduced the systemic production of CXCL13 and markedly reduced cerebral microgliosis, and, unexpectedly, a single high dose of 150 μg/kg of recombinant IL-10 significantly lowered the pathogen load in infected Igh6$^{-/-}$ mice. These results revealed several possible protective mechanisms for IL-10 during *Borrelia* infection including reduction of clinical disease, lowering of chemokine production, lessening of cellular inflammation and, at higher doses, antibody-independent improved pathogen clearance.

To provide further evidence of the protective role of IL-10, we used Rag2$^{-/-}$ (C57BL/10SgSnAi-[KO] RAG2) (RAG2$^{-/-}$) mice, with or without deficiency in IL-10 (Rag2/IL10$^{-/-}$). Severe morbidity and early mortality were observed in Rag2/IL10$^{-/-}$ mice inoculated with serotype 2 of *B. turicatae*. Macroscopic examination at necropsy revealed that the brain was the only organ in which haemorrhage was evident, despite the infection being systemic (Fig. 15.1). Microscopic examination of H&E stained sections revealed extensive subarachnoid and intracerebral haemorrhage. We also observed severe meningitis and infiltration of the cerebral microvessels by inflammatory cells, consistent with vasculitis. Bacteraemia was very high, suggesting that the absence of IL-10 in Rag2$^{-/-}$ mice resulted in even higher pathogen load leading to early and fatal damage to the cerebral microcirculation. Deficiency of two genes, one needed for adaptive immunity (Rag1) and one needed to control inflammation (IL-10), had turned a self-limited infection that spontaneously resolves into a rapidly fatal infectious disease with severe meningitis, leptomeningeal vasculitis, and subarachnoid and intraparenchymal haemorrhages and thrombosis.

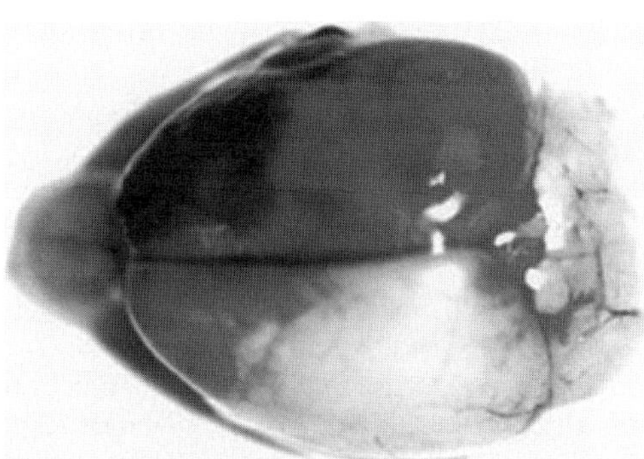

Fig. 15.1. Widespread subarachnoid haemorrhage in an IL-10-deficient mouse, 2 weeks after inoculation of the relapsing fever spirochaete *B. turicatae*. This is shown by the presence of large amounts of liquefied and coagulated blood covering the entire convexity of the right hemisphere and the anterior and medial dorsal aspect of the left hemisphere.

15.3.4 Inhibition of TNF-α by IL-10 during *Borrelia* meningitis

Previous studies in Igh6$^{-/-}$ and Rag1$^{-/-}$ mice infected with *B. turicatae* revealed a significant negative correlation between levels of IL-10 and TNF-α (Gelderblom *et al.*, 2007b). Similar results were obtained in infected Rag2/IL10$^{-/-}$ mice. To investigate this, we treated Rag2/IL10$^{-/-}$ mice infected with *B. turicatae* with a neutralizing antibody (MP6-XT22/11) to mouse TNF-α. Neutralization of TNF-α prevented the early mortality and lessened subarachnoid haemorrhage and leptomeningeal vasculitis, reduced bacteraemia and all the clinical manifestations of the infection, including vestibular dysfunction, and significantly increased systemic production of gamma interferon (IFN)-γ. Taken together, these results confirmed that IL-10 protects the host in *Borrelia* infection at least in part by inhibition of TNF-α.

15.3.5 IL-10 deficiency in immunocompetent mice

Previous studies in mice deficient in both B- and T-cells and IL-10 showed that they are unable to clear peak bacteraemia and rapidly succumb to brain haemorrhage. However, this is a situation that is less likely to occur in humans, whereas isolated IL-10 deficiency alone has been reported (de Lemos *et al.*, 2010). To investigate the protective role of IL-10 during *Borrelia* infection in immunocompetent mice, we inoculated mice deficient in IL-10 with *B. turicatae* and examined them during relapsing–remitting infection for up to 4 weeks (Londono *et al.*, 2011). Severe endothelial cell injury leading to haemorrhage in the brain and other organs occurred in IL-10-deficient mice, despite the production of serotype-specific antibodies that cleared peak bactaeremia. Studies *in vitro* showed that human brain microvascular endothelial cells (HBMECs) produce abundant pro-inflammatory mediators upon exposure to either intact borreliae or to purified lipoprotein. Notably, these HBMECs did not produce any detectable IL-10. Whole *Borrelia* and purified lipoprotein rapidly killed HBMECs by apoptosis in a time- and concentration-dependent manner. Importantly, exogenous IL-10 protected HBMECs from apoptosis. Apoptosis of HBMECs during exposure to a low pathogen load was associated with downregulation of TNF-α and TNFAIP3 and upregulation of BAX. By contrast, HBMEC apoptosis during exposure to high concentrations of purified lipoprotein was associated with marked upregulation of FAS, FAS ligand and the adaptor molecules RIPK1 and CFLAR (Londono *et al.*, 2011). Exogenous IL-10 reversed all the apoptotic signalling changes induced by whole borreliae or their purified lipoproteins. Thus, prominent brain endothelial cell apoptosis can occur during *Borrelia* infection in the absence of IL-10 and suggests a prominent role for borrelial lipoprotein-mediated activation of FAS and caspase-3 in this process.

15.4 Invasion Mechanisms into the Meninges

Borrelia meningitis results from invasion of the SAS and meninges by the pathogenic spirochaetes. Borreliae can be cultured from the CSF of humans with meningitis and have been identified in the meninges of experimentally infected animals (Cadavid and Barbour, 1998; Cadavid *et al.*, 2000). The evidence that *Borrelia* spirochaetes infect the brain parenchyma is less convincing. Spirochaetes were not found in the brain or spinal cord parenchyma of non-human primates experimentally infected with different genospecies of *B. burgdorferi*, even during immunosuppression (Cadavid *et al.*, 2000). Consistent with this observation is the fact that late manifestations of chronic progressive neuroborreliosis, unlike neurosyphilis, do not occur (Kruger *et al.*, 1989).

15.4.1 Neurotropism of borreliae

A characteristic feature of borreliae is the ability to disseminate to distant sites from their sites of inoculation in the skin. Their potential routes of dissemination include haematogenous and locally through the skin (Cadavid *et al.*, 2001). It is unclear whether borreliae cross cellular barriers intercellularly and/or transcellularly. Studies *in vitro* using human umbilical vein endothelial cells (HUVECs) infected with *B. burgdorferi* showed crossing of intercellular junctions of endothelial cells (Szczepanski *et al.*, 1990). However, *in vitro* borreliae have been shown to be internalized into endothelial cells (Ma *et al.*, 1991) and fibroblasts (Klempner *et al.*, 1993). We observed internalization of OM lipoproteins, but not intact spirochaetes in HBMECs (Sethi *et al.*, 2006). The association of *Borrelia* lipoproteins with brain endothelium was time dependent, saturable, required lipidation and was inhibited by incubation at lower temperature or with excess unlabelled lipidated protein (Gandhi *et al.*, 2010). One host factor that appears to help dissemination of *Borrelia* spirochaetes is the host's protease plasmin (Gebbia *et al.*, 1999; Coleman and Benach, 2000). It is likely that dissemination of borreliae into tissues is the result of specific interactions between their OM proteins and ligands on host cells. A role in adhesion to mammalian tissues has been shown for various *Borrelia* proteins including the variable major proteins of relapsing fever borreliae (Thomas *et al.*, 1994) and the Osp (Sadziene *et al.*, 1995) and decorin-binding proteins (Guo *et al.*, 1998) of Lyme disease borreliae. From the host, several molecules have been implicated in binding to borreliae to facilitate neuroinvasiveness, including integrins (Coburn *et al.*, 1993), glycolipids (Garcia Monco *et al.*, 1992), proteoglycans (Guo *et al.*, 1998) and GAGs (Leong *et al.*, 1998). Differences in binding of variable OM lipoproteins to components of host cell membranes or the ECM may explain differences in tissue tropism.

A notable feature of the genus *Borrelia* is neurotropism, meaning a propensity to invade the CNS. Both Lyme disease and relapsing fever can have prominent neurological complications including lymphocytic meningitis, radiculitis, cranial neuritis, myelitis and chronic encephalopathy, collectively referred to as neuroborreliosis. For unclear reasons, only up to 25% of patients with Lyme disease or relapsing fever develop neuroborreliosis. One possibility is that some borreliae are more neurotropic. This has been suggested for both Lyme disease (van Dam *et al.*, 1993) and tick-borne relapsing fever (Schuhardt and Hemphill, 1946). Prior to the discovery of penicillin, there was intense research into the phenomenon of neurotropism in relapsing fever (Cadavid and Barbour, 1998). Pioneers in the field noticed differences in the neurotropism of relapsing fever borreliae. Interest in this phenomenon decreased when effective treatment of relapsing fever with penicillin became available in the 1940s but returned in the 1980s when frequent neurological complications were recognized in Lyme disease (Reik *et al.*, 1979). A key step in *Borrelia* neuroinvasiveness is adhesion of circulating microbes to vascular surfaces in the face of the shear forces present in flowing blood (Moriarty *et al.*, 2012).

15.4.2 Serotype 1 of *Borrelia turicatae* is more neurotropic than isogenic serotype 2

The phenomenon of *Borrelia* tropism for the brain in relapsing fever was confirmed in Balb/c mice examined 3–5 days after intraperitoneal inoculation of *B. hermsii* serotype 7 (Cadavid *et al.*, 1993). Relapse serotypes were present in blood but not in the brain, implying that some *Borrelia* serotypes are better than others at infecting the brain. To confirm this observation, we turned to a strain (Oz1) of *B. turicatae* that had caused an outbreak of meningitis and cranial neuritis in visitors to a cave in Texas. One difficulty of working with immunocompetent mice was that the specific antibody response to the infection rapidly eliminated predominant serotypes from both blood and brain. To be able to study serotype neurotropism, we needed to eliminate immune selection by the host's antibody response. For this, we chose SCID mice that lack functional B- and T-cells and do not produce antibody needed to clear specific serotypes. In one of the four SCID mice originally inoculated with the Oz1 strain of *B. turicatae*, we found two serotypes in the blood, only one of which was also present in brain (Cadavid *et al.*, 1994). Several experiments confirmed that the serotype 1 strain was more neurotropic than the serotype 2 strain. Because serotype 2 was cultured from the brain after direct intracerebral inoculation, the difficulty seems to be with entering the brain rather than surviving or growing in it. This was surprising because serotype 2 was about tenfold more abundant in blood than serotype 1. This was the opposite of what occurs with most other neurotropic bacteria in which CNS invasion directly correlates with the intensity of bacteraemia. When the ratio of spirochaetes in the brain was compared with non-CNS tissue like the heart, serotype 1 was found to be 20 times more neurotropic than serotype 2. Because these results were obtained in SCID mice, we concluded that the higher neurotropism of serotype 1 represents niche selection and not merely increased survival in an immunologically privileged site like the brain. Infection of SCID mice with serotype 1 caused a 30-fold increase in macrophage infiltration/microglial activation in the CNS, compared with uninfected controls. Large numbers of macrophages/ramified microglia were seen along the leptomeninges and throughout the grey and white matter of the brain parenchyma in serotype 1-infected SCID mice. Mice infected with serotype 2 also had increased signal compared with uninfected controls but five-fold lower than in serotype 1-infected mice. Because the only discernible difference between serotypes 1 and 2 is the variable major protein they express (Vsp1 in serotype 1 and Vsp2 in serotype 2), these studies indicate that expression of abundant OM lipoproteins can profoundly influence neuroinvasiveness.

15.4.3 Localization of borreliae in the meninges and other tissues

We completed extensive studies of the localization of relapsing fever and Lyme disease borreliae in mammalian tissues using immunosuppressed animals (Cadavid *et al.*, 2000, 2001). For relapsing fever, we studied SCID mice inoculated intraperitoneally with serotypes 1 or 2 of *B. turicatae*. Examination of whole decalcified heads showed large numbers of spirochaetes in the skin, bone marrow, endomysium, dura mater, pia-arachnoid, SAS and middle and inner ear. Spirochaetes were rarely observed in the brain parenchyma itself and we estimated there were 100 times more leptomeningeal than brain parenchymal spirochaetes. Spirochaetes were not found in the choroid plexus or in salivary glands. In the leptomeninges they were free-floating in CSF or appeared attached to arachnoidal cells (Fig. 15.2). Spirochaetes were also observed intravascularly, despite extensive intracardiac perfusion with buffer at necropsy, and they appeared attached to or in the process of crossing microvascular endothelial cells to reach the SAS. Several tissues had large numbers of *B. turicatae* spirochaetes, including the heart, the joints, the liver and the mediastinum (Cadavid *et al.*, 1994; Pennington *et al.*, 1997, 1999). There were more serotype 1 than serotype 2 spirochaetes in the leptomeninges, even though the pathogen load in the blood was much larger with serotype 2 (Cadavid *et al.*, 2001). By contrast, the numbers of serotype 2 spirochaetes were much higher in non-CNS organs like the skin, the heart and the joints.

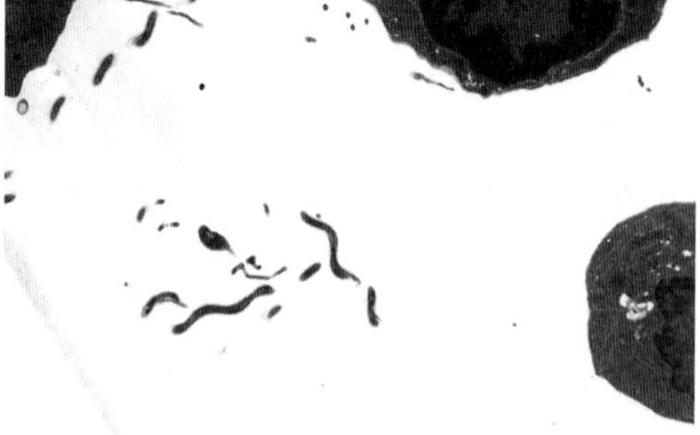

Fig. 15.2. Attachment of *B. turicatae* (denoted by arrow) to a human arachnoidal cell derived from a human meningioma (electron microscopy image).

A surprising observation was the finding of spirochaetes in the dura mater early after systemic inoculation; 3–4 days after intraperitoneal inoculation, the dura mater was the first tissue where spirochaetes were found outside the vasculature (Cadavid *et al.*, 2001). This suggests that early during *Borrelia* infection spirochaetes may gain access to the CNS not only by crossing the blood–brain barrier (BBB) from the cerebral microcirculation but also by crossing the barrier between the dura mater and the arachnoid anywhere along the neuroaxis. The high density of blood vessels and lymphatics in certain areas of the dura mater including nerve root entry/exit zones and arachnoid granulations may facilitate this early neuroinvasion. Studies of the localization of Lyme disease borreliae in steroid-immunosuppressed rhesus macaques inoculated with *B. burgdorferi* sensu stricto (N40 strain) revealed similar results, i.e. the preferred niche for *B. burgdorferi* in the CNS was the leptomeninges (Cadavid *et al.*, 2000). Also similar to relapsing fever borreliae, outside of the CNS, *B. burgdorferi* showed a predilection for the ECM of tissues like skin, heart, bladder, spinal nerve roots, peripheral nerves, nerve plexus and skeletal muscle (Cadavid *et al.*, 2000, 2003; Pachner *et al.*, 2004). The dorsal root ganglia were the only site where *B. burgdorferi* were found next to neurons. In immunocompetent rhesus macaques, the only tissue in which we were able to find spirochaetes microscopically was skin infected with *B. garinii* strains (Pachner *et al.*, 2004).

15.4.4 *Borrelia* lipoproteins can disseminate from the periphery to inflame the brain

The classic view is that bacteria need to enter the brain to cause cerebral inflammation and meningitis. However, in B-cell-deficient mice persistently infected with *B. turicatae,* we observed widespread cerebral microgliosis/macrophage infiltration despite a paucity of spirochaetes in the brain parenchyma. We therefore studied the possibility that *Borrelia* lipoproteins may be capable of disseminating from the periphery across the BBB into the brain to cause inflammation. To investigate this possibility, we injected wild-type and B-cell-deficient mice persistently infected with *B. turicatae* with purified lanthanide-labelled variable OM lipoproteins given intraperitoneally and measured their distribution in blood, various peripheral organs, and whole and capillary-depleted brain protein extracts at various intervals. The results showed that the Vsp1 and Vsp2 lipoproteins of *B. turicatae* were capable of disseminating to the brain and causing cerebral inflammation (as measured by amplification of genes encoding markers such as CXCL13) to different degrees. Vsp1 was better than Vsp2 and even superior to live serotype 1 spirochaetes at invading the brain from the blood. The dissemination of Vsp1 from the periphery to the brain occurred under normal conditions and to a much larger extent during infection. In contrast to Vsp1, Vsp2 disseminated better to peripheral organs than to the brain (Londono and Cadavid, 2010). This study for the first time provided experimental evidence that bacterial lipoproteins can disseminate from the periphery into the brain and cause inflammation.

15.4.5 BBB dysfunction during *Borrelia* meningitis

IL-10 deficiency during acute *Borrelia* infection results in markedly increased BBB permeability. By contrast, the absence of IL-10 in normal mice has no effect on BBB permeability, an indication that the biological role of IL-10 is needed at times of increased inflammation rather than under normal conditions. Microscopic examination of immunostained brains from infected wild-type and IL-10-deficient mice demonstrated several abnormalities in the BBB: these included fibrinogen leakage from blood to perivascular brain parenchyma, brain endothelial up-regulation of ICAM, VCAM and PCAM, disruption of tight junctions as evidenced by morphological alterations of ZO-1 staining, brain endothelial cell apoptosis, astrogliosis, loss of basement membrane integrity, and decreased expression of the water channel aquaporin 4 (D. Londono and D. Cadavid, 2012, unpublished observations) (Fig. 15.3). Importantly, we observed greater entry of albumin into the brain relative to blood during acute infection with serotype 1 than with serotype 2 of *B. turicatae*; this finding supports the view that the BBB is better protected during *B. turicatae* serotype 2 infection, probably as a result of greater production of IL-10 in response to the higher pathogen load characteristic of infection with this serotype (Cadavid *et al.*, 1994).

15.5 What Else We Need to Know

Much remains to be learned about *Borrelia* meningitis in both Lyme disease and relapsing fever. Due to the lack of good

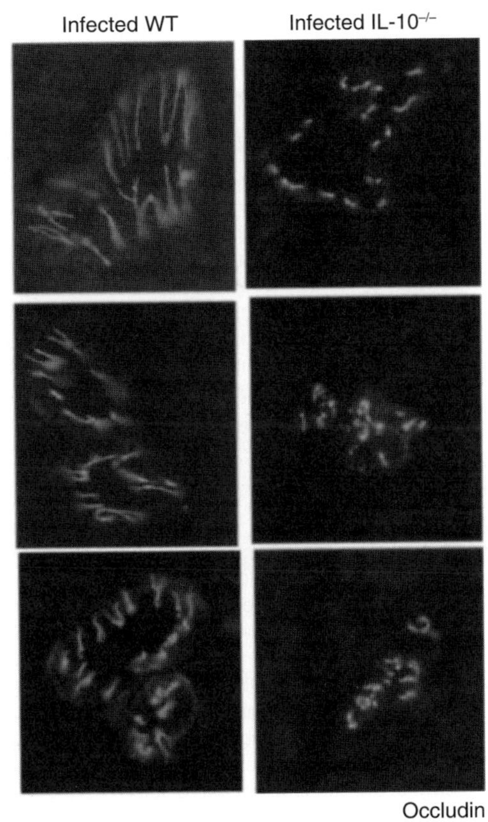

Fig. 15.3. Loss of tight junction proteins in the brain of mice deficient in IL-10 infected with *B. turicatae*. Immunofluorescence staining for the tight junction protein occludin. WT, wild type.

rodent models of *Borrelia* meningitis with *B. burgdorferi*, much of what we know at the experimental level has been learned using rodent models of relapsing fever. Although studies of the localization of *B. burgdorferi* in the CNS have been completed in rhesus macaques, it would be important to also investigate whether the key protective role of IL-10 in meningitis with relapsing fever spirochaetes is also important in Lyme meningitis. Another intriguing observation that needs attention is the lack of IL-10 production by human brain endothelial cells. Preliminary evidence suggests that IL-10 production may be detrimental to endothelial cells in the absence of inflammation. Also deserving further study is the issue of residual infection, i.e. whether it occurs following treatment of *B. burgdorferi* infection with antibiotics or following Lyme meningitis.

References

Bannwarth, A. (1941) Chronische lymphocytare meningitis, entzundliche polyneuritis und rheumatismus. *Archiv fur Pyschiatrie und Nervenkrankheiten* 113, 284–376.

Barbour, A.G. (1990) Antigenic variation of a relapsing fever *Borrelia* species. *Annual Reviews in Microbiology* 44, 155–171.

Barbour, A.G. (1993) Linear DNA of *Borrelia* species and antigenic variation. *Trends in Microbiology* 1, 236–239.

Barbour, A.G. and Hayes, S.F. (1986) Biology of *Borrelia* species. *Microbiology Reviews* 50, 381–400.

Behera, A.K., Hildebrand, E., Uematsu, S., Akira, S., Coburn, J. and Hu, L.T. (2006) Identification of a TLR-independent pathway for *Borrelia burgdorferi*-induced expression of matrix metalloproteinases and inflammatory mediators through binding to integrin $\alpha_3\beta_1$. *Journal of Immunology* 177, 657–664.

Bergstrom, S., Bundoc, V.G. and Barbour, A.G. (1989) Molecular analysis of linear plasmid-encoded major surface proteins, OspA and OspB, of the Lyme disease spirochaete *Borrelia burgdorferi*. *Molecular Microbiology* 3, 479–486.

Brissette, C.A., Haupt, K., Barthel, D., Cooley, A.E., Bowman, A., Skerka, C., Wallich, R., Zipfel, P.F., Kraiczy, P. and Stevenson, B. (2009) *Borrelia burgdorferi* infection-associated surface proteins ErpP, ErpA, and ErpC bind human plasminogen. *Infection and Immunity* 77, 300–306.

Brown, E.L., Wooten, R.M., Johnson, B.J., Iozzo, R.V., Smith, A., Dolan, M.C., Guo, B.P., Weis, J.J. and Hook, M. (2001) Resistance to Lyme disease in decorin-deficient mice. *Journal of Clinical Investigation* 107, 845–852.

Bulut, Y., Faure, E., Thomas, L., Equils, O. and Arditi, M. (2001) Cooperation of Toll-like receptor 2 and 6 for cellular activation by soluble tuberculosis factor and *Borrelia burgdorferi* outer surface protein A lipoprotein: role of Toll-interacting protein and IL-1 receptor signaling molecules in Toll-like receptor 2 signaling. *Journal of Immunology* 167, 987–994.

Burgdorfer, W., Barbour, A.G., Hayes, S.F., Benach, J.L., Grunwaldt, E. and Davis, J.P. (1982) Lyme disease – a tick-borne spirochetosis? *Science* 216, 1317–1319.

Cadavid, D. (2006) The mammalian host response to borrelia infection. *Wiener Klinische Wochenschrift* 118, 653–658.

Cadavid, D. and Barbour, A.G. (1998) Neuroborreliosis during relapsing fever: review of the clinical manifestations, pathology, and treatment of infections in humans and experimental animals. *Clinical Infectious Diseases* 26, 151–164.

Cadavid, D. and Londono, D. (2009) Understanding tropism and immunopathological mechanisms of relapsing fever spirochaetes. *Clinical Microbiology Infection* 15, 415–421.

Cadavid, D., Bundoc, V. and Barbour, A.G. (1993) Experimental infection of the mouse brain by a relapsing fever *Borrelia* species: a molecular analysis. *Journal of Infectious Diseases* 168, 143–151.

Cadavid, D., Thomas, D.D., Crawley, R. and Barbour, A.G. (1994) Variability of a bacterial surface protein and disease expression in a possible mouse model of systemic Lyme borreliosis. *Journal of Experimental Medicine* 179, 631–642.

Cadavid, D., Pennington, P.M., Kerentseva, T.A., Bergstrom, S. and Barbour, A.G. (1997) Immunologic and genetic analyses of VmpA of a neurotropic strain of *Borrelia turicatae*. *Infection and Immunity* 65, 3352–3360.

Cadavid, D., O'Neill, T., Schaefer, H. and Pachner, A.R. (2000) Localization of *Borrelia burgdorferi* in the nervous system and other organs in a nonhuman primate model of Lyme disease. *Laboratory Investigation* 80, 1043–1054.

Cadavid, D., Pachner, A.R., Estanislao, L., Patalapati, R. and Barbour, A.G. (2001) Isogenic serotypes of *Borrelia turicatae* show different localization in the brain and skin of mice. *Infection and Immunity* 69, 3389–3397.

Cadavid, D., Bai, Y., Dail, D., Hurd, M., Narayan, K., Hodzic, E., Barthold, S.W. and Pachner, A.R. (2003) Infection and inflammation in skeletal muscle from nonhuman primates infected with different genospecies of the Lyme disease spirochete *Borrelia burgdorferi*. *Infection and Immunity* 71, 7087–7098.

Cadavid, D., Sondey, M., Garcia, E. and Lawson, C.L. (2006) Residual brain infection in relapsing-fever borreliosis. *Journal of Infectious Diseases* 193, 1451–1458.

Christen, H.J. (1993) Bacterial meningitis and Lyme neuroborreliosis in childhood. *Current Opinion in Neurology and Neurosurgery* 6, 403–409.

Coburn, J., Leong, J.M. and Erban, J.K. (1993) Integrin $\alpha_{IIb}\beta_3$ mediates binding of the Lyme disease agent *Borrelia burgdorferi* to human platelets. *Proceedings of the National Academy of Sciences USA* 90, 7059–7063.

Coleman, J.L. and Benach, J.L. (2000) The generation of enzymatically active plasmin on the surface of spirochetes. *Methods* 21, 133–141.

Cooper, P.J., Fekade, D., Remick, D.G., Grint, P., Wherry, J. and Griffin, G.E. (2000) Recombinant human interleukin-10 fails to alter pro-inflammatory cytokine production or physiologic changes associated with the Jarisch–Herxheimer reaction. *Journal of Infectious Diseases* 181, 203–209.

de Lemos, R.C., Galle, P., Pedersen, B.K. and Hansen, M.B. (2010) A state of acquired IL-10 deficiency in 0.4% of Danish blood donors. *Cytokine* 51, 286–293.

Diterich, I., Rauter, C., Kirschning, C.J. and Hartung, T. (2003) *Borrelia burgdorferi*-induced tolerance as a model of persistence via immunosuppression. *Infection and Immunity* 71, 3979–3987.

Erdile, L.F. and Guy, B. (1997) OspA lipoprotein of *Borrelia burgdorferi* is a mucosal immunogen and adjuvant. *Vaccine* 15, 988–996.

Fischer, J.R., Parveen, N., Magoun, L. and Leong, J.M. (2003) Decorin-binding proteins A and B confer distinct mammalian cell type-specific attachment by *Borrelia burgdorferi*, the Lyme disease spirochete. *Proceedings of the National Academy of Sciences USA* 100, 7307–7312.

Fraser, C.M., *et al.* (1997) Genomic sequence of a Lyme disease spirochaete, *Borrelia burgdorferi*. *Nature* 390, 580–586.

Fuchs, H., Wallich, R., Simon, M.M. and Kramer, M.D. (1994) The outer surface protein A of the spirochete *Borrelia burgdorferi* is a plasmin(ogen) receptor. *Proceedings of the National Academy of Sciences USA* 91, 12594–12598.

Gandhi, G., Londono, D., Whetstine, C.R., Sethi, N., Kim, K.S., Zuckert, W.R. and Cadavid, D. (2010) Interaction of variable bacterial outer membrane lipoproteins with brain endothelium. *PLoS One* 5, e13257.

Garcia Monco, J.C., Fernandez, V.B., Rogers, R.C., Szczepanski, A., Wheeler, C.M. and Benach, J.L. (1992) *Borrelia burgdorferi* and other related spirochetes bind to galactocerebroside. *Neurology* 42, 1341–1348.

Gebbia, J.A., Monco, J.C., Degen, J.L., Bugge, T.H. and Benach, J.L. (1999) The plasminogen activation system enhances brain and heart invasion in murine relapsing fever borreliosis. *Journal of Clinical Investigation* 103, 81–87.

Gelderblom, H., Londono, D., Bai, Y., Cabral, E.S., Quandt, J., Hornung, R., Martin, R., Marques, A. and Cadavid, D. (2007a) High production of CXCL13 in blood and brain during persistent infection with the relapsing fever spirochete *Borrelia turicatae*. *Journal of Neuropathology and Experimental Neurology* 66, 208–217.

Gelderblom, H., Schmidt, J., Londono, D., Bai, Y., Quandt, J., Hornung, R., Marques, A., Martin, R. and Cadavid, D. (2007b) Role of interleukin 10 during persistent infection with the relapsing fever spirochete *Borrelia turicatae*. *American Journal of Pathology* 170, 251–262.

Giambartolomei, G.H., Dennis, V.A. and Philipp, M.T. (1998) *Borrelia burgdorferi* stimulates the production of interleukin-10 in peripheral blood mononuclear cells from uninfected humans and rhesus monkeys. *Infection and Immunity* 66, 2691–2697.

Good, C.D. and Jager, H.R. (2000) Contrast enhancement of the cerebrospinal fluid on MRI in two cases of spirochaetal meningitis. *Neuroradiology* 42, 448–450.

Grimm, D., Tilly, K., Byram, R., Stewart, P.E., Krum, J.G., Bueschel, D.M., Schwan, T.G., Policastro, P.F., Elias, A.F. and Rosa, P.A. (2004) Outer-surface protein C of the Lyme disease spirochete: a protein induced in ticks for infection of mammals. *Proceedings of the National Academy of Sciences USA* 101, 3142–3147.

Guo, B.P., Brown, E.L., Dorward, D.W., Rosenberg, L.C. and Hook, M. (1998) Decorin-binding adhesins from *Borrelia burgdorferi*. *Molecular Microbiology* 30, 711–723.

Hirschfeld, M., Kirschning, C.J., Schwandner, R., Wesche, H., Weis, J.H., Wooten, R.M. and Weis, J.J. (1999) Cutting edge: inflammatory signaling by *Borrelia burgdorferi* lipoproteins is mediated by Toll-like receptor 2. *Journal of Immunology* 163, 2382–2386.

Klempner, M.S., Noring, R. and Rogers, R.A. (1993) Invasion of human skin fibroblasts by the Lyme disease spirochete, *Borrelia burgdorferi*. *Journal of Infectious Diseases* 167, 1074–1081.

Kruger, H., Reuss, K., Pulz, M., Rohrbach, E., Pflughaupt, K.W., Martin, R. and Mertens, H.G. (1989) Meningoradiculitis and encephalomyelitis due to *Borrelia burgdorferi*: a follow-up study of 72 patients over 27 years. *Journal of Neurology* 236, 322–328.

Leong, J.M., Robbins, D., Rosenfeld, L., Lahiri, B. and Parveen, N. (1998) Structural requirements for glycosaminoglycan recognition by the Lyme disease spirochete, *Borrelia burgdorferi*. *Infection and Immunity* 66, 6045–6048.

Lisinski, T.J. and Furie, M.B. (2002) Interleukin-10 inhibits proinflammatory activation of endothelium in response to *Borrelia burgdorferi* or lipopolysaccharide but not interleukin-1β or tumor necrosis factor α. *Journal of Leukocyte Biology* 72, 503–511.

Londono, D. and Cadavid, D. (2010) Bacterial lipoproteins can disseminate from the periphery to inflame the brain. *American Journal of Pathology* 176, 2848–2857.

Londono, D., Bai, Y., Zuckert, W.R., Gelderblom, H. and Cadavid, D. (2005) Cardiac apoptosis in severe relapsing fever borreliosis. *Infection and Immunity* 73, 7669–7676.

Londono, D., Marques, A., Hornung, R.L. and Cadavid, D. (2008) Relapsing fever borreliosis in interleukin-10-deficient mice. *Infection and Immunity* 76, 5508–5513.

Londono, D., Carvajal, J., Strle, K., Kim, K.S. and Cadavid, D. (2011) IL-10 prevents apoptosis of brain endothelium during bacteremia. *Journal of Immunology* 186, 7176–7186.

Ma, Y., Sturrock, A. and Weis, J.J. (1991) Intracellular localization of *Borrelia burgdorferi* within human endothelial cells. *Infection and Immunity* 59, 671–678.

Moriarty, T.J., *et al.* (2012) Vascular binding of a pathogen under shear force through mechanistically distinct sequential interactions with host macromolecules. *Molecular Microbiology* 86, 1116–1131.

Nocton, J.J., Bloom, B.J., Rutledge, B.J., Persing, D.H., Logigian, E.L., Schmid, C.H. and Steere, A.C. (1996) Detection of *Borrelia burgdorferi* DNA by polymerase chain reaction in cerebrospinal fluid in Lyme neuroborreliosis. *Journal of Infectious Diseases* 174, 623–627.

Nordstrand, A., Shamaei-Tousi, A., Ny, A. and Bergstrom, S. (2001) Delayed invasion of the kidney and brain by *Borrelia crocidurae* in plasminogen-deficient mice. *Infection and Immunity* 69, 5832–5839.

Pachner, A.R. (1995) Early disseminated Lyme disease: Lyme meningitis. *American Journal of Medicine* 98, 30S–37S.

Pachner, A.R. and Steere, A.C. (1985) The triad of neurologic manifestations of Lyme disease: meningitis, cranial neuritis, and radiculoneuritis. *Neurology* 35, 47–53.

Pachner, A.R., Dail, D., Narayan, K., Dutta, K. and Cadavid, D. (2002) Increased expression of B-lymphocyte chemoattractant, but not pro-inflammatory cytokines, in muscle tissue in rhesus chronic Lyme borreliosis. *Cytokine* 19, 297–307.

Pachner, A.R., Dail, D., Bai, Y., Sondey, M., Pak, L., Narayan, K. and Cadavid, D. (2004) Genotype determines phenotype in experimental Lyme borreliosis. *Annals of Neurology* 56, 361–370.

Parveen, N., Caimano, M., Radolf, J.D. and Leong, J.M. (2003) Adaptation of the Lyme disease spirochaete to the mammalian host environment results in enhanced glycosaminoglycan and host cell binding. *Molecular Microbiology* 47, 1433–1444.

Pennington, P.M., Allred, C.D., West, C.S., Alvarez, R. and Barbour, A.G. (1997) Arthritis severity and spirochete burden are determined by serotype in the *Borrelia turicatae*–mouse model of Lyme disease. *Infection and Immunity* 65, 285–292.

Pennington, P.M., Cadavid, D. and Barbour, A.G. (1999) Characterization of VspB of *Borrelia turicatae*, a major outer membrane protein expressed in blood and tissues of mice. *Infection and Immunity* 67, 4637–4645.

Purser, J.E. and Norris, S.J. (2000) Correlation between plasmid content and infectivity in *Borrelia burgdorferi*. *Proceedings of the National Academy of Sciences USA* 97, 13865–13870.

Radolf, J.D., Arndt, L.L., Akins, D.R., Curetty, L.L., Levi, M.E., Shen, Y., Davis, L.S. and Norgard, M.V. (1995) *Treponema pallidum* and *Borrelia burgdorferi* lipoproteins and synthetic lipopeptides activate monocytes/macrophages. *Journal of Immunology* 154, 2866–2877.

Reik, L., Steere, A.C., Bartenhagen, N.H., Shope, R.E. and Malawista, S.E. (1979) Neurologic abnormalities of Lyme disease. *Medicine (Baltimore)* 58, 281–294.

Rupprecht, T.A., Pfister, H.W., Angele, B., Kastenbauer, S., Wilske, B. and Koedel, U. (2005) The chemokine CXCL13 (BLC): a putative diagnostic marker for neuroborreliosis. *Neurology* 65, 448–450.

Rupprecht, T.A., Kirschning, C.J., Popp, B., Kastenbauer, S., Fingerle, V., Pfister, H.W. and Koedel, U. (2007) *Borrelia garinii* induces CXCL13 production in human monocytes through Toll-like receptor 2. *Infection and Immunity* 75, 4351–4356.

Sadziene, A., Thomas, D.D. and Barbour, A.G. (1995) *Borrelia burgdorferi* mutant lacking Osp: biological and immunological characterization. *Infection and Immunity* 63, 1573–1580.

Schuhardt, V.T. and Hemphill, E.C. (1946) Brain involvement as a possible cause of relapse after treatment in spirochetal relapsing fever. *Science* 103, 422.

Seemanapalli, S.V., Xu, Q., McShan, K. and Liang, F.T. (2010) Outer surface protein C is a dissemination-facilitating factor of *Borrelia burgdorferi* during mammalian infection. *PLoS One* 5, e15830.

Sethi, N., Sondey, M., Bai, Y., Kim, K.S. and Cadavid, D. (2006) Interaction of a neurotropic strain of *Borrelia turicatae* with the cerebral microcirculation system. *Infection and Immunity* 74, 6408–6418.

Szczepanski, A., Furie, M.B., Benach, J.L., Lane, B.P. and Fleit, H.B. (1990) Interaction between *Borrelia burgdorferi* and endothelium *in vitro*. *Journal of Clinical Investigation* 85, 1637–1647.

Thomas, D.D., Cadavid, D. and Barbour, A.G. (1994) Differential association of *Borrelia* species with cultured neural cells. *Journal of Infectious Diseases* 169, 445–448.

Tumani, H. and Cadavid, D. (2011) Are high CSF levels of CXCL13 helpful for diagnosis of Lyme neuroborreliosis? *Neurology* 76, 1034–1035.

van Dam, A.P., Kuiper, H., Vos, K., Widjojokusumo, A., de Jongh, B.M., Spanjaard, L., Ramselaar, A.C., Kramer, M.D. and Dankert, J. (1993) Different genospecies of *Borrelia burgdorferi* are associated with distinct clinical manifestations of Lyme borreliosis. *Clinical Infectious Diseases* 17, 708–717.

Wallich, R., Pattathu, J., Kitiratschky, V., Brenner, C., Zipfel, P.F., Brade, V., Simon, M.M. and Kraiczy, P. (2005) Identification and functional characterization of complement regulator-acquiring surface protein 1 of the Lyme disease spirochetes *Borrelia afzelii* and *Borrelia garinii*. *Infection and Immunity* 73, 2351–2359.

Wilske, B., Preac-Mursic, V., Jauris, S., Hofmann, A., Pradel, I., Soutschek, E., Schwab, E., Will, G. and Wanner, G. (1993) Immunological and molecular polymorphisms of OspC, an immunodominant major outer surface protein of *Borrelia burgdorferi*. *Infection and Immunity* 61, 2182–2191.

Wooten, R.M., Modur, V.R., McIntyre, T.M. and Weis, J.J. (1996) *Borrelia burgdorferi* outer membrane protein A induces nuclear translocation of nuclear factor-κ B and inflammatory activation in human endothelial cells. *Journal of Immunology* 157, 4584–4590.

Yang, X.F., Pal, U., Alani, S.M., Fikrig, E. and Norgard, M.V. (2004) Essential role for OspA/B in the life cycle of the Lyme disease spirochete. *Journal of Experimental Medicine* 199, 641–648.

Zhang, J.R., Hardham, J.M., Barbour, A.G. and Norris, S.J. (1997) Antigenic variation in Lyme disease borreliae by promiscuous recombination of VMP-like sequence cassettes. *Cell* 89, 275–285.

16 Nosocomial Meningitis

Ronny Beer* and Bettina Pfausler
Innsbruck Medical University, Innsbruck, Austria

16.1 Introduction

Infectious complications in the neurological and neurosurgical patient population presenting as meningitis, ventriculitis, brain abscess, and subdural or epidural empyema are frequently associated with invasive procedures such as craniotomy or placement of intracranial devices necessary, for example, for intracranial pressure (ICP) monitoring or diversion of the cerebrospinal fluid (CSF) from an obstructed ventricular system (Ziai and Lewin, 2006; Beer *et al.*, 2008, 2010). In addition, intracranial infections may arise from other exogenous sources such as transmission of pathogens from healthcare personnel. Poor hand hygiene has been demonstrated to be one of the most important causes of hospital-acquired infections (Raad *et al.*, 2007). Hence, the majority of these infections must be considered nosocomial. Nosocomial meningitis is a potentially life-threatening condition that may contribute to a permanent adverse outcome of the patient. Reducing morbidity and mortality is strongly dependent on prompt diagnosis and on the institution of appropriate anti-infective therapy (Beer *et al.*, 2009; van de Beek *et al.*, 2010).

Although it has been established that nosocomial infections significantly alter therapeutic considerations and patient outcomes, stringent criteria for characterizing and diagnosing these diseases are still a matter of ongoing debate. It is worth noting that the term 'nosocomial' has been suggested to be replaced by 'healthcare-associated', a concept that might be useful for the categorization of infections occurring in the hospital setting (Lujan *et al.*, 2009). The National Healthcare Safety Network, Division of Healthcare Quality Promotion of the Centers for Disease Control and Prevention (CDC/NHSN) has published an update on the definition of the specific types of healthcare-associated infections in the acute care setting (Horan *et al.*, 2008). The definition of meningitis or ventriculitis according to CDC/NHSN is given in Table 16.1.

This overview will concentrate on nosocomial meningitis related to invasive neurosurgical procedures, because this infectious complication has been described as a distinct disease entity (Schade *et al.*, 2005; Weisfelt *et al.*, 2007).

16.2 Epidemiology

The true prevalence of healthcare-associated meningitis is difficult to estimate because epidemiological data are limited. Most

*ronny.beer@i-med.ac.at

Table 16.1. Definition of healthcare-associated meningitis or ventriculitis.

At least one of the following criteria must be met:
(1) Patient has organisms cultured from the CSF
(2) Patient has at least one of the following signs or symptoms with no other recognized cause: fever (>38°C), headache, meningeal signs (e.g. neck stiffness), cranial nerve signs or irritability, and at least one of the following:
(a) increased white cells, elevated protein and/or decreased glucose in the CSF;
(b) organisms seen on Gram stain of the CSF;
(c) organisms cultured from blood;
(d) positive antigen test of the CSF, blood or urine, and
(e) diagnostic single antibody titre (IgM) or fourfold increase in paired sera (IgG) for the pathogen; and if diagnosis is made ante mortem, the physician institutes appropriate anti-infective therapy

reports refer to post-neurosurgical (e.g. craniotomy and ventriculostomy) infectious complications (Leung *et al.*, 2007; Lo *et al.*, 2007; McClelland and Hall, 2007; Conen *et al.*, 2008; Hoefnagel *et al.*, 2008; Kim *et al.*, 2012). By contrast, only a few studies on the epidemiology of nosocomial intracranial infections secondary to penetrating traumatic brain injury (Baltas *et al.*, 1994) or systemic infections with secondary involvement of the subarachnoid space (SAS) (Frontera *et al.*, 2008) are available. Important risk factors for nosocomial meningitis are a history of neurosurgery, especially placement of intracranial devices such as ICP monitors or ventriculostomy catheters, history of recent head trauma with CSF leakage, presence of cranial or extracranial infectious foci such as otitis, sinusitis or pneumonia, and potentially an immunocompromised state (Weisfelt *et al.*, 2007; Conen *et al.*, 2008; Hoefnagel *et al.*, 2008; Kim *et al.*, 2012). The incidence of ventriculostomy-related infections ranges from 2% to 45% in the literature (Lyke *et al.*, 2001; Park *et al.*, 2004; Conen *et al.*, 2008), with an average rate of 9.5% calculated over the past 10 years (Kim *et al.*, 2012). A meta-analysis of 23 retrospective studies reported a cumulative rate of positive CSF cultures of 8.8% per patient and 8.1% per ventriculostomy catheter (Lozier *et al.*, 2002). It has been claimed that the majority of catheter-related nosocomial meningitis occurs within the first week after insertion, but recent studies identified a later peak of infection even after 2 weeks, particularly in patients with prolonged catheter placement due to severe intracranial disease (Lozier *et al.*, 2002; Lo *et al.*, 2007; Beer *et al.*, 2008). Other relevant predisposing factors for ventriculostomy-related meningitis are frequency of CSF sampling, catheter irrigation, intraventricular haemorrhage, subarachnoid haemorrhage, surgical technique and presence of other distant infections (Lozier *et al.*, 2002; Beer *et al.*, 2010; van de Beek *et al.*, 2010). The characteristics of nosocomial meningitis have also been evaluated in a prospective cohort study (Weisfelt *et al.*, 2007). Underlying conditions such as a history of neurosurgery or CSF leakage were present in 94% of the episodes and any kind of neurosurgical intervention accounted for 64% of the infections, whereas an immunocompromised state was present in 28% of the cohort, and a distant focus of infection was identified in 18% of the patients. In 28% of the study population, more than one risk factor could be identified. However, risk profiles have been inconsistently reported throughout the literature (Park *et al.*, 2004; Korinek *et al.*, 2005a, 2006). The incidence of bacterial meningitis after moderate or severe traumatic brain injury has been estimated to range between 1% and 2%, with CSF leakage as the major risk factor and fracture of the basal skull increasing the risk up to 25% (Baltas *et al.*, 1994).

16.3 Infection Versus Contamination and Colonization of Intracranial Devices

Regarding the frequent association of indwelling intracranial devices with nosocomial meningitis, efforts must be made to differentiate clinically relevant infections of the SAS that require immediate therapeutic attention from contamination and colonization of the abiotic device surface by a variety of microorganisms (Beer *et al.*, 2008). According to the criteria proposed by Lozier *et al.* (2002), contamination in the setting of ventriculostomy catheters constitutes an isolated positive CSF culture in the absence of abnormal CSF findings. In patients with the catheter *in situ*, colonization is defined by at least two positive CSF cultures with expected CSF profiles and lack of clinical signs other than fever. Pathological CSF findings, especially advancing pleocytosis, in the absence of positive CSF cultures, characterizes suspected device-related meningitis, whereas definite nosocomial meningitis is defined by positive CSF culture accompanied by abnormal CSF findings or appropriate clinical signs and symptoms. In addition, aseptic inflammation resulting from tissue response to brain injury or stimulation by non-infectious agents such as blood breakdown products or chemicals should be distinguished from infection (Zarrouk *et al.*, 2007).

16.4 Microbiology

Overall, Gram-positive organisms consistent with skin flora such as coagulase-negative staphylococci and *Staphylococcus aureus* are the most common pathogens involved in nosocomial meningitis (Lozier *et al.*, 2002; Bota *et al.*, 2005; Beer *et al.*, 2008; Conen *et al.*, 2008). These organisms account for approximately two-thirds of nosocomial CSF infections. Other Gram-positive bacteria traditionally isolated from nosocomial CSF infections are *Propionibacterium acnes* and enterococci. However, despite the predominance of Gram-positive species, an increasing proportion of Gram-negative nosocomial meningitis cases is being reported (Arabi *et al.*, 2005; Conen *et al.*, 2008; Camacho *et al.*, 2011). The spectrum of Gram-negative bacteria comprises Enterobacteriaceae such as *Escherichia coli* and *Klebsiella*, *Serratia* and *Enterobacter* spp. as well as non-fermenters such as *Pseudomonas aeruginosa* and *Acinetobacter baumanii*. Anaerobes and fungi, primarily *Candida* spp., are rarely identified (Dettenkofer *et al.*, 2001; Lozier *et al.*, 2002). Risk factors for fungal nosocomial CSF infections are broad-spectrum anti-infective therapy and compromised immune status (Korinek *et al.*, 2005a). Polymicrobial infections have been reported mainly in patients with ventriculoperitoneal shunts (Vinchon *et al.*, 2006) and are serious complications of intestinal perforation caused by the shunt tip (Fig. 16.1). Differences in microbiological profiles between studies might be attributed to differences in antibiotic usage and local flora. The aetiological microorganisms most frequently identified in nosocomial meningitis are listed in Table 16.2.

16.5 Pathogenesis with Special Emphasis on Biofilm Formation in *Staphylococcus* Infections

In general, infection should be envisaged as a spectrum of pathogenic mechanisms influenced by host–microbe interactions, microbe–microbe interactions, immunity-mediated antimicrobial host defences and environmental factors (Peters *et al.*, 2012). Imbalances in any of these interdependent factors can lead to the predisposition to or development of infection. A key step in the pathophysiology of meningitis is the invasion of pathogens through physiological barriers that protect the meningeal spaces to reach the CSF. Although recent findings have considerably expanded our understanding of the various strategies of certain pathogens to invade the SAS (as detailed throughout this book), the cellular and molecular mechanisms of nosocomial meningitis are still enigmatic in many circumstances.

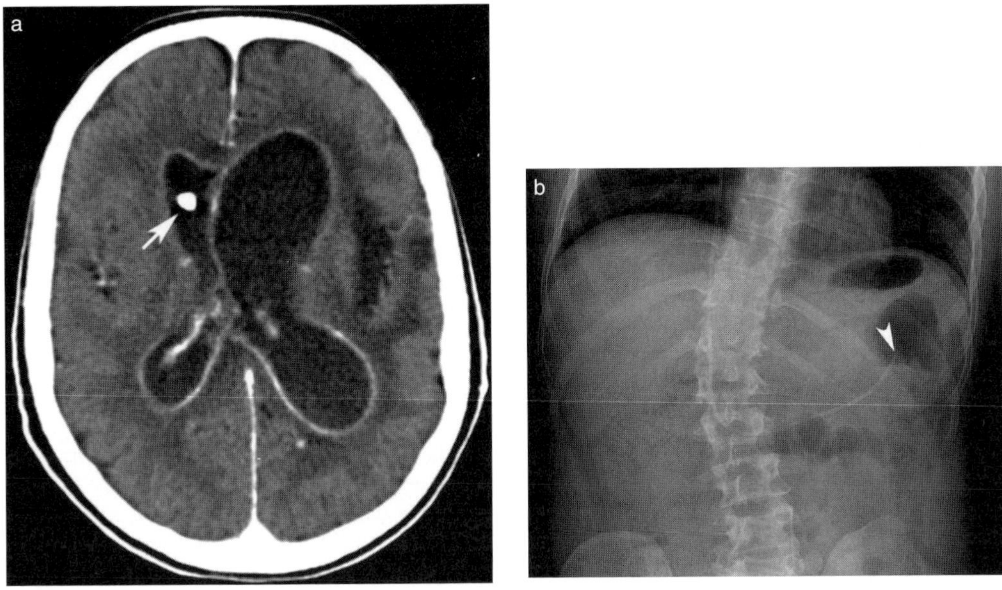

Fig. 16.1. (a) Representative contrast-enhanced cranial computed tomography scan of a patient with fulminant ventriculomeningitis illustrated by massive ependymal enhancement. Nosocomial meningitis originated from an ascending shunt system infection (arrow indicates proximal tip of the ventriculoperitoneal shunt in the right lateral ventricle). (b) Plain abdominal radiography of the same patient showing perforation of the left (splenic) flexure of the colon by the distal tip of the ventriculoperitoneal shunt (arrowhead). Cultures of CSF and shunt tips after system removal grew *Enterococcus faecalis* and *Escherichia coli* compatible with gut flora.

Table 16.2. Microbiology of nosocomial meningitis according to the literature (numbers rounded).

Organism	Percentage causation
Coagulase-negative staphylococci	47–65%
Staphylococcus aureus	12–29%
Propionibacterium acnes	1–14%
Gram-negative bacteria (e.g. *Escherichia coli, Pseudomonas aeruginosa*)	6–20%
Polymicrobial infections	~15%
Anaerobes	Rare
Candida sp.	Very rare

As in community-acquired meningitis, healthcare-associated meningitis can be caused by dissemination of blood-borne pathogens from a remote focus (Holloway *et al.*, 1996; Kim *et al.*, 2012) or contiguous spread from a neighbouring structure to the meningeal membranes. The latter mode of transmission is frequently encountered in patients with penetrating head injuries (Kourbeti *et al.*, 2012) or traumatic, spontaneous and iatrogenic CSF leaks (Horowitz *et al.*, 2011). However, in the case of nosocomial meningitis, another important pathomechanism must be taken into consideration. Currently, an overwhelming number of nosocomial CSF infections are propagated on abiotic surfaces such as ventriculostomy catheters or shunts. These devices are recognized as sources of chronic infection and can potentially serve as sites of inoculation into the SAS leading to meningitis. Importantly, abiotic medical materials bypass many of the mechanisms preventing microbial colonization of the CSF, because a number of innate immune defence mechanisms break down. The device itself acts both as a conduit through which microorganisms can migrate into the intracranial compartment from the external environment and as a convenient surface upon which biofilms can accumulate (Otto, 2012; Peters *et al.*, 2012). The increasing use of indwelling devices in various acute and chronic neurological diseases renders an understanding of the mechanisms behind and consequences of microbial colonization of biomaterials increasingly important (Arciola *et al.*, 2012).

Once the pathogens have gained access into the SAS, they take advantage of the immune privilege of the central nervous system to multiply and induce inflammation. The components of the host defence system that initiate the first line of immune response against invading pathogens have not been studied in detail in nosocomial meningitis. In compliance with the inflammatory response in community-acquired bacterial meningitis, it has been postulated that immune activation in the CSF is triggered by the recognition of different bacterial pathogen-associated molecular patterns by antigen-presenting cells present at low levels in the CSF or situated in the perivascular space or brain parenchyma as astrocytes and microglial cells (Weber and Tuomanen, 2007; Mook-Kanamori *et al.*, 2011). Soluble pattern recognition receptor (PRR) molecules involved in the pathophysiology of nosocomial meningitis include lipopolysaccharide-binding protein and members of the Toll-like receptor (TLR) family. Upon stimulation of these PRRs, an intracellular cascade is activated and leads to the production of inflammatory molecules, usually cytokines or chemokines, which modulate the immune response by activating or attracting specialized immune cells (see Christodoulides, Chapter 17, this volume). Importantly, deficiencies in the PRR downstream signalling pathway have been associated with healthcare-associated infections, including meningitis (Dziedzic *et al.*, 2004; Kumpf *et al.*, 2010).

16.5.1 Biofilm formation on intracranial devices

Most of the microorganisms associated with nosocomial meningitis rarely exist as single-species planktonic forms but are found thriving in a complex polymicrobial biofilm community attached to biotic and abiotic sites (Brogden *et al.*, 2005). The pathogens are either introduced during insertion of the device or derived from a temporary bacteraemia followed by adherence to the device surface and subsequent growth to form a biofilm. The pathophysiological importance of the availability of an artificial surface is supported by data from animal studies demonstrating that bacterial presence in the CSF can be transient if bacteraemia is not sustained, reflecting the fact that bacterial entry into the SAS may not always lead to meningitis. Biofilms can be defined as a varied collection of microorganisms (i.e. bacteria and fungi) encased in a self- and/or host-derived hydrated matrix (Arciola *et al.*, 2012). Depending on microbial characteristics and environmental conditions, the biofilm matrix consists of various substances such as polysaccharides, proteins, teichoic acids and extracellular DNA (Costerton *et al.*, 1999). Biofilms are able to resist anti-infective drugs, disinfectants and mechanisms of innate and adaptive host defence (Stewart and Costerton, 2001; Stewart, 2002). The mechanisms mediating the protective features of biofilms are multiple (Otto, 2012). For example, extracellular matrix (ECM) represents a mechanical barrier for immune cells. Further, limited diffusion through this matrix may contribute to the biofilm tolerance towards some antibiotics. In addition, biofilms can harbour pathogens that carry antibiotic resistance genes (Parsek and Singh, 2003) or show increased tolerance to antibiotics (also referred to as persister cells). Consequently, surface-associated biofilms act as a potential refuge and locus of recolonization after anti-infective therapy. Although the complex mechanisms required to form a functional biofilm are still under investigation, experimental data suggest a coordinated sequence of events (Mack *et al.*, 2004; Arciola *et al.*, 2012). Initial attachment of bacterial cells to the biotic or abiotic surface is followed by cell aggregation and accumulation in multiple bacterial layers. During this phase, the biofilm is progressively established on the colonized device. Subsequently, maturation of the biofilm takes place with development of characteristic structural features specific for the bacterial species. Once the biofilm reaches its final phase of maturation, dispersal of the micro-community is triggered, with detachment of bacteria from the matrix to initiate a new cycle of biofilm formation elsewhere or invasive infection.

16.5.2 *Staphylococcus epidermidis* biofilm formation and virulence factors

Staphylococcus epidermidis is an important member of the coagulase-negative staphylococci and one of the most abundant colonizers of human skin. Due to its identification as a major cause of device-related infections occurring in the healthcare setting, *S. epidermidis* is now recognized as a relevant opportunistic pathogen (Otto, 2012). In contrast to *S. aureus*, with its large arsenal of toxins developed for causing infection in the human host, *S. epidermidis* produces a series of molecules that provide protection from host defences and therefore appear to be necessary for the commensal lifestyle of this microorganism. However, some of these proteins and exopolymers may transform into virulence factors that facilitate the persistence of the bacteria after breaching the epithelial barrier of the host and establish invasive infection (Otto, 2009; Schoenfelder *et al.*, 2010). *S. epidermidis*, like many other coagulase-negative staphylococci, is an excellent biofilm former and, indeed, many features of biofilm pathophysiology have been first investigated in the 'slime' produced by *S. epidermidis* (Noble *et al.*, 1986; Rodgers *et al.*, 1994).

A selection of specific molecules involved in *Staphylococcus* adhesion, aggregation, biofilm structuring and detachment will be discussed (Arciola *et al.*, 2012; Otto, 2012). Adhesins represent an important group of virulence factors mediating surface adhesive interactions between microbial cells themselves, and between microorganisms and host cells and the ECM. They play a primary role in the early stages of infection, and in the pathogenesis of tissue tropism, surface adhesion and colonization. The adhesins group includes autolysins (Atls), which have been identified as specific proteins that mediate binding to the synthetic surface of indwelling medical devices. Further, accumulation in multiple bacterial layers is mediated by 'microbial surface components recognizing adhesive matrix molecules' (MSCRAMMs) and by intercellular adhesion (Speziale *et al.*, 2009). *S. epidermidis* has several MSCRAMMs for establishing tissue adhesion, via binding to fibronectin, vitronectin, collagen and fibrinogen (Williams *et al.*, 2002; Otto, 2012). Another important contribution to cell–cell adhesion is production of the polysaccharide intercellular adhesin (PIA). PIA synthesis is mediated by the intercellular adhesion (*icaADBC*) gene locus. Although several studies underscore the importance of PIA in infection, it still is a matter of ongoing debate whether PIA can be regarded as a virulence factor that clearly distinguishes invasive from colonizing *S. epidermidis* strains (Yao *et al.*, 2005). In addition, PIA has long been considered indispensible for *S. epidermidis* biofilm formation. In fact, the ECM of *Staphylococcus* biofilms also contains adhesive proteins (e.g. accumulation-associated protein, Aap, and biofilm-associated protein, Bap), which may functionally substitute for PIA (Kogan *et al.*, 2006). Interestingly, there is evidence that PIA-dependent biofilms are more robust than those exclusively formed by proteinaceous factors (Rohde *et al.*, 2007). In contrast to the cellular and molecular mechanisms underlying aggregation during biofilm development, cell–cell disruptive mechanisms have not been studied intensely. Recently, quorum sensing systems have been implicated in the control of *Staphylococcus* biofilm structuring (Boles and Horswill, 2011).

Also still under investigation are host defence mechanisms against bacteria organized in biofilms. Experimental data suggests that polymorphonuclear neutrophils (PMNs) surround biofilm and become activated. However, these cells do not migrate into the biofilm, probably because of a lack of chemotactic signals in addition to hindrance of migration into the matrix. In an attempt to kill bacteria, the PMNs release cytotoxic and proteolytic factors, thereby destroying the surrounding tissue. Thus, the infection persists or even progresses (Kristian *et al.*, 2008). In contrast to PMNs, macrophages appear to migrate into *Staphylococcus* biofilm, but these scavenging cells cannot resolve the infection as their bactericidal activity appears compromised (Thurlow *et al.*, 2011). With respect to biofilm clearance, it is worth mentioning that certain antibiotics such as rifampicin and daptomycin have been shown *in vitro* to diffuse easily into the biofilm matrix and to significantly reduce the number of *S. epidermidis* colony-forming units (Leite *et al.*, 2011).

Until recently, *S. epidermidis* has been regarded as relatively innocuous, partly due to the notion that it lacks secreted toxins as compared with *S. aureus*, whose virulence is based on a large repertoire of secreted molecules such as α-toxin, enterotoxins and leukocidins that are harmful to the host (Tong *et al.*, 2012). However, with identification and characterization of the phenol-soluble modulins (PSMs), the notion that *S. epidermidis* is virtually toxin-free had to be revised (Mehlin *et al.*, 1999). PSMs are peptides with cytolytic capacity, but are produced by *S. epidermidis* only at relatively low levels in accordance with the commonly limited aggressiveness of this opportunistic pathogen (Cheung *et al.*, 2010). It is worth noting that PSM peptides were also discovered in *S. aureus* and identified as virulence factors in bacteraemia and skin infections caused by community-associated methicillin-resistant *S. aureus* (Wang *et al.*, 2007). In addition, *S. epidermidis* produces a number of secreted proteases, which may also contribute to virulence by destruction of host proteins (Dubin *et al.*, 2001).

16.6 Clinical Features and Diagnosis

Any suspected intracranial infection must prompt an immediate diagnostic workup and the initiation of calculated empirical anti-microbial therapy. Fever and deterioration in the level of consciousness or an increase in ICP in the comatose or sedated patient are important early indicators of the potential presence of intracranial infections (Beer *et al.*, 2009). Neuroimaging and CSF analysis are the cornerstones in the diagnosis of nosocomial meningitis. It should be emphasized that performance of such examinations must not delay initiation of appropriate anti-infective therapy. In many cases, lumbar puncture may be contraindicated due to intracranial hypertension; however, CSF recovery may be possible through ventricular catheters. One has to bear in mind that analysis of ventricular CSF does not always allow the diagnosis of meningitis, because CSF circulation and thereby spread of the infection might be blocked with blood or expanding masses. The presence of a focal collection of pus (e.g. abscess, empyema) warrants immediate neurosurgical evacuation, both to reduce ICP and to allow for microbiological analysis of the purulent collection. In addition, cultures from blood and other body fluids as secretions from paranasal sinus must be obtained (Ziai and Lewin, 2006; van de Beek *et al.*, 2010). However, cultures may require prolonged incubation times and the result may be negative in patients with prior antibiotic therapy. A study comparing the results from Gram stains and CSF cultures demonstrated that Gram staining had a very high specificity but an unacceptably low sensitivity of 18% in screening for device-related bacterial meningitis (Schade *et al.*, 2006).

In every patient with a history of neurosurgery or head trauma, there must be a high level of suspicion of intracranial infectious complications, in case of the development of systemic inflammatory response syndrome. On the other hand, clinical and biochemical parameters such as fever or an increase in acute phase proteins may also be a manifestation of the underlying neurological disease (Diringer *et al.*, 2004). Moreover, monitoring of inflammatory parameters does not allow discrimination between systemic or intracranial infection in these patients (Martinez *et al.*, 2002). Studies investigating the value of CSF biochemical parameters, such as CSF leucocyte count, CSF protein, increased CSF lactate and a decreased CSF/serum glucose ratio, conclude that no single parameter can reliably predict or exclude nosocomial intracranial infection (Conen *et al.*, 2008; Muttaiyah *et al.*, 2008). In addition, CSF analysis might be of limited value in identifying intracranial infections due to aseptic inflammation in the case of haemorrhagic CSF. In this setting, calculation of the so-called cell index (ratio of leucocytes and erythrocytes in CSF divided by the ratio of leucocytes and erythrocytes in peripheral blood) may confirm intracranial infection (Pfausler *et al.*, 2004; Beer *et al.*, 2009). Furthermore, inflammation of meninges and ventricular ependyma may be less pronounced when caused by staphylococci. The presence of such a low-grade infection illustrates the challenges of diagnosing nosocomial meningitis and explains the need for additional diagnostic means, because prompt initiation of appropriate anti-infective therapy is associated with improved outcome and reduction in the length of stay at the intensive care unit and hospital (Houck *et al.*, 2004; Proulx *et al.*, 2005; Lepur and Barsić, 2007).

16.7 Therapeutic Considerations

Calculated antimicrobial therapy of nosocomial meningitis must consider the most likely pathogens involved, local resistance patterns, underlying disease and patient factors such as age, co-morbidities and immune status (Beer *et al.*, 2010; van de Beek *et al.*, 2010). Recommendations for empiric anti-infective therapy for bacterial intracranial infections in adults according to risk factor are presented in Table 16.3.

The anti-infectives selected must adequately penetrate the blood–brain barrier and blood–CSF barrier. Because nosocomial intracranial infections can be caused by multidrug-resistant Gram-positive and Gram-negative pathogens, initial empiric treatment with the glycopeptide antibiotic vancomycin, in combination with a cephalosporin with anti-pseudomonal activity or a carbapenem, is recommended, until culture results provide information to adapt antimicrobial therapy according to resistance testing (Ziai and Lewin, 2006; Beer *et al.*, 2008; van de Beek *et al.*, 2010). In patients with a contraindication for systemic vancomycin administration in whom an external ventriculostomy catheter is placed, vancomycin can be safely administered intrathecally (Pfausler *et al.*, 2003; Ziai and

Table 16.3. Calculated antibiotic therapy for bacterial intracranial infections in adults according to risk factor. (Adapted from Beer *et al.*, 2010.)

Risk factor	Common pathogens	Preferred antimicrobial therapy
Post-craniotomy	Staphylococci (e.g. *S. aureus*, *S. epidermidis*), Gram-negative bacilli	Vancomycin[a] or linezolid[b] plus third[c] (or fourth[d]) generation cephalosporin or meropenem[e]
Penetrating head injury	Staphylococci (e.g. *S. aureus*, *S. epidermidis*), Gram-negative bacilli	Vancomycin[a] or linezolid[b] plus third[c] (or fourth[d]) generation cephalosporin or meropenem[e]
Basal skull fracture (early)	*Streptococcus pneumoniae*, haemolytic streptococci, anaerobes (i.e. microbial oral flora)	Third[c] generation cephalosporin plus vancomycin[a] or linezolid[b] (plus metronidazole)

Suggested daily dosing in adult patients with normal renal and/or hepatic function:
[a]Vancomycin 15 mg/kg every 8 h to maintain a serum trough concentration of 15–20 mg/l.
[b]Linezolid 600 mg every 12 h.
[c]Cefotaxime 2 g every 4–6 h (antimicrobial coverage should be based on local antimicrobial susceptibility).
[d]Cefepime 2 g every 4–6 h (antimicrobial coverage should be based on local antimicrobial susceptibility).
[e]Meropenem 2 g every 8 h.

Lewin, 2009). For patients with severe allergy to β-lactam antibiotics, moxifloxacin might prove an alternative (Kanellakopoulou *et al.*, 2008). The efficacy of linezolid for the treatment of nosocomial Gram-positive ventriculomeningitis has been demonstrated (Myrianthefs *et al.*, 2006; Beer *et al.*, 2007). Nosocomial meningitis due to antibiotic-resistant *Acinetobacter* spp. is becoming an increasingly common clinical entity. In these cases, combination therapy of systemic and intrathecally administered polymyxins plus removal of infected devices is suggested (Kim *et al.*, 2009).

Recommendations on the duration of antimicrobial therapy of nosocomial meningitis have not been studied rigorously. Mostly, treatment is continued for 10–14 days. If repeated CSF cultures are negative, some experts have suggested shorter durations (Brown *et al.*, 2000). However, it needs to be stressed that therapy of nosocomial CSF infections must be individualized, because some patients with preceding or concurrent anti-infective therapy may need appropriate empiric antimicrobial treatment, despite negative microbiological CSF testing (Beer *et al.*, 2008). While the routine prophylactic exchange of non-infected indwelling devices is still controversial (Lo *et al.*, 2007), there is consensus on the timely removal of neurosurgical hardware infected with pathogens capable of biofilm formation (Vajramani *et al.*, 2005). Importantly, catheter removal requires concomitant antimicrobial therapy (Ziai and Lewin, 2006). Recurrence of nosocomial CSF infections is reported in 25% of cases (Kestle *et al.*, 2006). Therefore, a high level of suspicion needs to be maintained after termination of antimicrobial therapy.

16.8 Prevention

Because of potential pitfalls in early diagnosis and subsequent delayed initiation of the appropriate antimicrobial therapy, prevention of nosocomial meningitis is of paramount importance. Special emphasis should be placed on the avoidance of modifiable risk factors (Korinek *et al.*, 2005b). Preventative measures include adequate surgical techniques and hygiene as well as the prophylactic administration of antibiotics in patients undergoing neurosurgery (Korinek *et al.*, 2005a; Barker, 2007). However, the benefit of periprocedural antibiotics may be outweighed by predisposing the patient to infections by more resistant pathogens with a higher mortality rate. Available data suggest that prophylactic exchange of indwelling devices does not significantly reduce the incidence of nosocomial meningitis, as infection may be acquired by introduction of bacteria following insertion of a new catheter (Arabi *et al.*, 2005; Lo *et al.*, 2007). The insertion of antimicrobial-impregnated ventriculostomy catheters has been proposed to prevent bacterial colonization along the catheter surface, thereby reducing the risk of device-related meningitis (Abla *et al.*, 2011; Sonabend *et al.*, 2011; Thomas *et al.*, 2012). However, the possible induction of antimicrobial resistance, leading to major healthcare problems, is a significant concern (Pople *et al.*, 2012). A relatively new option that may overcome this disadvantage is the introduction of intracranial devices impregnated with silver nanoparticles. Two prospective studies and a retrospective analysis found reduced infection rates with the use of silver nanoparticle-bearing external ventricular drain catheters (Lackner *et al.*, 2008; Fichtner *et al.*, 2010; Keong *et al.*, 2012).

16.9 Summary

Nosocomial meningitis remains a serious complication of invasive neurosurgical procedures and a variety of severe brain injuries and is associated with significant morbidity and mortality. Patients requiring indwelling intracranial devices to restore neurological function are extremely vulnerable to the development of nosocomial meningitis. Mounting evidence suggests that nosocomial meningitis in such cases is the result of biofilm formation on the device and is often caused by coagulase-negative staphylococci, with *S. epidermidis* isolated most frequently. However, the cellular and molecular mechanisms involved in nosocomial meningitis caused by these organisms are still very poorly understood. The emergence of multidrug-resistant pathogens contributes to the complexity of the management of nosocomial meningitis. Continuous surveillance, including systematic collection and analysis of data on the occurrence and microbiology of nosocomial meningitis, is warranted. Specific risk factors such as neurosurgical intervention, presence of biotic or abiotic medical devices or distant foci of infection must be assessed. Timely diagnosis and prompt initiation of appropriate anti-infective therapy is of utmost importance, being associated with improved patient outcomes. Furthermore, the identification of potential targets for the inhibition of biofilm development may ultimately provide means to modify microbial colonization of biological or synthetic materials and thus reduce the impact of healthcare-associated meningitis on human health. In line with this, the ongoing characterization of the constituents and of the architecture of staphylococcal biofilm will allow the development of treatment strategies to disrupt biofilm formation. Materials loaded with antibacterial substances, or coated with anti-adhesive agents or nanostructures, have already shown promising results.

References

Abla, A.A., Zabramski, J.M., Jahnke, H.K., Fusco, D. and Nakaji, P. (2011) Comparison of two antibiotic-impregnated ventricular catheters: a prospective sequential series trial. *Neurosurgery* 68, 437–442.

Arabi, Y., Memish, Z.A., Balkhy, H.H., Francis, C., Ferayan, A., Al Shimemeri, A. and Almuneef, M.A. (2005) Ventriculostomy-associated infections: incidence and risk factors. *American Journal of Infection Control* 33, 137–143.

Arciola, C.R., Campoccia, D., Speziale, P., Montanaro, L. and Costerton, J.W. (2012) Biofilm formation in *Staphylococcus* implant infections. A review of molecular mechanisms and implications for biofilm-resistant materials. *Biomaterials* 33, 5967–5982.

Baltas, I., Tsoulfa, S., Sakellariou, P., Vogas, V., Fylaktakis, M. and Kondodimou, A. (1994) Posttraumatic meningitis: bacteriology, hydrocephalus, and outcome. *Neurosurgery* 35, 422–426.

Barker, F.G., 2nd (2007) Efficacy of prophylactic antibiotics against meningitis after craniotomy: a meta-analysis. *Neurosurgery* 60, 887–894.

Beer, R., Engelhardt, K.W., Pfausler, B., Broessner, G., Helbok, R., Lackner, P., Brenneis, C., Kaehler, S.T., Georgopoulos, A. and Schmutzhard, E. (2007) Pharmacokinetics of intravenous linezolid in cerebrospinal fluid and plasma in neurointensive care patients with staphylococcal ventriculitis associated with external ventricular drains. *Antimicrobial Agents and Chemotherapy* 51, 379–382.

Beer, R., Lackner, P., Pfausler, B. and Schmutzhard, E. (2008) Nosocomial ventriculitis and meningitis in neurocritical care patients. *Journal of Neurology* 255, 1617–1624.

Beer, R., Pfausler, B. and Schmutzhard, E. (2009) Management of nosocomial external ventricular drain-related ventriculomeningitis. *Neurocritical Care* 10, 363–367.

Beer, R., Pfausler, B. and Schmutzhard, E. (2010) Infectious intracranial complications in the neuro-ICU patient population. *Current Opinion in Critical Care* 16, 117–122.

Boles, B.R. and Horswill, A.R. (2011) Staphylococcal biofilm disassembly. *Trends in Microbiology* 19, 449–455.

Bota, D.P., Lefranc, F., Vilallobos, H.R., Brimioulle, S. and Vincent, J.L. (2005) Ventriculostomy-related infections in critically ill patients: a 6-year experience. *Journal of Neurosurgery* 103, 468–472.

Brogden, K.A., Guthmiller, J.M. and Taylor, C.E. (2005) Human polymicrobial infections. *Lancet* 365, 253–255.

Brown, E.M., de Louvois, J., Bayston, R., Lees, P.D. and Pople, I.K. (2000) The management of neurosurgical patients with postoperative bacterial or aseptic meningitis or external ventricular drain-associated ventriculitis. Infection in Neurosurgery Working Party of the British Society for Antimicrobial Chemotherapy. *British Journal of Neurosurgery* 14, 7–12.

Camacho, E.F., Boszczowski, I., Basso, M., Jeng, B.C., Freire, M.P., Guimarães, T., Teixeira, M.J. and Costa, S.F. (2011) Infection rate and risk factors associated with infections related to external ventricular drain. *Infection* 39, 47–51.

Cheung, G.Y., Rigby, K., Wang, R., Queck, S.Y., Braughton, K.R., Whitney, A.R., Teintze, M., DeLeo, F.R. and Otto, M. (2010) *Staphylococcus epidermidis* strategies to avoid killing by human neutrophils. *PLoS Pathogens* 6, e1001133.

Conen, A., Walti, L.N., Merlo, A., Fluckiger, U., Battegay, M. and Trampuz, A. (2008) Characteristics and treatment outcome of cerebrospinal fluid shunt-associated infections in adults: a retrospective analysis over an 11-year period. *Clinical Infectious Diseases* 47, 73–82.

Costerton, J.W., Stewart, P.S. and Greenberg, E.P. (1999) Bacterial biofilms: a common cause of persistent infections. *Science* 284, 1318–1322.

Dettenkofer, M., Ebner, W., Els, T., Babikir, R., Lucking, C., Pelz, K., Rüden, H. and Daschner, F. (2001) Surveillance of nosocomial infections in a neurology intensive care unit. *Journal of Neurology* 248, 959–964.

Diringer, M.N., Reaven, N.L., Funk, S.E. and Uman, G.C. (2004) Elevated body temperature independently contributes to increased length of stay in neurologic intensive care unit patients. *Critical Care Medicine* 32, 1489–1495.

Dubin, G., Chmiel, D., Mak, P., Rakwalska, M., Rzychon, M. and Dubin, A. (2001) Molecular cloning and biochemical characterisation of proteases from *Staphylococcus epidermidis*. *Biological Chemistry* 382, 1575–1582.

Dziedzic, T., Slowik, A. and Szczudlik, A. (2004) Nosocomial infections and immunity: lesson from brain-injured patients. *Critical Care* 8, 266–270.

Fichtner, J., Güresir, E., Seifert, V. and Raabe, A. (2010) Efficacy of silver-bearing external ventricular drainage catheters: a retrospective analysis. *Journal of Neurosurgery* 112, 840–846.

Frontera, J.A., Fernandez, A., Schmidt, J.M., Claassen, J., Wartenberg, K.E., Badjatia, N., Parra, A., Connolly, E.S. and Mayer, S.A. (2008) Impact of nosocomial infectious complications after subarachnoid hemorrhage. *Neurosurgery* 62, 80–87.

Hoefnagel, D., Dammers, R., Ter Laak-Poort, M.P. and Avezaat, C.J. (2008) Risk factors for infections related to external ventricular drainage. *Acta Neurochirurgica (Wien)* 150, 209–214.

Holloway, K.L., Barnes, T., Choi, S., Bullock, R., Marshall, L.F., Eisenberg, H.M., Jane, J.A., Ward, J.D., Young, H.F. and Marmarou, A. (1996) Ventriculostomy infections: the effect of monitoring duration and catheter exchange in 584 patients. *Journal of Neurosurgery* 85, 419–424.

Horan, T.C., Andrus, M. and Dudeck, M.A. (2008) CDC/NHSN surveillance definition of health care-associated infection and criteria for specific types of infections in the acute care setting. *American Journal of Infection Control* 36, 309–332.

Horowitz, G., Fliss, D.M., Margalit, N., Wasserzug, O. and Gil, Z. (2011) Association between cerebrospinal fluid leak and meningitis after skull base surgery. *Otolaryngology – Head and Neck Surgery* 145, 689–693.

Houck, P.M., Bratzler, D.W., Nsa, W., Ma, A. and Bartlett, J.G. (2004) Timing of antibiotic administration and outcomes for Medicare patients hospitalized with community-acquired pneumonia. *Archives of Internal Medicine* 164, 637–644.

Kanellakopoulou, K., Pagoulatou, A., Stroumpoulis, K., Vafiadou, M., Kranidioti, H., Giamarellou, H. and Giamarellos-Bourboulis, E.J. (2008) Pharmacokinetics of moxifloxacin in non-inflamed cerebrospinal fluid of humans: implication for a bactericidal effect. *Journal of Antimicrobial Chemotherapy* 61, 1328–1331.

Keong, N.C., Bulters, D.O., Richards, H.K., Farrington, M., Sparrow, O.C., Pickard, J.D., Hutchinson, P.J. and Kirkpatrick, P.J. (2012) The SILVER (Silver Impregnated Line Versus EVD Randomized trial): a double-blind, prospective, randomized, controlled trial of an intervention to reduce the rate of external ventricular drain infection. *Neurosurgery* 71, 394–403.

Kestle, J.R., Garton, H.J., Whitehead, W.E., Drake, J.M., Kulkarni, A.V., Cochrane, D.D., Muszynski, C. and Walker, M.L. (2006) Management of shunt infections: a multicenter pilot study. *Journal of Neurosurgery: Pediatrics* 105, 177–181.

Kim, B.N., Peleg, A.Y., Lodise, T.P., Lipman, J., Li, J., Nation, R. and Paterson, D.L. (2009) Management of meningitis due to antibiotic-resistant *Acinetobacter* species. *Lancet Infectious Diseases* 9, 245–255.

Kim, J.H., Desai, N.S., Ricci, J., Stieg, P.E., Rosengart, A.J., Härtl, R. and Fraser, J.F. (2012) Factors contributing to ventriculostomy infection. *World Neurosurgery* 77, 135–140.

Kogan, G., Sadovskaya, I., Chaignon, P., Chokr, A. and Jabbouri, S. (2006) Biofilms of clinical strains of *Staphylococcus* that do not contain polysaccharide intercellular adhesin. *FEMS Microbiology Letters* 255, 11–16.

Korinek, A.M., Golmard, J.L., Elcheick, A., Bismuth, R., van Effenterre, R., Coriat, P. and Puybasset, L. (2005a) Risk factors for neurosurgical site infections after craniotomy: a critical reappraisal of antibiotic prophylaxis on 4,578 patients. *British Journal of Neurosurgery* 19, 155–162.

Korinek, A.M., Reina, M., Boch, A.L., Rivera, A.O., De Bels, D. and Puybasset, L. (2005b) Prevention of external ventricular drain-related ventriculitis. *Acta Neurochirurgica (Wien)* 147, 39–45.

Korinek, A.M., Baugnon, T., Golmard, J.L., van Effenterre, R., Coriat, P. and Puybasset, L. (2006) Risk factors for adult nosocomial meningitis after craniotomy: role of antibiotic prophylaxis. *Neurosurgery* 59, 126–133.

Kourbeti, I.S., Vakis, A.F., Papadakis, J.A., Karabetsos, D.A., Bertsias, G., Filippou, M., Ioannou, A., Neophytou, C., Anastasaki, M. and Samonis, G. (2012) Infections in traumatic brain injury patients. *Clinical Microbiology and Infection* 18, 359–364.

Kristian, S.A., Birkenstock, T.A., Sauder, U., Mack, D., Götz, F. and Landmann, R. (2008) Biofilm formation induces C3a release and protects *Staphylococcus epidermidis* from IgG and complement deposition and from neutrophil-dependent killing. *Journal of Infectious Diseases* 197, 1028–1035.

Kumpf, O., *et al.* (2010) Influence of genetic variations in *TLR4* and *TIRAP/Mal* on the course of sepsis and pneumonia and cytokine release: an observational study in three cohorts. *Critical Care* 14, R103.

Lackner, P., Beer, R., Broessner, G., Helbok, R., Galiano, K., Pleifer, C., Pfausler, B., Brenneis, C., Huck, C., Engelhardt, K., Obwegeser, A.A. and Schmutzhard, E. (2008) Efficacy of silver nanoparticles-impregnated external ventricular drain catheters in patients with acute occlusive hydrocephalus. *Neurocritical Care* 8, 360–365.

Leite, B., Gomes, F., Teixeira, P., Souza, C., Pizzolitto, E. and Oliveira, R. (2011) In vitro activity of daptomycin, linezolid and rifampicin on *Staphylococcus epidermidis* biofilms. *Current Microbiology* 63, 313–317.

Lepur, D. and Barsić, B. (2007) Community-acquired bacterial meningitis in adults: antibiotic timing in disease course and outcome. *Infection* 35, 225–231.

Leung, G.K., Ng, K.B., Taw, B.B. and Fan, Y.W. (2007) Extended subcutaneous tunnelling technique for external ventricular drainage. *British Journal of Neurosurgery* 21, 359–364.

Lo, C.H., Spelman, D., Bailey, M., Cooper, D.J., Rosenfeld, J.V. and Brecknell, J.E. (2007) External ventricular drain infections are independent of drain duration: an argument against elective revision. *Journal of Neurosurgery* 106, 378–383.

Lozier, A.P., Sciacca, R.R., Romagnoli, M.F. and Connolly, E.S., Jr (2002) Ventriculostomy-related infections: a critical review of the literature. *Neurosurgery* 51, 170–181.

Lujan, M., Gallego, M. and Rello, J. (2009) Healthcare-associated infections. A useful concept? *Current Opinion in Critical Care* 15, 419–424.

Lyke, K.E., Obasanjo, O.O., Williams, M.A., O'Brien, M., Chotani, R. and Perl, T.M. (2001) Ventriculitis complicating use of intraventricular catheters in adult neurosurgical patients. *Clinical Infectious Diseases* 33, 2028–2033.

Mack, D., Becker, P., Chatterjee, I., Dobinsky, S., Knobloch, J.K., Peters, G., Rohde, H. and Herrmann, M. (2004) Mechanisms of biofilm formation in *Staphylococcus epidermidis* and *Staphylococcus aureus*: functional molecules, regulatory circuits, and adaptive responses. *International Journal of Medical Microbiology* 294, 203–212.

Martínez, R., Gaul, C., Buchfelder, M., Erbguth, F. and Tschaikowsky, K. (2002) Serum procalcitonin monitoring for differential diagnosis of ventriculitis in adult intensive care patients. *Intensive Care Medicine* 28, 208–210.

McClelland, S., 3rd and Hall, W.A. (2007) Postoperative central nervous system infection: incidence and associated factors in 2111 neurosurgical procedures. *Clinical Infectious Diseases* 45, 55–59.

Mehlin, C., Headley, C.M. and Klebanoff, S.J. (1999) An inflammatory polypeptide complex from *Staphylococcus epidermidis*: isolation and characterization. *Journal of Experimental Medicine* 189, 907–918.

Mook-Kanamori, B.B., Geldhoff, M., van der Poll, T. and van de Beek, D. (2011) Pathogenesis and pathophysiology of pneumococcal meningitis. *Clinical Microbiology Reviews* 24, 557–591.

Muttaiyah, S., Ritchie, S., Upton, A. and Roberts, S. (2008) Clinical parameters do not predict infection in patients with external ventricular drains: a retrospective observational study of daily cerebrospinal fluid analysis. *Journal of Medical Microbiology* 57, 207–209.

Myrianthefs, P., Markantonis, S.L., Vlachos, K., Anagnostaki, M., Boutzouka, E., Panidis, D. and Baltopoulos, G. (2006) Serum and cerebrospinal fluid concentrations of linezolid in neurosurgical patients. *Antimicrobial Agents and Chemotherapy* 50, 3971–3976.

Noble, M.A., Reid, P.E., Park, C.M. and Chan, V.Y. (1986) Inhibition of human neutrophil bacteriocidal activity by extracellular substance from slime-producing *Staphylococcus epidermidis*. *Diagnostic Microbiology and Infectious Disease* 4, 335–339.

Otto, M. (2009) *Staphylococcus epidermidis* – the 'accidental' pathogen. *Nature Reviews Microbiology* 7, 555–567.

Otto, M. (2012) Molecular basis of *Staphylococcus epidermidis* infections. *Seminars in Immunopathology* 34, 201–214.

Park, P., Garton, H.J., Kocan, M.J. and Thompson, B.G. (2004) Risk of infection with prolonged ventricular catheterization. *Neurosurgery* 55, 594–599.

Parsek, M.R., and Singh, P.K. (2003) Bacterial biofilms: an emerging link to disease pathogenesis. *Annual Review of Microbiology* 57, 677–701.

Peters, B.M., Jabra-Rizk, M.A., O'May, G.A., Costerton, J.W. and Shirtliff, M.E. (2012) Polymicrobial interactions: impact on pathogenesis and human disease. *Clinical Microbiology Reviews* 25, 193–213.

Pfausler, B., Spiss, H., Beer, R., Kampfl, A., Engelhardt, K., Schober, M. and Schmutzhard, E. (2003) Treatment of staphylococcal ventriculitis associated with external cerebrospinal fluid drains: a prospective randomized trial of intravenous compared with intraventricular vancomycin therapy. *Journal of Neurosurgery* 98, 1040–1044.

Pfausler, B., Beer, R., Engelhardt, K., Kemmler, G., Mohsenipour, I. and Schmutzhard, E. (2004) Cell index – a new parameter for the early diagnosis of ventriculostomy (external ventricular drainage)-related ventriculitis in patients with intraventricular hemorrhage? *Acta Neurochirurgica (Wien)* 146, 477–481.

Pople, I., *et al.* (2012) Comparison of infection rate with the use of antibiotic-impregnated vs standard extraventricular drainage devices: a prospective, randomized controlled trial. *Neurosurgery* 71, 6–13.

Proulx, N., Fréchette, D., Toye, B., Chan, J. and Kravcik, S. (2005) Delays in the administration of antibiotics are associated with mortality from adult acute bacterial meningitis. *QJM: An International Journal of Medicine* 98, 291–298.

Raad, I., Hanna, H. and Maki, D. (2007) Intravascular catheter-related infections: advances in diagnosis, prevention, and management. *Lancet Infectious Diseases* 7, 645–657.

Rodgers, J., Phillips, F. and Olliff, C. (1994) The effects of extracellular slime from *Staphylococcus epidermidis* on phagocytic ingestion and killing. *FEMS Immunology and Medical Microbiology* 9, 109–115.

Rohde, H., *et al.* (2007) Polysaccharide intercellular adhesin or protein factors in biofilm accumulation of *Staphylococcus epidermidis* and *Staphylococcus aureus* isolated from prosthetic hip and knee joint infections. *Biomaterials* 28, 1711–1720.

Schade, R.P., Schinkel, J., Visser, L.G., Van Dijk, J.M., Voormolen, J.H. and Kuijper, E.J. (2005) Bacterial meningitis caused by the use of ventricular or lumbar cerebrospinal fluid catheters. *Journal of Neurosurgery* 102, 229–234.

Schade, R.P., Schinkel, J., Roelandse, F.W., Geskus, R.B., Visser, L.G., van Dijk, J.M., Voormolen, J.H., Van Pelt, H. and Kuijper, E.J. (2006) Lack of value of routine analysis of cerebrospinal fluid for prediction and diagnosis of external drainage-related bacterial meningitis. *Journal of Neurosurgery* 104, 101–108.

Schoenfelder, S.M., Lange, C., Eckart, M., Hennig, S., Kozytska, S. and Ziebuhr, W. (2010) Success through diversity – how *Staphylococcus epidermidis* establishes as a nosocomial pathogen. *International Journal of Medical Microbiology* 300, 380–386.

Sonabend, A.M., Korenfeld, Y., Crisman, C., Badjatia, N., Mayer, S.A. and Connolly, E.S., Jr (2011) Prevention of ventriculostomy-related infections with prophylactic antibiotics and antibiotic-coated external ventricular drains: a systematic review. *Neurosurgery* 68, 996–1005.

Speziale, P., Pietrocola, G., Rindi, S., Provenzano, M., Provenza, G., Di Poto, A., Visai, L. and Arciola, C.R. (2009) Structural and functional role of *Staphylococcus aureus* surface components recognizing adhesive matrix molecules of the host. *Future Microbiology* 4, 1337–1352.

Stewart, P.S. (2002) Mechanisms of antibiotic resistance in bacterial biofilms. *International Journal of Medical Microbiology* 292, 107–113.

Stewart, P.S. and Costerton, J.W. (2001) Antibiotic resistance of bacteria in biofilms. *Lancet* 358, 135–138.

Thomas, R., Lee, S., Patole, S. and Rao, S. (2012) Antibiotic-impregnated catheters for the prevention of CSF shunt infections: a systematic review and meta-analysis. *British Journal of Neurosurgery* 26, 175–184.

Thurlow, L.R., Hanke, M.L., Fritz, T., Angle, A., Aldrich, A., Williams, S.H., Engebretsen, I.L., Bayles, K.W., Horswill, A.R. and Kielian, T. (2011) *Staphylococcus aureus* biofilms prevent macrophage phagocytosis and attenuate inflammation in vivo. *Journal of Immunology* 186, 6585–6596.

Tong, S.Y., Chen, L.F. and Fowler, V.G., Jr (2012) Colonization, pathogenicity, host susceptibility, and therapeutics for *Staphylococcus aureus*: what is the clinical relevance? *Seminars in Immunopathology* 34, 185–200.

Vajramani, G.V., Jones, G., Bayston, R. and Gray, W.P. (2005) Persistent and intractable ventriculitis due to retained ventricular catheters. *British Journal of Neurosurgery* 19, 496–501.

van de Beek, D., Drake, J.M. and Tunkel, A.R. (2010) Nosocomial bacterial meningitis. *New England Journal of Medicine* 362, 146–154.

Vinchon, M., Baroncini, M., Laurent, T. and Patrick, D. (2006) Bowel perforation caused by peritoneal shunt catheters: diagnosis and treatment. *Neurosurgery* 58 (Suppl 1), ONS76–ONS82.

Wang, R., Braughton, K.R., Kretschmer, D., Bach, T.H., Queck, S.Y., Li, M., Kennedy, A.D., Dorward, D.W., Klebanoff, S.J., Peschel, A., DeLeo, F.R. and Otto, M. (2007) Identification of novel cytolytic peptides as key virulence determinants for community-associated MRSA. *Nature Medicine* 13, 1510–1514.

Weber, J.R. and Tuomanen, E.I. (2007) Cellular damage in bacterial meningitis: an interplay of bacterial and host driven toxicity. *Journal of Neuroimmunology* 184, 45–52.

Weisfelt, M., van de Beek, D., Spanjaard, L. and de Gans, J. (2007) Nosocomial bacterial meningitis in adults: a prospective series of 50 cases. *Journal of Hospital Infection* 66, 71–78.

Williams, R.J., Henderson, B., Sharp, L.J. and Nair, S.P. (2002) Identification of a fibronectin-binding protein from *Staphylococcus epidermidis*. *Infection and Immunity* 70, 6805–6810.

Yao, Y., Sturdevant, D.E., Villaruz, A., Xu, L., Gao, Q. and Otto, M. (2005) Factors characterizing *Staphylococcus epidermidis* invasiveness determined by comparative genomics. *Infection and Immunity* 73, 1856–1860.

Zarrouk, V., Vassor, I., Bert, F., Bouccara, D., Kalamarides, M., Bendersky, N., Redondo, A., Sterkers, O. and Fantin, B. (2007) Evaluation of the management of postoperative aseptic meningitis. *Clinical Infectious Diseases* 44, 1555–1559.

Ziai, W.C. and Lewin, J.J., 3rd (2006) Advances in the management of central nervous system infections in the ICU. *Critical Care Clinics* 22, 661–694.

Ziai, W.C. and Lewin, J.J., 3rd (2009) Improving the role of intraventricular antimicrobial agents in the management of meningitis. *Current Opinion in Neurology* 22, 277–282.

17 Inflammation in the Subarachnoid Space

Myron Christodoulides*
University of Southampton Faculty of Medicine, Southampton General Hospital, Southampton, UK

17.1 Introduction

Classical pyogenic leptomeningitis is an acute, compartmentalized intracranial inflammatory response induced in the cerebrospinal fluid (CSF)-filled spaces of the subarachnoid space (SAS) and is characterized by the upregulated accumulation of a wide variety of host response factors and the production of 'pus'. In this chapter, the molecular and cellular composition of this meningeal pus is described.

After entry into the CSF, leptomeningitis is established as a consequence of bacterial growth without immune restriction (Simberkoff *et al.*, 1980) and the direct interactions of pathogens with the different cell types present in the SAS. Meningeal irritation involves the stimulation of endothelial cells, the leptomeninges, macrophages, dendritic cells, infiltrating polymorphonuclear leucocytes (PMNLs) and monocytes, and cortical astrocytes and microglia. The major pyogenic and neonatal meningeal pathogens all show a specific predilection for binding to microvascular endothelial cells and also to cells of the leptomeninges, which represent the largest surface area of cells in the SAS. The leptomeninges play a fundamental role in host cell defence and inflammation within the SAS. Animal models and *in vitro* cell culture models have been described for studying the pathological consequences that occur following the interactions between bacteria and the blood–brain barrier (BBB)/blood–cerebrospinal fluid barrier (BCSFB) and the leptomeninges (Koedel and Pfister, 1999; Hardy *et al.*, 2000; Siddiqui *et al.*, 2012).

The major component of Gram-negative pyogenic bacteria that can induce inflammation is lipopolysaccharide (LPS) endotoxin. Other modulins can trigger cytokine release in manners distinct from LPS, and they include outer-membrane proteins, lipid A-associated proteins, porins and chaperonins of Gram-negative bacteria; lipoteichoic acid (LTA), heat-shock proteins, glycoproteins, lipoproteins and peptides of Gram-positive bacteria; extracellular products including toxins, superantigens and IgA protease; polysaccharides; DNA; and cell-wall and membrane-associated components including fimbriae, pili, muramyl dipeptide and peptidoglycan (Plata-Salaman *et al.*, 1998; Wilson *et al.*, 1998; Moreillon and Majcherczyk, 2003).

*mc4@soton.ac.uk

17.2 Cytokines in Leptomeningitis

17.2.1 Pro-inflammatory cytokines

The cytokines interleukin (IL)-1β, IL-6 and tumour necrosis factor (TNF)-α are early pro-inflammatory mediators in meningitis. High levels of these cytokines are observed in the CSF of patients with bacterial meningitis, but not in patients with viral meningitis or controls (Leist *et al.*, 1988; Arditi *et al.*, 1990; van Furth *et al.*, 1995). The role of LPS in stimulating cytokine production in the CSF during leptomeningitis has been studied comprehensively by Brandtzaeg and van Deuren (2012). Concentrations of LPS in the CSF of patients with meningococcal leptomeningitis correlate positively with increasing levels of TNF-α, IL-1 and IL-6 in the CSF and increased clinical severity and poor neurological outcome.

The meninges do not secrete IL-1α, IL-1β or TNF-α following challenge with *Neisseria meningitidis, Haemophilus influenzae, Streptococcus pneumoniae, Escherichia coli* K1 or Group B *Streptococcus* (GBS) (Fowler *et al.*, 2004; Alkuwaity *et al.*, 2012). In patients with bacterial meningitis, TNF-α mRNA was detected in CSF PMNLs during the early phase of infection and in mononuclear cells in the later stages (Ossege *et al.*, 1996). Infiltrating blood monocytes secrete TNF-α in experimental animal models of meningitis (Bitsch *et al.*, 1997), as do ependymal cells lining the ventricles and choroid plexus epithelium (Tarlow *et al.*, 1993). In addition, endothelial cells challenged *in vivo* and *in vitro* with meningeal pathogens also secrete TNF-α (Sharief *et al.*, 1992). In GBS meningitis induced in infant rats, TNF-α and IL-1β expression is seen in the ependyma and the meninges at 4 h and within the brain parenchyma by 12 h (Kim *et al.*, 2004). The most likely cellular sources of IL-1β in the CSF in leptomeningitis are infiltrating monocytes, resident meningeal macrophages, endothelial cells and neutrophils. Caspase 1 plays a pivotal role in generating mature IL-1β and elevated levels of both molecules in the CSF of patients with acute bacterial meningitis correlate with adverse clinical outcome (Koedel *et al.*, 2002). IL-1β production may also be dependent on the NOD-like receptor family, pyrin domain containing 3 (NLRP3) inflammasome in pneumococcal infection (Witzenrath *et al.*, 2011).

Infection of meningeal cell lines with *N. meningitidis* and *H. influenzae* induced significant IL-6 protein secretion (Fowler *et al.*, 2004). This is consistent with observations *in vivo* that suggest IL-6 production by cells within the SAS, because elevated levels of IL-6 occur in the CSF before leucocytes migrate from the blood and cytokine levels are higher than in serum (Waage *et al.*, 1989). High levels of IL-12 are also found in the CSF of patients with meningitis, and the presence of both IL-6 and IL-12 can be used as indicators of meningeal irritation (Hsieh *et al.*, 2009). Pathophysiological concentrations of IL-6 can also be produced by vascular endothelial cells, infiltrating macrophages and T-cells and also by astrocytes, microglia, neurons and oligodendrocytes within the brain parenchyma (Gruol and Nelson, 1997). In addition, both microglia and astrocytes can secrete TNF-α and IL-1β during meningitis.

17.2.2 Chemokines

Members of the CXC chemokine subfamily are predominantly neutrophil attractants and activators but can also attract activated T-cells and natural killer (NK) cells. In the CC subfamily, chemokines attract mainly monocytes and T-lymphocytes, and to a lesser extent basophils, eosinophils and NK cells. At the onset of pyogenic meningitis (*N. meningitidis, S. pneumoniae* and *H. influenzae*), PMNLs are characteristically found in the SAS, and during the reconstitution phase the pattern of cell infiltration gradually changes to mononuclear cells consisting mainly of monocytes/macrophages and lymphocytes (Lahrtz *et al.*, 1998). Significantly elevated levels of the CXC chemokines IL-8 and CXCL1-related oncogene (growth-related oncogene (GRO)-α) (Seki *et al.*, 1993; Lopez-Cortes *et al.*, 1995; Spanaus *et al.*, 1997) and CC chemokines MCP-1, MIP-1α and MIP-1β (Sprenger *et al.*, 1996; Inaba *et al.*, 1997) can be detected in the CSF of patients with bacterial meningitis, but the levels of RANTES are lower. Indeed, in the principal bacterial meningitides, the levels of IL-8, MCP-1 and MIP-1α in CSF are remarkably similar (Mastroianni *et al.*, 1998).

The cellular sources of chemokines during bacterial meningitis are not clear. It is likely that cells within the SAS, including activated inflammatory cells, are responsible for the local production of chemokines, rather than chemokines entering from the circulation where they can be readily scavenged by high-affinity erythrocyte chemokine receptors. Infection of meningioma cells with *N. meningitidis* and *H. influenzae* induces significant secretion of IL-8, MCP-1 and RANTES and the cytokine growth factor granuloctye–macrophage colony-stimulating factor (GM-CSF) (Fowler *et al.*, 2004). Elevated levels of GM-CSF and related molecules G-CSF and M-CSF have all been detected in the CSF of patients with infectious meningitis (Gallo *et al.*, 1990; Shimoda *et al.*, 1991). In contrast, the meninges do not secrete MIP-1α or MIP-1β in response to bacterial infection.

In addition to the leptomeninges, other cells within the SAS are likely to produce CXC and CC chemokines in response to meningeal pathogens. Macrophages are classical producers of IL-8, MCP-1 and MIP-1α (Maurer and von Stebut, 2004; Deshmane *et al.*, 2009), and endothelial cells also contribute to IL-8 secretion. It is also possible that astrocytes in the *glia limitans superficilias* may be stimulated to produce IL-8 and MCP-1 by bacterial cell-wall products or pro-inflammatory cytokines (Deshmane *et al.*, 2009) that may diffuse across the pia mater. In addition, brain microglia can also produce MCP-1 in response to LPS. Expression of RANTES, although classically produced by lymphocytes, has also been localized to both astrocytes and microglia in experimental animal models of meningitis. However, the contribution of astrocytes and microglia to chemokine synthesis during leptomeningitis *in vivo* is not known.

Other cytokines with chemotactic activity have been identified in the CSF of patients with meningitis, including IL-16 (Suzuki *et al.*, 2003), CXCL16 (Woehrl *et al.*, 2010) and CXCL5 (epithelial-cell-derived neutrophil-activating protein (ENA)-78) (Zwijnenburg *et al.*, 2003a). The chemokine B lymphocyte chemoattractant (BLC), CXCR3 chemokine CXCL11 (I-TAC), CXCL4, stromal derived factor-1α (SDF-1α) and IL-4 have also been observed in patients with neuroborreliosis (Rupprecht *et al.*, 2005a,b). A protein array analysis of the CSF of patients with meningitis and controls identified further new factors, such as macrophage inflammatory protein-lδ (CCL15) and neutrophil-activating peptide-2 (CXCL7) (Kastenbauer *et al.*, 2005). In pneumococcal meningitis patients, new observations included monocyte chemoattractant protein-2 (CCL8), pulmonary and activation-regulated chemokine (CCL18), macrophage inflammatory protein-3α (CCL20) and several growth factors (Kastenbauer *et al.*, 2005). In murine pneumococcal meningitis, the upregulation of new proteins lymphotactin (XCL-1), MIP-1γ (CCL9) and MCP-5 (CCL12), cytokine responsive gene-2 (CRG-2/CXCLIO) and CXCL16, insulin-like growth factor binding protein 3 (IGFBP3), T-cell activation-3 (TCA-3/CCLI) and platelet factor-4 (PF-4/C1) was observed in addition to the classical profile of IL-1β, IL-6, KC, MIP-2 and MCP-1/CCL2 (Klein *et al.*, 2006).

17.2.3 Effects of cytokine release in the CNS

IL-6, IL-1β and TNF-α play central roles in the pathophysiology of leptomeningitis. IL-6 induces acute-phase proteins and leucocytosis, activates the complement and clotting cascades and the stress-response system in the CNS and CSF via central monoaminergic pathways, and regulates the hypothalamus–pituitary–adrenal axis (Mihara *et al.*, 2012). There is a strong correlation between LPS and IL-6 levels and fever, and IL-1β-mediated fever may be dependent on the expression of IL-6 in the SAS and CNS (Conti *et al.*, 2004). Both TNF-α and IL-1β play synergistic roles in initiating leptomeningeal inflammation (Ramilo *et al.*, 1990), and are associated with prolonged fever, seizures and spasticity, with high levels in the CSF correlating positively with mortality (Waage *et al.*, 1987; Glimaker *et al.*, 1993). In addition, they trigger the release of other cytokines and inflammatory mediators, cooperate in promoting increases in the permeability of blood vessels both in the brain and the CSF, and influence the transport of compounds and cells into the CSF (Pan *et al.*, 2011). The significant increases in levels of IL-1β and TNF-α in the SAS are likely to contribute to the massive recruitment of PMNLs into the CSF during meningitis through the upregulation of endothelial-derived adhesion molecules such as P- and E-selectins (Tang *et al.*, 1996). Furthermore, the cooperative interactions of cytokines with matrix metalloproteinases (MMPs) have also been suggested as aids to leucocyte recruitment (Van Lint and Libert, 2007). Recent studies have shown a correlation between high levels of TNF-α and a predominance of PMNLs in the CSF of patients in the acute phase of bacterial meningitis: this was a consequence of rapid death of lymphocytes and monocytes and concomitant PMNL survival (Kawakami *et al.*, 2011).

In children with meningitis, high levels of the immunomodulatory cytokine IL-16 secreted in the CSF also correlate with meningism (Suzuki *et al.*, 2003). IL-16 exhibits chemotactic behaviour and may cooperate with other pro-inflammatory cytokines to promote meningitis. In addition, endogenous IL-18 production has been shown to contribute to a detrimental inflammatory response during experimental pneumococcal meningitis (Zwijnenburg *et al.*, 2003b).

In response to pneumococci, C-reactive protein (CRP) binding to the phosphocholine residues on bacterial cell walls increases the production of TNF-α and IL-1β (Mold and Du Clos, 2006). The role of CRP is protective, by increasing complement-dependent clearance and killing of bacteria. The cytokine IL-17 is also significantly elevated in the CSF of children with bacterial meningitis, where it is believed to play a role in neutrophil infiltration and neuronal protection (Asano *et al.*, 2010). The production of TNF-α and gamma interferon (IFN-γ) is associated with tissue necrosis in tuberculous meningitis, and elevated levels of these two cytokines correlate positively with disease severity (Babu *et al.*, 2008). Further evidence of the role of these cytokines in necrosis is shown by infection of neonatal rats with GBS and pneumococci, which leads to meningitis characterized by increases in the levels of CINC-1, IL-1β, IL-6, IL-10, TNF-α and myeloperoxidase. Expression of these cytokines was elevated in the CSF, hippocampus and cortex and their concerted activities were associated with a breakdown of the BBB (Barichello *et al.*, 2010, 2011). In mice infected with pneumococci, the barrier can also be disrupted by the action of TNF-α (Tsao *et al.*, 2002). In addition, the cooperative effects of nitric oxide (NO), TNF-α and IL-1β, secreted by glial cells that have been activated by LTA from Gram-positive organisms, also open the BBB (Boveri *et al.*, 2006).

The CXC and CC chemokines found in the CSF of patients with meningitis contribute to the observed CSF-mediated chemotaxis of neutrophils and monocyte/macrophages *in vivo* and *in vitro* (Spanaus *et al.*, 1997; Lahrtz *et al.*, 1998). IL-8, MCP-1, RANTES, MIP-1α and MIP-1β all upregulate cell adhesion molecules on endothelia, which is required for PMNL trafficking through veins into the SAS. In addition, MIP-1α, in cooperation with IL-8 and G-CSF, induces the accumulation of neutrophils into the CSF from the blood (Inaba *et al.*, 1997). Upregulation of CXCL16 in the CSF of patients with pneumococcal meningitis implicates this chemokine as an additional neutrophil chemoattractant during disease (Woehrl *et al.*, 2010). Expression of CXCL16 is induced by IFN-γ and TNF-α and is dependent on Toll-like receptor (TLR) 2/TLR4 and MyD88 signalling. The neutrophil chemoattractant CXCL5 is also elevated in the CSF of patients with bacterial meningitis (Zwijnenburg *et al.*, 2003a). MCP-1 is the major chemoattractant for monocytes and macrophages in leptomeningitis, but the coordinated chemotactic activity of MIP-1α and M-CSF may also contribute to monocyte accumulation in the SAS. In addition, CXCL11 has been reported to stimulate chemotaxis of mononuclear cells in neuroborreliosis (Rupprecht *et al.*, 2005a). GM-CSF, which is required primarily for PMNL maturation in the SAS, may also function as a chemoattractant. In addition, GM-CSF secreted by activated endothelial cells can delay the constitutive apoptosis of neutrophils during experimental meningitis induced in mice (Coxon *et al.*, 1999).

In contrast to the active role of the leptomeninges and activated inflammatory cells in the removal of pathogens in the SAS, the reactions induced by chemokines and PMNLs also cause significant cell and tissue injury in areas surrounding inflammatory foci. IL-8 stimulates the production of reactive oxygen species (ROS) and the release of degrading enzymes via exocytosis of granules from PMNLs (Geiser *et al.*, 1993), as well as inducing additional pro-inflammatory factors including platelet activating factor (PAF) and leukotriene B_4 (LTB_4). In addition, MCP-1 causes the release of lysosomal enzymes and induces respiratory burst in monocytes (Rollins *et al.*, 1991). The production of anti-inflammatory cytokines during lepto-meningitis contributes to the complex network of cytokines that have stimulatory and inhibitory effects on progression of the inflammatory response (Tansey and Wyss-Coray, 2008). High levels of IL-10 and transforming growth factor (TGF)-β have been observed in the CSF of patients with bacterial meningitis (Kornelisse *et al.*, 1996; Huang *et al.*, 1997). The main cellular sources of IL-10 and TGF-β in the CSF are most likely resident macrophages, infiltrating monocytes and T-lymphocytes and not the leptomeninges. Numerous other cell types including activated B-cells, neutrophils and endothelial cells (Konkel and Chen, 2012) may also secrete TGF-β during leptomeningeal inflammation. Both IL-10 and TGF-β may be physiologically involved in the course of leptomeningitis as negative feedback signals to limit the production and effects of TNF-α, IL-1 and IL-6; in addition, both cytokines can downregulate the increase in IL-8 production from human brain tissue treated with LPS, IL-1β or TNF-α (Sabat *et al.*, 2010; Konkel and Chen, 2012). Other anti-inflammatory activities of IL-10 include the inhibition of chemokine production by PMNLs, macrophages and endothelial cells, and downregulation of ICAM-1 expression. TGF-β can also reduce any increases in regional cerebral blood flow, intracranial pressure and brain oedema formation during experimental pneumococcal meningitis in the rat (Pfister *et al.*, 1992). The biological activities of pro-inflammatory cytokines within the CSF may also be attenuated by the presence of soluble cytokine receptors, such as the IL-1 receptor antagonist and TNF receptors; or, conversely, they may exacerbate the inflammatory response by prolonging the biological half-lives of these mediators (Tauber and Moser, 1999). Consequently, the roles of these antagonistic molecules in leptomeningitis are unclear.

TNF-α-induced IFN-γ production in cooperation with IL-12 has been suggested to contribute to natural immunity against bacteria in the CSF (Kornelisse *et al.*, 1997). Patients suffering from meningitis show increased levels of TRAIL, the TNF-related apoptosis-inducing ligand; in experimental animals, TRAIL modifies the inflammatory response and reduces neuronal cell death in the hippocampus (Hoffmann *et al.*, 2007).

17.2.4 Downregulation of the CSF inflammatory response

Although meningitis is the overwhelming response of the host to bacterial presence in the SAS, there are instances in which bacteria can suppress inflammation to enable survival and growth of the pathogen during the early stages of the disease. Whereas meningococci and *H. influenzae* stimulate strong inflammatory cytokine release from meningeal cells, pneumococci, *E. coli* K1 and GBS do not (Fowler *et al.*, 2004; Alkuwaity *et al.*, 2012). Inhibition of cytokine release is a consequence of pathogen-induced cell death and/or active inhibitory mechanisms related to virulence factor expression. Inhibition of inflammatory responses is not limited only to the meninges: infection of monocytes with *E. coli* K1 suppresses the production of TNF-α, RANTES, MIP-1β, IL-1β and IL-8 by preventing nuclear factor (NF)-κB activation (Selvaraj and Prasadarao, 2005). *M. tuberculosis* infection of microglia has been reported to inhibit IL-1 and IL-10 production *in vitro* (Curto *et al.*, 2004). In addition, the production of a serine protease by *S. suis* leads to the degradation of IL-8 secreted by brain microvascular endothelial cells (BMECs), thereby delaying the recruitment of neutrophils and enabling the pathogen to invade the CSF (Vanier *et al.*, 2009). GBS also produce a serine protease, CspA, which is active against chemokines (Bryan and Shelver, 2009) and proteolytic inactivation of cytokines has also been described for *Streptococcus pyogenes* (Kaur *et al.*, 2007). Other mechanisms could include escape from antimicrobial peptide lysis, e.g. by CRAMP, the activation of host endogenous degradative enzymes, the alteration of expression of chemokines or chemokine receptors, the ability to block chemokine receptor signalling pathways or possibly through the transient production of anti-chemokine antibodies (Liston and McColl, 2003).

17.3 The Nature and Role of Other Molecules in Leptomeningitis

Without doubt, the generation of cytokines and chemokines by leptomeningeal cells and immune effector cells is critical in leptomeningitis; however, other equally important host defence mechanisms and pathophysiological mediators of injury are also apparent in the progression of the disease. The identities of other molecules found in the CSF of patients with meningitis (of broad bacterial aetiology) are shown in Fig. 17.1. Among all these, NO and ROS play important roles in the pathophysiology of bacterial meningitis and are discussed in detail elsewhere (see Klein *et al.* Chapter 6, this volume). The production of MMPs also contributes significantly to the damage observed during meningitis. Elevated levels of MMP-9 and endogenous TIMP-1 (tissue inhibitor of MMP) are observed in patients with bacterial meningitis (Leppert *et al.*, 2000; Tsai *et al.*, 2011). MMP-8 and -13 are also detectable (Lindberg *et al.*, 2006). The sources of MMPs during meningitis are likely to be infiltrating PMNLs and macrophages, the meninges, endothelial cells and cytokine-stimulated astrocytes and microglia. Studies with autopsy tissues have shown that endothelial cells are strongly positive for MMP-9 during meningitis (Sulik and Chyczewski, 2008). Expression of TIMP-1, TIMP-2 and MMP-9 is also observed in PMNLs. Moreover, MMP-9 levels decrease in astrocytes as TIMP-1 levels increase. MMPs are multifunctional molecules: they process TNF-α to its soluble form, and levels of MMP-9 correlate with levels of this cytokine in the CSF. During meningococcal infection *in vitro*, MMP-8 cleaves the tight junction protein occludin between human BMECs, leading to disassembly of the cell junction and cell matrix adhesion. This not only leads to bacterial penetration of the BCSFB but allows extravasation of leucocytes through vessel walls (Paul *et al.*, 1998; Leib *et al.*, 2000). In addition, increased levels of serum MMP-2 in patients with bacterial meningitis are an indicator of damage to the BCSFB (Kanoh *et al.*, 2008). Elevated levels of MMP-9 are a risk factor for the development of neurological deficits following meningitis. In the infant rat model of pneumococcal meningitis, cortical damage is associated with gelatinolytic activity in the parenchyma and with degradation of type IV collagen. An imbalance between MMP-9 and TIMP-1 was strongly associated with this increased gelatinolysis (Sellner and Leib, 2006).

17.4 Inflammation Beyond the CSF

It is clear from post-mortem studies that the bacterial growth and inflammatory exudate/pus are largely confined to the SAS and subpial space. Despite the high levels of adherence of the major pyogenic and neonatal pathogens to meningeal cells, these organisms invade poorly by the intracellular route (Fowler *et al.*, 2004; Alkuwaity *et al.*, 2012). The lack of bacterial internalization is not due to an inability to internalize foreign material (Weller, 2005), suggesting the absence of host cell-surface receptors that may be required for mediating transcellular passage of meningeal pathogens. However, whereas meningococci and *H. influenzae* type B do not readily penetrate the pia mater by intercellular or intracellular routes, pneumococci, *E. coli* K1 and GBS can rapidly induce pia mater cell death and gain access to the subpial space (Fowler *et al.*, 2004; Alkuwaity *et al.*, 2012). The pia mater provides a barrier to the spread of particulate matter such as erythrocytes in subarachnoid haemorrhage, but inflammatory cells readily penetrate this layer (Weller, 2005).

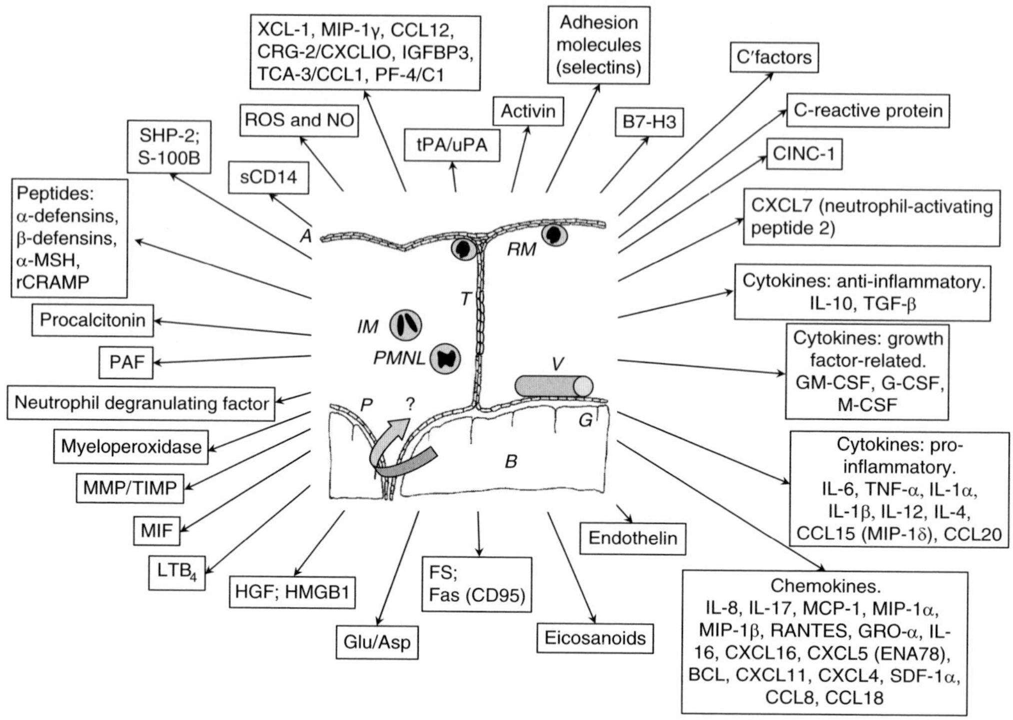

Fig. 17.1. The 'inflammatory soup': a diagrammatic representation of the molecules that are produced in the SAS in response to invading bacteria. In addition to cytokines, chemokines, ROS, NO and MMPs, a plethora of other molecules have been identified in the CSF of patients with bacterial meningitis. These include activin, adhesion molecules (ICAM-1 and ELAM-1), complement factors (C3, factor B and C5a and C3a receptor), co-stimulatory molecule B7-H3, the antimicrobial peptides rCRAMP (LL-37), α-defensins and β-defensins (HBD-1, HBD-2), degranulating factor for neutrophils, eicosanoids (e.g. prostaglandin E2), endothelin, excitatory amino acids (e.g. glutamate and aspartate), follistatin (FS), hepatocyte growth factor (HGF), high mobility group box 1 (HMGB1), heat shock protein 72 (Hsp72), leukotriene (LT) B_4, α-melanocyte stimulating hormone (α-MSH), macrophage migration inhibitory factor (MIF), platelet activating factor (PAF), procalcitonin, protein tyrosine phosphatase SHP2, S-100B, soluble (s)CD14, soluble Fas, (CD95), tissue-type plasminogen activator (tPA) and urokinase-type plasminogen activator (uPA). A, arachnoid mater; B, brain; P, pia mater; RM, resident macrophage; V, blood vessel; T, trabeculae; G, glia limitans; PMNL, neutrophils; IM, infiltrating monocytes. For additional details and a comprehensive bibliography for these molecules, see the blog at myronchristodoulides.wordpress.com.

Underlying the pia mater in the subpial space are layers of collagen bundles and arterioles and veins crossing the space as they enter or leave the brain. Limiting the subpial space is the basement membrane of the *glia limitans superficialis,* which coats compacted layers of astrocyte processes (Kreutzberg *et al.*, 1997). The *glia limitans* appears to be a major barrier to the entry of cells and probably fluid into the brain and is also likely to further limit the spread of bacteria and inflammation into CNS tissue.

Cortical cell and neuron death associated with leptomeningitis results predominantly from infarction due to occlusion by thrombus of inflamed vessels in the SAS. Reactive microglia and astrocytosis may be seen in the *glia limitans* and superficial layers of the brain. Animal models and *in vitro* cell culture models have suggested that neurological damage might be due, in part, to the effects of IL-1, IL-6 and TNF-α (Gibson *et al.*, 2004; Sriram and O'Callaghan, 2007; Spooren *et al.*, 2011) on the brain parenchyma. In addition, apoptosis of neurons in the dentate gyrus of the hippocampus of humans, mediated by bacterial virulence factors, occurs and is discussed elsewhere in this book. Studies have also shown that bacterial pathogens can induce cytokine release by astrocytes, microglia and neurons (Prinz *et al.*, 1999; Al Jindan *et al.*, 2008). Binding of Gram-positive LTA to TLR2 on microglia and astrocytes triggers signalling through ERK1/2 (extracellular-signal-regulated kinase 1/2) and p38 MAPKs (mitogen-activated protein kinases) to activate NF-κB and induce cytokine production (Neher and Brown, 2007). These activated microglia can subsequently induce neuronal apoptosis via NO-dependent mechanisms. LTA can also induce MMP-9 expression in rat brain astrocytes via PDGF receptors and NF-κB (Hsieh *et al.*, 2010). Gram-negative pathogens such as *E. coli* induce cytokine production by astrocytes through activation of the TRAF, NIK, IKK and NF-κB signal pathways (Kim *et al.*, 2005). Primary cultures of murine microglia and astrocytes that are exposed to bacterial antigens also show an increase in the association of nucleotide-binding oligomerization domain-2 (NOD2) with its downstream effector molecule, Rip2 kinase (Chauhan *et al.*, 2009). NOD2 is an important receptor in the *in vitro* inflammatory response of glial cells to meningococcal and *Borrelia burgdorferi* antigens, including muramyl dipeptide. NOD2 also appears to be associated with pathogen-induced astrogliosis, demyelination, behavioural changes and elevated inflammatory cytokine levels. Astrocytes are also a major source of MMPs: human brain biopsies show that MMP-9 secretion by astrocytes is a predominant feature in CNS infection by *Mycobacterium tuberculosis* and could contribute to morbidity and mortality by supporting matrix degradation (Harris *et al.*, 2007). Infection with meningococci or *Borrelia* also delays production of the anti-inflammatory cytokine IL-10 by microglia and astrocytes (Rasley *et al.*, 2006). Nevertheless, IL-10 secretion potentially limits damaging inflammation within the CNS in response to meningeal pathogens. Moreover, glial cell production of IL-10 could be involved in downregulation of the inflammatory response in the brain parenchyma during chronic bacterial infections.

17.5 Conclusions

Despite the presence of the BBB and BCSFB, the CNS is not sheltered from infectious disease. It is patently clear that an extraordinarily diverse range of bacteria can cause infections of the CNS, and the host immune response to these pathogens is largely innate and dependent on multiple receptors enabling 'pattern recognition' of the pathogen(s) by cells within the SAS. Indeed, *S. pneumoniae*, *H. influenzae* and *N. meningitidis* activate several TLR molecules in species-specific patterns (Mogensen *et al.*, 2006). Bacteria that enter the SAS cause leptomeningitis, which is characterized by the production and accumulation of an extraordinary pool of biological molecules (Fig. 17.1). Although leptomeningitis serves to limit bacterial spread, it is at the expense of the host, leading to gross cell and tissue necrosis. If untreated, bacterial leptomeningitis is invariably fatal; for survivors, permanent neurological damage is common. What is clear from the preceding chapters is that the pathogen(s)–host interactions during meningitis are complex, and it is essential to understand the mechanisms involved at the cellular and molecular levels in order to develop more effective treatments for improving patient care and reducing the incidence of neurological sequelae.

References

Al Jindan, R., Vallely, P. and Klapper, P. (2008) Cytokine release by microglia, astrocytes, neurons and a mixed culture in a pneumococcal meningitis culture model. *Journal of Neuroimmunology* 203, 225.

Alkuwaity, K., Taylor, A., Heckels, J., Doran, K. and Christodoulides, M. (2012) Group B *Streptococcus* interactions with human meningeal cells and astrocytes *in vitro*. *PloS ONE* 7, e42660.

Arditi, M., Manogue, K.R., Caplan, M. and Yogev, R. (1990) Cerebrospinal fluid cachectin tumor necrosis factor-α and platelet activating factor concentrations and severity of bacterial meningitis in children. *Journal of Infectious Diseases* 162, 139–147.

Asano, T., Ichiki, K., Koizumi, S., Kaizu, K., Hatori, T., Fujino, O., Mashiko, K., Sakamoto, Y., Miyasho, T. and Fukunaga, Y. (2010) IL-17 is elevated in cerebrospinal fluids in bacterial meningitis in children. *Cytokine* 51, 101–106.

Babu, G., Kumaf, A., Kalita, J. and Misra, U. (2008) Proinflammatory cytokine levels in the serum and cerebrospinal fluid of tuberculous meningitis patients. *Neuroscience Letters* 436, 48–51.

Barichello, T., dos Santos, I., Savi, G.D., Simoes, L.R., Silvestre, T., Comim, C.M., Sachs, D., Teixeira, M.M., Teixeira, A.L. and Quevedo, J. (2010) TNF-α, IL-1β, IL-6, and cinc-1 levels in rat brain after meningitis induced by *Streptococcus pneumoniae*. *Journal of Neuroimmunology* 221, 42–45.

Barichello, T., Lemos, J.C., Generoso, J.S., Cipriano, A.L., Milioli, G.L., Marcelino, D.M., Vuolo, F., Petronilho, F., Dal-Pizzol, F., Vilela, M.C. and Teixeira, A.L. (2011) Oxidative stress, cytokine/chemokine and disruption of blood–brain barrier in neonate rats after meningitis by *Streptococcus agalactiae*. *Neurochemical Research* 36, 1922–1930.

Bitsch, A., Trostdorf, F., Bruck, W., Schmidt, H., Fischer, F.R. and Nau, R. (1997) Central nervous system TNFα-mRNA expression during rabbit experimental pneumococcal meningitis. *Neuroscience Letters* 237, 105–108.

Boveri, M., Kinsner, A., Berezowski, V., Lenfant, A.M., Draing, C., Cecchelli, R., Dehouck, M.P., Hartung, T., Prieto, P. and Bal-Price, A. (2006) Highly purified lipoteichoic acid from Gram-positive bacteria induces in vitro blood–brain barrier disruption through glia activation: role of pro-inflammatory cytokines and nitric oxide. *Neuroscience* 137, 1193–1209.

Brandtzaeg, P. and van Deuren, M. (2012) Classification and pathogenesis of meningococcal infections. In: Christodoulides, M. (ed.) *Neisseria Meningitidis: Advanced Methods and Protocols*. Humana Press, New York, pp. 21–35.

Bryan, J.D. and Shelver, D.W. (2009) *Streptococcus agalactiae* CspA is a serine protease that inactivates chemokines. *Journal of Bacteriology* 191, 1847–1854.

Chauhan, V.S., Sterka, D.G., Furr, S.R., Young, A.B. and Marriott, I. (2009) NOD2 plays an important role in the inflammatory responses of microglia and astrocytes to bacterial CNS pathogens. *Glia* 57, 414–423.

Conti, B., Tabarean, I., Andrei, C. and Bartfai, T. (2004) Cytokines and fever. *Frontiers in Bioscience* 9, 1433–1449.

Coxon, A., Tang, T. and Mayadas, T.N. (1999) Cytokine-activated endothelial cells delay neutrophil apoptosis in vitro and in vivo: a role for granulocyte/macrophage colony-stimulating factor. *Journal of Experimental Medicine* 190, 923–933.

Curto, M., Reali, C., Palmieri, G., Scintu, F., Schivo, M.L., Sogos, V., Marcialis, M.A., Ennas, M.G., Schwarz, H., Pozzi, G. and Gremo, F. (2004) Inhibition of cytokines expression in human microglia infected by virulent and non-virulent mycobacteria. *Neurochemistry International* 44, 381–392.

Deshmane, S.L., Kremlev, S., Amini, S. and Sawaya, B.E. (2009) Monocyte chemoattractant protein-1 (MCP-1): an overview. *Journal of Interferon and Cytokine Research* 29, 313–326.

Fowler, M.I., Weller, R.O., Heckels, J.E. and Christodoulides, M. (2004) Different meningitis-causing bacteria induce distinct inflammatory responses on interaction with cells of the human meninges. *Cellular Microbiology* 6, 555–567.

Gallo, P., Pagni, S., Giometto, B., Piccinno, M.G., Bozza, F., Argentiero, V. and Tavolato, B. (1990) Macrophage-colony stimulating factor (M-CSF) in the cerebrospinal fluid. *Journal of Neuroimmunology* 29, 105–112.

Geiser, T., Dewald, B., Ehrengruber, M.U., Clark-Lewis, I. and Baggiolini, M. (1993) The interleukin-8-related chemotactic cytokines Gro-α, Gro-β, and Gro-γ activate human neutrophil and basophil leukocytes. *Journal of Biological Chemistry* 268, 15419–15424.

Gibson, R.M., Rothwell, N.J. and Le Feuvre, R.A. (2004) CNS injury: the role of the cytokine IL-1. *Veterinary Journal* 168, 230–237.

Glimaker, M., Kragsbjerg, P., Forsgren, M. and Olcen, P. (1993) Tumor necrosis factor-α (TNF-α) in cerebrospinal fluid from patients with meningitis of different etiologies – high levels of TNF-α indicate bacterial meningitis. *Journal of Infectious Diseases* 167, 882–889.

Gruol, D.L. and Nelson, T.E. (1997) Physiological and pathological roles of interleukin-6 in the central nervous system. *Molecular Neurobiology* 15, 307–339.

Hardy, S.J., Christodoulides, M., Weller, R.O. and Heckels, J.E. (2000) Interactions of *Neisseria meningitidis* with cells of the human meninges. *Molecular Microbiology* 36, 817–829.

Harris, J.E., Nuttall, R.K., Elkington, P.T., Green, J.A., Horncastle, D.E., Graeber, M.B., Edwards, D.R. and Friedland, J.S. (2007) Monocyte–astrocyte networks regulate matrix metalloproteinase gene expression and secretion in central nervous system tuberculosis in vitro and in vivo. *Journal of Immunology* 178, 1199–1207.

Hoffmann, O., Priller, J., Prozorovski, T., Schulze-Topphoff, U., Baeva, N., Lunemann, J.D., Aktas, O., Mahrhofer, C., Stricker, S., Zipp, F. and Weber, J.R. (2007) TRAIL limits excessive host immune responses in bacterial meningitis. *Journal of Clinical Investigation* 117, 2004–2013.

Hsieh, C.C., Lu, J.H., Chen, S.J., Lan, C.C., Chow, W.C. and Tang, R.B. (2009) Cerebrospinal fluid levels of interleukin-6 and interleukin-12 in children with meningitis. *Child's Nervous System* 25, 461–465.

Hsieh, H.L., Wang, H.H., Wu, C.Y., Tung, W.H. and Yang, C.M. (2010) Lipoteichoic acid induces matrix metalloproteinase-9 expression via transactivation of PDGF receptors and NF-kappa B activation in rat brain astrocytes. *Neurotoxicity Research* 17, 344–359.

Huang, C.C., Chang, Y.C., Chow, N.H. and Wang, S.T. (1997) Level of transforming growth factor β1 is elevated in cerebrospinal fluid of children with acute bacterial meningitis. *Journal of Neurology* 244, 634–638.

Inaba, Y., Ishiguro, A. and Shimbo, T. (1997) The production of macrophage inflammatory protein-1α in the cerebrospinal fluid at the initial stage of meningitis in children. *Pediatric Research* 42, 788–793.

Kanoh, Y., Ohara, T., Kanoh, M. and Akahoshi, T. (2008) Serum matrix metalloproteinase-2 levels indicate blood–CSF barrier damage in patients with infectious meningitis. *Inflammation* 31, 99–104.

Kastenbauer, S., Angele, B., Sporer, B., Pfister, H.W. and Koedel, U. (2005) Patterns of protein expression in infectious meningitis: a cerebrospinal fluid protein array analysis. *Journal of Neuroimmunology* 164, 134–139.

Kaur, S., Talay, S., Graham, R., Frank, R., Hanski, E. and Chhatwal, G. (2007) Functional studies on the IL-8 degrading surface protease of *Streptococcus pyogenes. International Journal of Medical Microbiology* 297, 121.

Kawakami, Y., Tsukimoto, M., Kuwabara, K., Fujita, T., Fujino, O., Kojima, S. and Fukunaga, Y. (2011) Tumor necrosis factor-α-induced mononuclear cell death may contribute to polymorphonuclear cell predominance in the cerebrospinal fluid of patients with bacterial meningitis. *Journal of Nippon Medical School* 78, 360–366.

Kim, J.M., Oh, Y.K., Lee, J.H., Im, D.Y., Kim, Y.J., Youn, J., Lee, C.H., Son, H., Lee, Y.S., Park, J.Y. and Choi, I.H. (2005) Induction of proinflammatory mediators requires activation of the TRAF, NIK, IKK and NF-κ B signal transduction pathway in astrocytes infected with *Escherichia coli. Clinical and Experimental Immunology* 140, 450–460.

Kim, Y.S., Honkaniemi, J., Sharp, F.R. and Tauber, M.G. (2004) Expression of proinflammatory cytokines tumor necrosis factor-α and interleukin-1β in the brain during experimental Group B streptococcal meningitis. *Molecular Brain Research* 128, 95–102.

Klein, M., Paul, R., Angele, B., Popp, B., Pfister, H.W. and Koedel, U. (2006) Protein expression pattern in experimental pneumococcal meningitis. *Microbes and Infection* 8, 974–983.

Koedel, U. and Pfister, H.W. (1999) Models of experimental bacterial meningitis – role and limitations. *Infectious Disease Clinics of North America* 13, 549–577.

Koedel, U., Winkler, F., Angele, B., Fontana, A., Flavell, R.A. and Pfister, H.W. (2002) Role of caspase-1 in experimental pneumococcal meningitis: evidence from pharmacologic caspase inhibition and caspase-1-deficient mice. *Annals of Neurology* 51, 319–329.

Konkel, J.E. and Chen, W. (2012) Role of TGF-β in immune suppression and inflammation. In: Wang, R.F. (ed.) *Innate Immune Regulation and Cancer Immunotherapy*. Springer, New York, pp. 289–301.

Kornelisse, R.F., Savelkoul, H.J., Mulder, P.G., Suur, M.H., van der Straaten, P.J.C., van der Heijden, A.J., Sukhai, R.N., Hahlen, K., Neijens, H.J. and deGroot, R. (1996) Interleukin-10 and soluble tumor necrosis factor receptors in cerebrospinal fluid of children with bacterial meningitis. *Journal of Infectious Diseases* 173, 1498–1502.

Kornelisse, R.F., Hack, C.E., Savelkoul, H.F.J., Raan, T.C.T.M., Hop, W.C.J., vanMierlo, G., Suur, M.H., Neijens, H.J. and deGroot, R. (1997) Intrathecal production of interleukin-12 and gamma interferon in patients with bacterial meningitis. *Infection and Immunity* 65, 877–881.

Kreutzberg, G.W., Blakemore, W.F. and Graeber, M.B. (1997) Cellular pathology of the central nervous system. In: Graham, D.I. and Lantos, P.L. (eds) *Greenfield's Neuropathology*. Edward Arnold, London, pp. 85–156.

Lahrtz, F., Piali, L., Spanaus, K.S., Seebach, J. and Fontana, A. (1998) Chemokines and chemotaxis of leukocytes in infectious meningitis. *Journal of Neuroimmunology* 85, 33–43.

Leib, S.L., Leppert, D., Clements, J. and Tauber, M.G. (2000) Matrix metalloproteinases contribute to brain damage in experimental pneumococcal meningitis. *Infection and Immunity* 68, 615–620.

Leist, T.P., Frei, K., Kamhansen, S., Zinkernagel, R.M. and Fontana, A. (1988) Tumor necrosis factor-α in cerebrospinal fluid during bacterial, but not viral, meningitis – evaluation in murine model infections and in patients. *Journal of Experimental Medicine* 167, 1743–1748.

Leppert, D., Leib, S.L., Grygar, C., Miller, K.M., Schaad, U.B. and Hollander, G.A. (2000) Matrix metalloproteinase (MMP)-8 and MMP-9 in cerebrospinal fluid during bacterial meningitis: Association with blood–brain barrier damage and neurological sequelae. *Clinical Infectious Diseases* 31, 80–84.

Lindberg, R.L.P., Sorsa, T., Tervahartiala, T., Hoffmann, F., Mellanen, L., Kappos, L., Schaad, U.B., Leib, S.L. and Leppert, D. (2006) Gelatinase B [matrix metalloproteinase (MMP)-9] and collagenases (MMP-8/-13) are upregulated in cerebrospinal fluid during aseptic and bacterial meningitis in children. *Neuropathology and Applied Neurobiology* 32, 304–317.

Liston, A. and McColl, S. (2003) Subversion of the chemokine world by microbial pathogens. *Bioessays* 25, 478–488.

Lopez-Cortes, L.F., Cruz-Ruiz, M., Gomez-Mateos, J., Viciana-Fernandez, P., Martinez-Marcos, F.J. and Pachon, J. (1995) Interleukin-8 in cerebrospinal fluid from patients with meningitis of different etiologies – its possible role as neutrophil chemotactic factor. *Journal of Infectious Diseases* 172, 581–584.

Mastroianni, C.M., Lancella, L., Mengoni, F., Lichtner, M., Santopadre, P., D'Agostino, C., Ticca, F. and Vullo, V. (1998) Chemokine profiles in the cerebrospinal fluid (CSF) during the course of pyogenic and tuberculous meningitis. *Clinical and Experimental Immunology* 114, 210–214.

Maurer, M. and von Stebut, E. (2004) Macrophage inflammatory protein-1. *International Journal of Biochemistry & Cell Biology* 36, 1882–1886.

Mihara, M., Hashizume, M., Yoshida, H., Suzuki, M. and Shiina, M. (2012) IL-6/IL-6 receptor system and its role in physiological and pathological conditions. *Clinical Science* 122, 143–159.

Mogensen, T.H., Paludan, S.R., Kilian, M. and Ostergaard, L. (2006) Live *Streptococcus pneumoniae, Haemophilus influenzae*, and *Neisseria meningitidis* activate the inflammatory response through Toll-like receptors 2, 4, and 9 in species-specific patterns. *Journal of Leukocyte Biology* 80, 267–277.

Mold, C. and Du Clos, T.W. (2006) C-reactive protein increases cytokine responses to *Streptococcus pneumoniae* through interactions with Fcγ receptors. *Journal of Immunology* 176, 7598–7604.

Moreillon, P. and Majcherczyk, P.A. (2003) Proinflammatory activity of cell-wall constituents from Gram-positive bacteria. *Scandinavian Journal of Infectious Diseases* 35, 632–641.

Neher, J. and Brown, G. (2007) Neurodegeneration in models of Gram-positive bacterial infections of the central nervous system. *Biochemical Society Transactions* 35, 1166–1167.

Ossege, L.M., Sindern, E., Voss, B. and Malin, J.P. (1996) Expression of tumor necrosis factor-α and transforming growth factor-β 1 in cerebrospinal fluid cells in meningitis. *Journal of the Neurological Sciences* 144, 1–13.

Pan, W., Stone, K.P., Hsuchou, H., Manda, V.K., Zhang, Y. and Kastin, A.J. (2011) Cytokine signaling modulates blood–brain barrier function. *Current Pharmaceutical Design* 17, 3729–3740.

Paul, R., Lorenzl, S., Koedel, U., Sporer, B., Vogel, U., Frosch, M. and Pfister, H.W. (1998) Matrix metalloproteinases contribute to the blood–brain barrier disruption during bacterial meningitis. *Annals of Neurology* 44, 592–600.

Pfister, H.W., Frei, K., Ottnad, B., Koedel, U., Tomasz, A. and Fontana, A. (1992) Transforming growth factor β_2 inhibits cerebrovascular changes and brain edema formation in the tumor necrosis factor α-independent early phase of experimental pneumococcal meningitis. *Journal of Experimental Medicine* 176, 265–268.

Plata-Salaman, C.R., Ilyin, S.E., Gayle, D. and Flynn, M.C. (1998) Gram-negative and Gram-positive bacterial products induce differential cytokine profiles in the brain: analysis using an integrative molecular–behavioral in vivo model. *International Journal of Molecular Medicine* 1, 387–397.

Prinz, M., Kann, O., Draheim, H.J., Schumann, R.R., Kettenmann, H., Weber, J.R. and Hanisch, U.K. (1999) Microglial activation by components of Gram-positive and -negative bacteria: distinct and common routes to the induction of ion channels and cytokines. *Journal of Neuropathology and Experimental Neurology* 58, 1078–1089.

Ramilo, O., Saez-Llorens, X., Mertsola, J., Jafari, H., Olsen, K.D., Hansen, E.J., Yoshinaga, M., Ohkawara, S., Nariuchi, H. and McCracken, G.H. (1990) Tumor necrosis factor-α cachectin and interleukin-1β initiate meningeal inflammation. *Journal of Experimental Medicine* 172, 497–507.

Rasley, A., Tranguch, S.L., Rati, D.M. and Marriott, I. (2006) Murine glia express the immunosuppressive cytokine, interleukin-10, following exposure to *Borrelia burgdorferi* or *Neisseria meningitidis*. *Glia* 53, 583–592.

Rollins, B.J., Walz, A. and Baggiolini, M. (1991) Recombinant human MCP-1/JE induces chemotaxis, calcium flux, and the respiratory burst in human monocytes. *Blood* 78, 1112–1116.

Rupprecht, T.A., Koedel, U., Muhlberger, B., Wilske, B., Fontana, A. and Pfister, H.W. (2005a) CXCL11 is involved in leucocyte recruitment to the central nervous system in neuroborreliosis. *Journal of Neurology* 252, 820–823.

Rupprecht, T.A., Pfister, H.W., Angele, B., Kastenbauer, S., Wilske, B. and Koedel, U. (2005b) The chemokine CXCL13 (BLC): a putative diagnostic marker for neuroborreliosis. *Neurology* 65, 448–450.

Sabat, R., Gruetz, G., Warszawska, K., Kirsch, S., Witte, E., Wolk, K. and Geginat, J. (2010) Biology of interleukin-10. *Cytokine & Growth Factor Reviews* 21, 331–344.

Seki, T., Joh, K. and Ohishi, T. (1993) Augmented production of interleukin-8 in cerebrospinal fluid in bacterial meningitis. *Immunology* 80, 333–335.

Sellner, J. and Leib, S.L. (2006) In bacterial meningitis cortical brain damage is associated with changes in parenchymal MMP-9/TIMP-1 ratio and increased collagen type IV degradation. *Neurobiology of Disease* 21, 647–656.

Selvaraj, S.K. and Prasadarao, N.V. (2005) *Escherichia coli* K1 inhibits proinflammatory cytokine induction in monocytes by preventing NF-κ B activation. *Journal of Leukocyte Biology* 78, 544–554.

Sharief, M.K., Ciardi, M. and Thompson, E.J. (1992) Blood–brain barrier damage in patients with bacterial meningitis – association with tumor necrosis factor-α but not interleukin-1-β. *Journal of Infectious Diseases* 166, 350–358.

Shimoda, K., Okamura, S., Omori, F., Mizuno, Y., Hara, T., Aoki, T., Ueda, K. and Niho, Y. (1991) Granulocyte colony-stimulating factor in cerebrospinal fluid from patients with meningitis. *Blood* 77, 2214–2217.

Siddiqui, R., Edwards-Smallbone, J., Flynn, R. and Khan, N.A. (2012) Next generation of non-mammalian blood–brain barrier models to study parasitic infections of the central nervous system. *Virulence* 3, 159–163.

Simberkoff, M.S., Moldover, N.H. and Rahall, J.J. (1980) Absence of detectable bactericidal and opsonic activities in normal and infected human cerebrospinal fluids. *Journal of Laboratory and Clinical Medicine* 95, 362–372.

Spanaus, K.S., Nadal, D., Pfister, H.W., Seebach, J., Widmer, U., Frei, K., Gloor, S. and Fontana, A. (1997) C-X-C and C-C chemokines are expressed in the cerebrospinal fluid in bacterial meningitis and mediate chemotactic activity on peripheral blood-derived polymorphonuclear and mononuclear cells in vitro. *Journal of Immunology* 158, 1956–1964.

Spooren, A., Kolmus, K., Laureys, G., Clinckers, R., De Keyser, J., Haegeman, G. and Gerlo, S. (2011) Interleukin-6, a mental cytokine. *Brain Research Reviews* 67, 157–183.

Sprenger, H., Rosler, A., Tonn, P., Braune, H.J., Huffmann, G. and Gemsa, D. (1996) Chemokines in the cerebrospinal fluid of patients with meningitis. *Clinical Immunology and Immunopathology* 80, 155–161.

Sriram, K. and O'Callaghan, J.P. (2007) Divergent roles for tumor necrosis factor-α in the brain. *Journal of Neuroimmune Pharmacology* 2, 140–153.

Sulik, A. and Chyczewski, L. (2008) Immunohistochemical analysis of MMP-9, MMP-2 and TIMP-1, TIMP-2 expression in the central nervous system following infection with viral and bacterial meningitis. *Folia Histochemica et Cytobiologica* 46, 437–442.

Suzuki, T., Ishiguro, A. and Shimbo, T. (2003) Transient elevation of interleukin-16 levels at the initial stage of meningitis in children. *Clinical and Experimental Immunology* 131, 484–489.

Tang, T., Frenette, P.S., Hynes, R.O., Wagner, D.D. and Mayadas, T.N. (1996) Cytokine-induced meningitis is dramatically attenuated in mice deficient in endothelial selectins. *Journal of Clinical Investigation* 97, 2485–2490.

Tansey, M.G. and Wyss-Coray, T. (2008) Cytokines in CNS inflammation and disease. In: Lane, T.E., Carson, M., Bergmann, C. and Wyss-Coray, T. (eds) *Central Nervous System Diseases and Inflammation*. Springer, New York, pp. 59–106.

Tarlow, M.J., Jenkins, R., Comis, S.D., Osborne, M.P., Stephens, S., Stanley, P. and Crocker, J. (1993) Ependymal cells of the choroid plexus express tumor necrosis factor-α. *Neuropathology and Applied Neurobiology* 19, 324–328.

Tauber, M.G. and Moser, B. (1999) Cytokines and chemokines in meningeal inflammation: biology and clinical implications. *Clinical Infectious Diseases* 28, 1–12.

Tsai, H., Shi, M., Lee, S., Wann, S., Tai, M. and Chen, Y. (2011) Expression of matrix metalloproteinases and their tissue inhibitors in the serum and cerebrospinal fluid of patients with meningitis. *Clinical Microbiology and Infection* 17, 780–784.

Tsao, N., Chang, W.W., Liu, C.C. and Lei, H.Y. (2002) Development of hematogenous pneumococcal meningitis in adult mice: the role of TNF-α. *FEMS Immunology and Medical Microbiology* 32, 133–140.

van Furth, A.M., Seijmonsbergen, E.M., Langermans, J.A.M., Groeneveld, P.H.P., Debel, C.E. and van Furth, R. (1995) High levels of interleukin-10 and tumor necrosis factor-α in cerebrospinal fluid during the onset of bacterial meningitis. *Clinical Infectious Diseases* 21, 220–222.

Van Lint, P. and Libert, C. (2007) Chemokine and cytokine processing by matrix metalloproteinases and its effect on leukocyte migration and inflammation. *Journal of Leukocyte Biology* 82, 1375–1381.

Vanier, G., Segura, M., Lecours, M.P., Grenier, D. and Gottschalk, M. (2009) Porcine brain microvascular endothelial cell-derived interleukin-8 is first induced and then degraded by *Streptococcus suis*. *Microbial Pathogenesis* 46, 135–143.

Waage, A., Halstensen, A. and Espevik, T. (1987) Association between tumour necrosis factor in serum and fatal outcome in patients with meningococcal disease. *Lancet* 1, 355–357.

Waage, A., Halstensen, A. and Shalaby, R. (1989) Local production of tumor necrosis factor factor α, interleukin 1 and interleukin 6 in meningococcal meningitis. *Journal of Experimental Medicine* 170, 1859–1867.

Weller, R. (2005) Microscopic morphology and histology of the human meninges. *Morphologie* 89, 22–34.

Wilson, M., Seymour, R. and Henderson, B. (1998) Bacterial perturbation of cytokine networks. *Infection and Immunity* 66, 2401–2409.

Witzenrath, M., *et al.* (2011) The NLRP3 inflammasome is differentially activated by pneumolysin variants and contributes to host defense in pneumococcal pneumonia. *Journal of Immunology* 187, 434–440.

Woehrl, B., Klein, M., Rupprecht, T.A., Schmetzer, H., Angele, B., Haecker, H., Haecker, G., Pfister, H.W. and Koedel, U. (2010) CXCL16 contributes to neutrophil recruitment to cerebrospinal fluid in pneumococcal meningitis. *Journal of Infectious Diseases* 202, 1389–1396.

Zwijnenburg, P.J.G., De Bie, H.M.A., Roord, J.J., van der Poll, T. and van Furth, A.M. (2003a) Chemotactic activity of CXCL5 in cerebrospinal fluid of children with bacterial meningitis. *Journal of Neuroimmunology* 145, 148–153.

Zwijnenburg, P.J.G., van der Poll, T., Florquin, S., Akira, S., Takeda, K., Roord, J.J. and van Furth, A.M. (2003b) Interleukin-18 gene-deficient mice show enhanced defense and reduced inflammation during pneumococcal meningitis. *Journal of Neuroimmunology* 138, 31–37.

Index

Page numbers in **bold** refer to figures and tables